Contents

Contents

Guideline Development Group membership and acknowledgements

Guideline Development Group

Peter Brocklehurst	Group Leader
Belinda Ackerman	Midwife
Brian Cook	General Practitioner
Joanie Dimavicius	Consumer
Helen Edwards	Radiographer
Gill Gyte	Consumer
Shahid Husain	Neonatologist
Gwyneth Lewis	Confidential Enquiry into Maternal Deaths
Tim Overton	Obstetrician
Gill Roberts	RCOG Patient Information Specialist
Stephen Robson	Obstetrician
Julia Sanders	Midwife
Anne White	General Practitioner
Jane Thomas	Director NCC-WCH
Sue Lee	Research Fellow NCC-WCH
Jennifer Gray	Informatics Specialist NCC-WCH
Natalie Terry	Administrative support NCC-WCH
Hannah Rose Douglas	Health Economist, London School of Hygiene and Tropical Medicine
Dimitra Lambrelli	Health Economist London School of Hygiene and Tropical Medicine

Acknowledgments

Additional support was also received from:

- David Asomani, Anna Burt, Heather Brown, Susan Davidson, Gregory Eliovson, Susan Murray and Alex McNeil at the National Collaborating Centre for Women's and Children's Health.
- Stravros Petrou at the National Perinatal Epidemiology Unit and Kirsten Duckitt at the John Radcliffe Hospital, Oxford.
- Members of the previous Antenatal Care Guideline Development Group: John Spencer (Chairman), J Bradley, Jean Chapple, R Cranna, Marion Hall, Marcia Kelson, Catherine McCormack, Ralph Settatree, Lindsay Smith, L Turner, Martin Whittle, Julie Wray.
- The Patient Involvement Unit, whose glossary we have amended for use in this guideline.
- The Three Centres Consensus Guidelines on Antenatal Care, Mercy Hospital for Women, Monash Medical Centre (Southern Health) and The Royal Women's Hospital (Women's & Children's Health), Melbourne 2001, whose work we benefited from in the development of this guideline.

Stakeholder organisations

- Action on Pre-Eclampsia (APEC)
- Antenatal Results and Choices

- Association for Continence Advice (ACA)
- Association for Improvements in Maternity Services (AIMS)
- Association of Radical Midwives
- Association of the British Pharmaceuticals Industry (ABPI)
- Aventis Pasteur MSD
- Brighton Healthcare NHS Trust
- British Association of Paediatric Surgeons
- British Association of Perinatal Medicine
- British Dietetic Association
- British Maternal and Fetal Medicine Society
- British Medical Association
- British National Formulary
- British Psychological Society
- BUPA
- Chartered Society of Physiotherapy
- CIS'ters
- Department of Health
- Evidence based Midwifery Network
- Faculty of Public Health Medicine
- Gateshead Primary Care Trust
- General Medical Council
- Group B Strep Support
- Health Development Agency
- Hospital Infection Society
- Isabel Medical Charity
- Maternity Alliance
- Mental Health Foundation
- Monmouthshire Local Health Group
- National Childbirth Trust
- NHS Quality Improvement Scotland
- Nottingham City Hospital
- Obstetric Anaesthetists Association
- Royal College of General Practitioners
- Royal College of General Practitioners Wales
- Royal College of Midwives
- Royal College of Nursing
- Royal College of Obstetricians and Gynaecologists
- Royal College of Paediatrics and Child Health
- Royal College of Pathologists
- Royal College of Psychiatrists
- Royal College of Radiologists
- Royal Pharmaceutical Society of Great Britain
- Royal Society of Medicine
- Scottish Intercollegiate Guidelines Network (SIGN)
- Sickle Cell Society
- Society and College of Radiographers
- STEPS
- Survivors Trust
- Twins and Multiple Births Association (TAMBA)
- UK Coalition of People Living with HIV and AIDS
- UK National Screening Committee
- UK Pain Society
- United Kingdom Association of Sonographers
- Victim Support
- Welsh Assembly Government (formerly National Assembly for Wales)
- West Gloucestershire Primary Care Trust
- Young Minds

Peer reviewers

Susan Bewley, Leanne Bricker, Howard Cuckle, Andrew Dawson, Viv Dickinson, Grace Edwards, Jason Gardosi, Duncan Irons, Deirdre Murphy, Tim Reynolds, Jilly Rosser, Lindsay Smith, John Spencer, Pat Tookey, Derek Tuffnell, Gavin Young.

Abbreviations

ACOG	American College of Obstetricians and Gynecologists
ACTH	adrenocorticotrophic hormone
AFP	alphafetoprotein
AIDS	acquired immunodeficiency syndrome
ANC	antenatal care
APEC	Action on Pre-eclampsia
ASB	asymptomatic bacteriuria
BMI	body mass index
BP	blood pressure
BV	bacterial vaginosis
CAMP	Christie, Atkinson, Munch, Peterson test
CDSC	Communicable Disease Surveillance Centre
cfu/ml	colony-forming units per millilitre
CI	confidence interval
CINAHL	Cumulative Index to Nursing and Allied Health Literature
CMV	cytomegalovirus
CNS	central nervous system
CS	caesarean section
CTG	cardiotocography
DA	direct agglutination test
DARE	Database of Abstracts and Reviews of Effectiveness
DNA	deoxyribonucleic acid
eAg	hepatitis e antigen
ECV	external cephalic version
EEA	European Economic Area
EIA	enzyme immunoassay
ELISA	enzyme-linked immunosorbent assay
EOGBS	early-onset group B streptococcus
EPDS	Edinburgh Postnatal Depression Scale
EPIC	external intermittent pneumatic compression
EU	European Union
FBG	fasting plasma glucose
FGM	female genital mutilation
FTA-abs	fluorescent treponemal antibody – absorbed test
GBS	group B streptococcus
GCT	glucose challenge test
GDG	Guideline Development Group
GDM	gestational diabetes mellitus
GPP	good practice point
GTT	glucose tolerance test
Hb	haemoglobin
HBIG	hepatitis B immune globulin
HBsAg	hepatitis B surface antigen
HBV	hepatitis B virus
hCG	human chorionic gonadotrophin (can be total or free beta)
HCV	hepatitis C virus
HDN	haemolytic disease of the newborn
HEED	Health Economic Evaluations Database
HELLP	haemolysis, elevated liver enzymes and low platelet count
HIV	human immunodeficiency virus
HPA	Health Protection Agency
HPLC	high-performance liquid chromatography

HTA	Health Technology Assessment
ICD-9	International Classification of Diseases, 9th edition
IU	international units
IUGR	intrauterine growth restriction
LA	latex agglutination test
LE	leucocyte esterase
LGA	large for gestational age
LMP	last menstrual period
LSHTM	London School of Hygiene and Tropical Medicine
MCH	mean corpuscular haemoglobin
MeSH	medical subject headings
MIDIRS	Midwives Information and Resource Service
MTCT	mother-to-child transmission
NCC-WCH	National Collaborating Centre for Women's and Children's Health
NCRSP	National Congenital Rubella Surveillance Programme
NHS	National Health Service
NHS EED	NHS Economic Evaluations Database
NICE	National Institute for Clinical Excellence
NICU	neonatal intensive care unit
NNT	number needed to treat
NPV	negative predictive value
NS	not significant
NSC	(UK) National Screening Committee
NSF	National Service Framework
NT	nuchal translucency
ONS	Office for National Statistics
OR	odds ratio
OTC	over-the-counter
PAPP-A	plasma protein A
PCR	polymerase chain reaction
PCT	primary care trust
PHLS	Public Health Laboratory Service
PIH	pregnancy-induced hypertension
PPI	proton pump inhibitor
PPV	positive predictive value
RCOG	Royal College of Obstetricians and Gynaecologists
RCT	randomised controlled trial
RhD	rhesus D
RIBA	recombinant immunoblot assay
RNA	ribonucleic acid
RPG	random plasma glucose
RPR	rapid plasmin reagin test
RR	relative risk
RST	reagent strip testing
SD	standard deviation
SFH	symphysis–fundal height
SGA	small for gestational age
SIGN	Scottish Intercollegiate Guidelines Network
SPD	symphysis pubis dysfunction
TPHA	*Treponema pallidum* haemagglutination assay
uE_3	unconjugated oestriol
UK	United Kingdom
US CDC	United States Centers for Disease Control and Prevention
USS	ultrasound scan
UTI	urinary tract infection
VDRL	Venereal Disease Research Laboratory (test for syphilis)
VE	vaginal examination
WHO	World Health Organization
WMD	weighted mean difference

Glossary of terms

Bias
Influences on a study that can lead to invalid conclusions about a treatment or intervention. Bias in research can make a treatment look better or worse than it really is. Bias can even make it look as if the treatment works when it actually doesn't. Bias can occur by chance or as a result of systematic errors in the design and execution of a study. Bias can occur at different stages in the research process, e.g. in the collection, analysis, interpretation, publication or review of research data.

Blinding or masking
The practice of keeping the investigators or subjects of a study ignorant of the group to which a subject has been assigned. For example, a clinical trial in which the participating patients or their doctors are unaware of whether they (the patients) are taking the experimental drug or a placebo (dummy treatment). The purpose of 'blinding' or 'masking' is to protect against **bias**. See also **Double blind study**.

Case—control study
A study that starts with the identification of a group of individuals sharing the same characteristics (e.g. people with a particular disease) and a suitable comparison (control) group (e.g. people without the disease). All subjects are then assessed with respect to things that happened to them in the past, e.g. things that might be related to getting the disease under investigation. Such studies are also called **retrospective** as they look back in time from the outcome to the possible causes.

Case report (or case study)
Detailed report on one patient (or case), usually covering the course of that person's disease and their response to treatment.

Case series
Description of several cases of a given disease, usually covering the course of the disease and the response to treatment. There is no comparison (**control**) group of patients.

Clinical trial
A research study conducted with patients which tests out a drug or other intervention to assess its effectiveness and safety. Each trial is designed to answer scientific questions and to find better ways to treat individuals with a specific disease. This general term encompasses **controlled clinical trials** and **randomised controlled trials**.

Cohort
A group of people sharing some common characteristic (e.g. patients with the same disease), followed up in a research study for a specified period of time.

Cohort study
An observational study that takes a group (cohort) of patients and follows their progress over time in order to measure outcomes such as disease or mortality rates and make comparisons according to the treatments or interventions that patients received. Thus within the study group, subgroups of patients are identified (from information collected about patients) and these groups are compared with respect to outcome, e.g. comparing mortality between one group that received a specific treatment and one group which did not (or between two groups that received different levels of treatment). Cohorts can be assembled in the present and followed into the future (a 'concurrent' or 'prospective' cohort study) or identified from past records and followed forward from that time up to the present (a 'historical' or 'retrospective' cohort study). Because patients are not randomly allocated to subgroups, these subgroups may be quite different in their characteristics and some adjustment must be made when analysing the results to ensure that the comparison between groups is as fair as possible.

Confidence interval A way of expressing certainty about the findings from a study or group of studies, using statistical techniques. A confidence interval describes a range of possible effects (of a treatment or intervention) that is consistent with the results of a study or group of studies. A wide confidence interval indicates a lack of certainty or precision about the true size of the clinical effect and is seen in studies with too few patients. Where confidence intervals are narrow they indicate more precise estimates of effects and a larger sample of patients studied. It is usual to interpret a '95%' confidence interval as the range of effects within which we are 95% confident that the true effect lies.

Control group A group of patients recruited into a study that receives no treatment, a treatment of known effect, or a placebo (dummy treatment), in order to provide a comparison for a group receiving an experimental treatment, such as a new drug.

Controlled clinical trial (CCT) A study testing a specific drug or other treatment involving two (or more) groups of patients with the same disease. One (the experimental group) receives the treatment that is being tested, and the other (the comparison or control group) receives an alternative treatment, a placebo (dummy treatment) or no treatment. The two groups are followed up to compare differences in outcomes to see how effective the experimental treatment was. A CCT where patients are randomly allocated to treatment and comparison groups is called a **randomised controlled trial**.

Cost benefit analysis A type of economic evaluation where both costs and benefits of healthcare treatment are measured in the same monetary units. If benefits exceed costs, the evaluation would recommend providing the treatment.

Cost effectiveness A type of economic evaluation that assesses the additional costs and benefits of doing something different. In cost effectiveness analysis, the costs and benefits of different treatments are compared. When a new treatment is compared with current care, its additional costs divided by its additional benefits is called the cost effectiveness ratio. Benefits are measured in natural units, for example, cost per additional heart attack prevented.

Cost utility analysis A special form of **cost effectiveness** analysis where benefit is measured in quality adjusted life years. A treatment is assessed in terms of its ability to extend or improve the quality of life.

Crossover study design A study comparing two or more interventions in which the participants, upon completion of the course of one treatment, are switched to another. For example, for a comparison of treatments A and B, half the participants are randomly allocated to receive them in the order A, B and half to receive them in the order B, A. A problem with this study design is that the effects of the first treatment may carry over into the period when the second is given. Therefore a crossover study should include an adequate 'wash-out' period, which means allowing sufficient time between stopping one treatment and starting another so that the first treatment has time to wash out of the patient's system.

Cross-sectional study The observation of a defined set of people at a single point in time or time period – a snapshot. (This type of study contrasts with a **longitudinal study**, which follows a set of people over a period of time.)

Double blind study A study in which neither the subject (patient) nor the observer (investigator or clinician) is aware of which treatment or intervention the subject is receiving. The purpose of blinding is to protect against bias.

Evidence based The process of systematically finding, appraising and using research findings as the basis for clinical decisions.

Evidence-based clinical practice Evidence-based clinical practice involves making decisions about the care of individual patients based on the best research evidence available rather than basing decisions on personal opinions or common practice (which may not always be evidence based). Evidence-based clinical practice therefore involves integrating individual clinical expertise and patient preferences with the best available evidence from research.

Evidence table　　A table summarising the results of a collection of studies which, taken together, represent the evidence supporting a particular recommendation or series of recommendations in a guideline.

Exclusion criteria　　See **Selection criteria**.

Experimental study　　A research study designed to test whether a treatment or intervention has an effect on the course or outcome of a condition or disease, where the conditions of testing are to some extent under the control of the investigator. **Controlled clinical trial** and **randomised controlled trial** are examples of experimental studies.

Gold standard　　A method, procedure or measurement that is widely accepted as being the best available.

Gravid　　Pregnant.

Health economics　　A field of conventional economics which examines the benefits of healthcare interventions (e.g. medicines) compared with their financial costs.

Heterogeneity　　Or lack of **homogeneity**. The term is used in **meta-analyses** and **systematic reviews** when the results or estimates of effects of treatment from separate studies seem to be very different, in terms of the size of treatment effects, or even to the extent that some indicate beneficial and others suggest adverse treatment effects. Such results may occur as a result of differences between studies in terms of the patient populations, outcome measures, definition of **variables** or duration of follow up.

Homogeneity　　This means that the results of studies included in a **systematic review** or **meta-analysis** are similar and there is no evidence of **heterogeneity**. Results are usually regarded as homogeneous when differences between studies could reasonably be expected to occur by chance. See also **Consistency**.

Inclusion criteria　　See **Selection criteria**.

Intervention　　Healthcare action intended to benefit the patient, e.g. drug treatment, surgical procedure, psychological therapy.

Longitudinal study　　A study of the same group of people at more than one point in time. (This type of study contrasts with a **cross-sectional study**, which observes a defined set of people at a single point in time.)

Masking　　See **Blinding**.

Meta-analysis　　Results from a collection of independent studies (investigating the same treatment) are pooled, using statistical techniques to synthesise their findings into a single estimate of a treatment effect. Where studies are not compatible, e.g. because of differences in the study populations or in the outcomes measured, it may be inappropriate or even misleading to statistically pool results in this way. See also **Systematic review** and **Heterogeneity**.

Multiparous　　Having carried more than one pregnancy to a viable stage.

Non-experimental study　　A study based on subjects selected on the basis of their availability, with no attempt having been made to avoid problems of bias.

Nulliparous　　Having never given birth to a viable infant.

Number needed to treat (NNT)　　This measures the impact of a treatment or intervention. It states how many patients need to be treated with the treatment in question in order to prevent an event that would otherwise occur; e.g. if the NNT = 4, then four patients would have to be treated to prevent one bad outcome. The closer the NNT is to one, the better the treatment is. Analogous to the NNT is the number needed to harm (NNH), which is the number of patients that would need to receive a treatment to cause one additional adverse event. e.g. if the NNH = 4, then four patients would have to be treated for one bad outcome to occur.

Observational study

In research about diseases or treatments, this refers to a study in which nature is allowed to take its course. Changes or differences in one characteristic (e.g. whether or not people received a specific treatment or intervention) are studied in relation to changes or differences in other(s) (e.g. whether or not they died), without the intervention of the investigator. There is a greater risk of selection bias than in **experimental studies**.

Odds ratio

Odds are a way of representing probability, especially familiar from betting. In recent years odds ratios have become widely used in reports of clinical studies. They provide an estimate (usually with a **confidence interval**) for the effect of a treatment. Odds are used to convey the idea of 'risk' and an odds ratio of one between two treatment groups would imply that the risks of an adverse outcome were the same in each group. For rare events the odds ratio and the **relative risk** (which uses actual risks and not odds) will be very similar. See also **Relative risk**, **Risk ratio**.

Parous

Having borne at least one viable offspring (usually more than 24 weeks of gestation).

Peer review

Review of a study, service or recommendations by those with similar interests and expertise to the people who produced the study findings or recommendations. Peer reviewers can include professional, patient and carer representatives.

Pilot study

A small-scale 'test' of the research instrument. For example, testing out (piloting) a new questionnaire with people who are similar to the population of the study, in order to highlight any problems or areas of concern, which can then be addressed before the full-scale study begins.

Placebo

Placebos are fake or inactive treatments received by participants allocated to the **control group** in a clinical trial, which are indistinguishable from the active treatments being given in the experimental group. They are used so that participants are ignorant of their treatment allocation in order to be able to quantify the effect of the experimental treatment over and above any **placebo effect** due to receiving care or attention.

Placebo effect

A beneficial (or adverse) effect produced by a **placebo** and not due to any property of the placebo itself.

Power

See **Statistical power**.

Prospective study

A study in which people are entered into the research and then followed up over a period of time with future events recorded as they happen. This contrasts with studies that are **retrospective**.

p value

If a study is done to compare two treatments then the p value is the probability of obtaining the results of that study, or something more extreme, if there really was no difference between treatments. (The assumption that there really is no difference between treatments is called the 'null hypothesis'.) Suppose the p-value was 0.03. What this means is that, if there really was no difference between treatments, there would only be a 3% chance of getting the kind of results obtained. Since this chance seems quite low we should question the validity of the assumption that there really is no difference between treatments. We would conclude that there probably is a difference between treatments. By convention, where the value of p is below 0.05 (i.e. less than 5%) the result is seen as statistically significant. Where the value of p is 0.001 or less, the result is seen as highly significant. p values just tell us whether an effect can be regarded as statistically significant or not. In no way do they relate to how big the effect might be, for which we need the **confidence interval**.

Qualitative research

Qualitative research is used to explore and understand people's beliefs, experiences, attitudes, behaviour and interactions. It generates non-numerical data, e.g. a patient's description of their pain rather than a measure of pain. In health care, qualitative techniques have been commonly used in research documenting the experience of chronic illness and in studies about the functioning of organisations. Qualitative research techniques such as focus groups and in-depth interviews have been used in one-off projects commissioned by guideline development groups to find out more about the views and experiences of patients and carers.

Quantitative research

Research that generates numerical data or data that can be converted into numbers, for example clinical trials or the National Census, which counts people and households.

Random allocation or randomisation

A method that uses the play of chance to assign participants to comparison groups in a research study; for example, by using a random numbers table or a computer-generated random sequence. Random allocation implies that each individual (or each unit in the case of cluster randomisation) being entered into a study has the same chance of receiving each of the possible interventions.

Randomised controlled trial

A study to test a specific drug or other treatment in which people are randomly assigned to two (or more) groups: one (the experimental group) receiving the treatment that is being tested, and the other (the comparison or control group) receiving an alternative treatment, a placebo (dummy treatment) or no treatment. The two groups are followed up to compare differences in outcomes to see how effective the experimental treatment was. (Through randomisation, the groups should be similar in all aspects apart from the treatment they receive during the study.)

Relative risk

A summary measure which represents the ratio of the risk of a given event or outcome (e.g. an adverse reaction to the drug being tested) in one group of subjects compared with another group. When the 'risk' of the event is the same in the two groups the relative risk is 1. In a study comparing two treatments, a relative risk of 2 would indicate that patients receiving one of the treatments had twice the risk of an undesirable outcome than those receiving the other treatment. Relative risk is sometimes used as a synonym for **risk ratio**.

Reliability

Reliability refers to a method of measurement that consistently gives the same results. For example, someone who has a high score on one occasion tends to have a high score if measured on another occasion very soon afterwards. With physical assessments it is possible for different clinicians to make independent assessments in quick succession and if their assessments tend to agree then the method of assessment is said to be reliable.

Retrospective study

A retrospective study deals with the present and past and does not involve studying future events. This contrasts with studies that are **prospective**.

Risk ratio

Ratio of the risk of an undesirable event or outcome occurring in a group of patients receiving experimental treatment compared with a comparison (control) group. The term **relative risk** is sometimes used as a synonym of risk ratio.

Sample

A part of the study's target population from which the subjects of the study will be recruited. If subjects are drawn in an unbiased way from a particular population, the results can be generalised from the sample to the population as a whole.

Screening	The presumptive identification of an unrecognised disease or defect by means of tests, examinations or other procedures that can be applied rapidly. Screening tests differentiate apparently well persons who may have a disease from those who probably have not. A screening test is not intended to be diagnostic but should be sufficiently **sensitive** and **specific** to reduce the proportion of false results, positive or negative, to acceptable levels. Persons with positive or suspicious findings must be referred to the appropriate healthcare provider for diagnosis and necessary treatment.
Selection criteria	Explicit standards used by guideline development groups to decide which studies should be included and excluded from consideration as potential sources of evidence.
Sensitivity	In diagnostic testing, this refers to the chance of having a positive test result given that you have the disease. 100% sensitivity means that all those with the disease will test positive, but this is not the same the other way around. A patient could have a positive test result but not have the disease — this is called a 'false positive'. The sensitivity of a test is also related to its 'negative predictive value' (true negatives) – a test with a sensitivity of 100% means that all those who get a negative test result do not have the disease. To fully judge the accuracy of a test, its **specificity** must also be considered.
Specificity	In diagnostic testing, this refers to the chance of having a negative test result given that you do not have the disease. 100% specificity means that all those without the disease will test negative, but this is not the same the other way around. A patient could have a negative test result yet still have the disease – this is called a 'false negative'. The specificity of a test is also related to its 'positive predictive value' (true positives) – a test with a specificity of 100% means that all those who get a positive test result definitely have the disease. To fully judge the accuracy of a test, its **sensitivity** must also be considered.
Statistical power	The ability of a study to demonstrate an association or causal relationship between two **variables**, given that an association exists. For example, 80% power in a clinical trial means that the study has a 80% chance of ending up with a P value of less than 5% in a statistical test (i.e. a statistically significant treatment effect) if there really was an important difference (e.g. 10% versus 5% mortality) between treatments. If the statistical power of a study is low, the study results will be questionable (the study might have been too small to detect any differences). By convention, 80% is an acceptable level of power. See also **p value**.
Systematic review	A review in which evidence from scientific studies has been identified, appraised and synthesised in a methodical way according to predetermined criteria. May or may not include a **meta-analysis**.
Validity	Assessment of how well a tool or instrument measures what it is intended to measure.
Variable	A measurement that can vary within a study, e.g. the age of participants. Variability is present when differences can be seen between different people or within the same person over time, with respect to any characteristic or feature that can be assessed or measured.

1. Introduction

1.1 Aim of the guideline

The ethos of this guideline is that pregnancy is a normal physiological process and that, as such, any interventions offered should have known benefits and be acceptable to pregnant women. The guideline has been developed with the following aims: to offer information on best practice for baseline clinical care of all pregnancies and comprehensive information on the antenatal care of the healthy woman with an uncomplicated singleton pregnancy. It provides evidence-based information for clinicians and pregnant women to make decisions about appropriate treatment in specific circumstances. The guideline will complement the Children's National Service Frameworks (England and Wales), which is in development and which will produce standards for service configuration, with emphasis on how care is delivered and by whom, including issues of ensuring equity of access to care for disadvantaged women and women's views about service provision (For more information, see www.doh.gov.uk/nsf/children.htm for England and www.wales.nhs.uk/sites/page.cfm?orgid=334&pid=934 for Wales). The guideline has also drawn on the evidence-based recommendations of the UK National Screening Committee (NSC).

The *Changing Childbirth* report explicitly confirmed that women should be the focus of maternity care.[1] Care during pregnancy should enable a woman to make informed decisions, based on her needs, having discussed matters fully with the professionals involved.

Reviews of women's views on antenatal care suggest that key aspects of care valued by women are respect, competence, communication, support and convenience.[2] Access to information and provision of care by the same small group of people are also key aspects of care that lend themselves to a pregnant woman feeling valued as an individual and more in control.[3]

Current models of antenatal care originated in the early decades of the 20th century. The pattern of visits recommended at that time (monthly until 30 weeks, then fortnightly to 36 weeks and then weekly until delivery) is still recognisable today. It has been said that antenatal care has escaped critical assessment.[4] Both the individual components and composite package of antenatal care should conform to the criteria for a successful screening programme, namely that:

- the condition being screened for is an important health problem
- the screening test (further diagnostic test and treatment) is safe and acceptable
- the natural history of the condition is understood
- early detection and treatment has benefit over later detection and treatment
- the screening test is valid and reliable
- there are adequate facilities for confirming the test results and resources for treatment
- the objectives of screening justify the costs.

A complete list of the NSC criteria for screening can be found in the NSC online library (www.nsc.nhs.uk/library/lib_ind.htm) under the title, *The UK National Screening Committee's criteria for appraising the viability, effectiveness and appropriateness of a screening programme.*

1.2 Areas outside the remit of the guideline

The guideline will not produce standards for service configuration, which are being addressed by the Children's National Service Frameworks (England and Wales), nor will it address quality standard issues (such as laboratory standards), which are addressed by the National Screening Committee.[5]

Although the guideline addresses screening for many of the complications of pregnancy, it does not include information on the investigation and appropriate ongoing management of these complications if they arise in pregnancy (for example, the management of pre-eclampsia, fetal anomalies and multiple pregnancies).

Any aspect of intrapartum and postpartum care has not been included in this guideline. This includes preparation for birth and parenthood, risk factor assessment for intrapartum care, breastfeeding and postnatal depression. These topics will be addressed in future National Institute for Clinical Excellence (NICE) guidelines on intrapartum and postpartum care.

The guideline offers recommendations on baseline clinical care for all pregnant women but it does not offer information on the additional care that some women will require. Pregnant women with the following conditions usually require care additional to that detailed in this guideline:

- cardiac disease, including hypertension
- renal disease
- endocrine disorder or diabetes requiring insulin
- psychiatric disorder (on medication)
- haematological disorder, including thromboembolic disease, autoimmune diseases such as antiphospholipid syndrome
- epilepsy requiring anticonvulsant drugs
- malignant disease
- severe asthma
- drug use such as heroin, cocaine (including crack cocaine) and ecstasy
- HIV or hepatitis B virus (HBV) infected
- autoimmune disorders
- obesity (body mass index, BMI, 35 or more at first contact) or underweight (BMI less than 18 at first contact)
- women who may be at higher risk of developing complications e.g. women 40 years and older and women who smoke
- women who are particularly vulnerable (e.g. teenagers) or who lack social support.

Women who have experienced any of the following in previous pregnancies:

- recurrent miscarriage (three or more consecutive pregnancy losses) or a mid-trimester loss
- severe pre-eclampsia, HELLP syndrome or eclampsia
- rhesus isoimmunisation or other significant blood group antibodies
- terine surgery including caesarean section, myomectomy or cone biopsy
- antenatal or postpartum haemorrhage on two occasions
- retained placenta on two occasions
- puerperal psychosis
- grand multiparity (more than six pregnancies)
- a stillbirth or neonatal death
- a small-for-gestational-age infant (less than fifth centile)
- a large-for-gestational-age infant (greater than 95th centile)
- a baby weighing less than 2500 g or more than 4500 g
- a baby with a congenital anomaly (structural or chromosomal).

1.3   For whom is the guideline intended?

This guideline is of relevance to those who work in or use the National Health Service (NHS) in England and Wales:

- professional groups who share in caring for pregnant women, such as obstetricians, midwives, radiographers, physiotherapists, anaesthetists, general practitioners, paediatricians and others
- those with responsibilities for commissioning and planning maternity services, such as primary care trusts in England, Health Commission Wales, public health and trust managers
- pregnant women.

A version of this guideline for pregnant women, their partners and the public is available, entitled *Routine antenatal care for healthy pregnant women. Understanding NICE guidance: information for pregnant women, their families and the public* (reproduced in Appendix 1). It can be downloaded from the NICE website (www.nice.org.uk) or ordered via the NHS Response Line (0870 1555 455; quote reference number N0310 for an English version and N0311 for an English and Welsh version).

1.4 Who has developed the guideline?

The Guideline was developed by a multiprofessional and lay working group (the Guideline Development Group) convened by the National Collaborating Centre for Women's and Children's Health (NCC-WCH). Membership included:

- two consumers
- two general practitioners
- two midwives
- two obstetricians
- a radiographer
- a neonatologist
- a representative from the Confidential Enquiries from Maternal Deaths (CEMD).

Staff from NCC-WCH provided methodological support for the guideline development process, undertook the systematic searches, retrieval and appraisal of the evidence and wrote successive drafts of the document.

In accordance with the NICE guideline development process,[6] all guideline development group members have made and updated any declarations of interest.

1.5 Guideline methodology

The development of the guideline was commissioned by the National Institute for Clinical Excellence (NICE) and developed in accordance with the guideline development process outlined in *The Guideline Development Process – Information for National Collaborating Centres and Guideline Development Groups*, available from the NICE website (www.nice.org.uk).[6]

Literature search strategy

The aim of the literature review was to identify and synthesise relevant evidence within the published literature, in order to answer the specific clinical questions. Searches were performed using generic and specially developed filters, relevant MeSH (medical subject headings) terms and free-text terms. Details of all literature searches are available upon application to the NCC-WCH.

Guidelines by other development groups were searched for on the National Guidelines Clearinghouse database, the TRIP database and OMNI service on the Internet. The reference lists in these guidelines were checked against the searches to identify any missing evidence.

Searches were carried out for each topic of interest. The Cochrane Database of Systematic Reviews, up to Issue 3, 2003, was searched to identify systematic reviews of randomised controlled trials, with or without meta-analyses and randomised controlled trials. The electronic database, MEDLINE (Ovid version for the period January 1966 to April 2003), EMBASE (Ovid version from January 1980 to April 2003), MIDIRS (Midwives Information and Resource Service), CINAHL (Cumulative Index to Nursing and Allied Health Literature), the British Nursing Index (BNI) and PsychInfo were also searched.

The Database of Abstracts and Reviews of Effectiveness (DARE) was searched. Reference lists of non-systematic review articles and studies obtained from the initial search were reviewed and journals in the RCOG library were hand-searched to identify articles not yet indexed. There was no systematic attempt to search the 'grey literature' (conferences, abstracts, theses and unpublished trials).

A preliminary scrutiny of titles and abstracts was undertaken and full papers were obtained if they appeared to address the Guideline Development Group's (GDG) question relevant to the topic. Following a critical review of the full version of the study, articles not relevant to the subject in question were excluded. Studies that did not report on relevant outcomes were also excluded. Submitted evidence from stakeholders was included where the evidence was relevant to the GDG clinical question and when it was either better or equivalent in quality to the research identified in the literature searches.

The economic evaluation included a search of:

- NHS Economic Evaluations Database (NHS EED)
- www.ohe-heed.com http://nhscrd.york.ac.uk/nhsdhp.htm
- Cochrane Database of Systematic Reviews, Issue 3, 2003
- MEDLINE January 1966 to April 2003
- EMBASE 1980 to April 2003.

Relevant experts in the field were contacted for further information.

The search strategies were designed to find any economic study related to specific antenatal screening programmes. Abstracts and database reviews of papers found were reviewed by the health economist and were discarded if they appeared not to contain any economic data or if the focus of the paper did not relate to the precise topic or question being considered (i.e. to screening strategy alternatives that were not relevant to this guideline). Relevant references in the bibliographies of reviewed papers were also identified and reviewed. These were assessed by the health economists against standard criteria.

Clinical effectiveness

For all the subject areas, evidence from the study designs least subject to sources of bias was included. Where possible, the highest levels of evidence were used, but all papers were reviewed using established guides (see below). Published systematic reviews or meta-analyses were used if available. For subject areas where neither was available, other appropriate experimental or observational studies were sought.

Identified articles were assessed methodologically and the best available evidence was used to form and support the recommendations. The highest level of evidence was selected for each clinical question. Using the evidence-level structure shown in Table 1.1, the retrieved evidence was graded accordingly.

Hierarchy of evidence

The clinical question dictates the highest level of evidence that should be sought. For issues of therapy or treatment, the highest level of evidence is meta-analyses of randomised controlled trials or randomised controlled trials themselves. This would equate to a grade A recommendation.

For issues of prognosis, a cohort study is the best level of evidence available. The best possible level of evidence would equate to a grade B recommendation. It should not be interpreted as an inferior grade of recommendation, as it represents the highest level of evidence attainable for that type of clinical question.

Table 1.1 Structure of evidence levels

Level	Definition
1a	Systematic review and meta-analysis of randomised controlled trials
1b	At least one randomised controlled trial
2a	At least one well-designed controlled study without randomisation
2b	At least one other type of well-designed quasi-experimental study
3	Well-designed non-experimental descriptive studies, such as comparative studies, correlation studies or case studies
4	Expert committee reports or opinions and/or clinical experience of respected authorities

For diagnostic tests, test evaluation studies examining the performance of the test were used if the efficacy of the test was required. Where an evaluation of the effectiveness of the test on management and outcome was required, evidence from randomised controlled trials or cohort studies was sought.

All retrieved articles have been appraised methodologically using established guides. Where appropriate, if a systematic review, meta-analysis or randomised controlled trial existed in relation to a topic, studies of a weaker design were not sought.

The evidence was synthesised using qualitative methods. These involved summarising the content of identified papers in the form of evidence tables and agreeing brief statements that accurately reflect the relevant evidence. Quantitative techniques (meta-analyses) were performed if appropriate and necessary.

For the purposes of this guideline, data are presented as relative risk (RR) where relevant (i.e. in RCTs and cohort studies) or as odds ratios (OR) where relevant (i.e. in systematic reviews of RCTs). Where these data are statistically significant they are also presented as numbers needed to treat (NNT), if relevant.

Health economics

In antenatal care, there is a relatively large body of economic literature that has considered the economic costs and consequences of different screening programmes and considered the organisation of antenatal care. The purpose of including economic evidence in a clinical guideline is to allow recommendations to be made not just on the clinical effectiveness of different forms of care, but on the cost effectiveness as well. The aim is to produce guidance that uses scarce health service resources efficiently; that is, providing the best possible care within resource constraints.

The economic evidence is focused around the different methods of screening, although some work has been undertaken to examine the cost effectiveness of different patterns of antenatal care (the number of antenatal appointments) and to explore women's preferences for different aspects of their antenatal care. The economic evidence presented in this guideline is not a systematic review of all the economic evidence around antenatal care. It was decided that the health economic input into the guideline should focus on specific topics where the guideline development group thought that economic evidence would help them to inform their decisions. This approach was made on pragmatic grounds (not all the economic evidence could be reviewed with the resources available) and on the basis that economic evidence should not be based only on the economic literature, but should be consistent with the clinical effectiveness evidence presented in the guideline. Some of the economic evaluation studies did not address the specific alternatives (say, for screening) that were addressed in the guideline. Therefore, for each of the specific topic areas where the economic evidence was reviewed, a simple economic model was developed in order to present the guideline development group with a coherent picture of the costs and consequences of the decisions based on the clinical and economic evidence. The role of the health economist in this guideline was to review the literature in these specific areas and obtain cost data considered to be the closest to current UK opportunity cost (the value of the resources used, rather than the price or charge).

The approach adopted for this guideline was for the health economic analysis to focus on specific areas. Topics for economic analysis were selected on the following basis by the guideline development group.

- Does the proposed topic have major resource implications?
- Is there a change of policy involved?
- Are there sufficient data of adequate quality to allow useful review or modelling?
- Is there a lack of consensus among clinicians?
- Is there a particular area with a large amount of uncertainty?

Where the above answers were "yes", this indicated that further economic analysis including modelling is more likely to be useful.

The Guideline Development Group identified six areas where the potential impact of alternative strategies could be substantial and where the health economics evidence should focus. These were: screening for asymptomatic bacteriuria, screening for group B streptococcus, screening for syphilis, screening for sickle cell and thalassaemia, ultrasound screening for structural abnormalities and Down's syndrome screening.

For all these topics, a review of the economic evidence was undertaken, followed by simple economic modelling of the cost effectiveness in England and Wales of different strategies.

The review of the economic evaluation studies included cost-effectiveness studies (only those where an incremental cost-effectiveness ratio had been determined or could be determined from the data presented). The topic had to focus on the appropriate alternatives (the appropriate clinical question), preferably able to be generalised to the England and Wales setting, and therefore be useful in constructing a simple decision model. The review of the evidence included cost-effectiveness studies, cost-consequence studies (cost of present and future costs only) and high-quality systematic reviews of the evidence. A narrative review of all the evidence is not presented in the main guideline. Appendix 2 shows the way the models have been constructed, the economic and clinical parameters incorporated into each model, the sources of data that have been used (cost data and clinical data), the results of the baseline model and the sensitivity analysis.

Evidence on the cost consequences associated with alternative screening strategies was obtained from various published sources that addressed these issues. The purpose was to obtain good quality cost data judged by the health economist to be as close as possible to the true opportunity cost of the intervention (screening programme).

The key cost variables considered were:

- the cost of a screening programme (the cost of different screening interventions and the cost of expanding and contracting a screening programme)
- the cost of treatment of women found to be carriers of a disease
- the cost of any adverse or non-therapeutic effects of screening or treatment to the woman
- the cost of the consequences of screening and not screening to the fetus and infant, including fetal loss, ending pregnancy, and the lifetime costs of caring for infants born with disabilities.

Cost data not available from published sources were obtained from the most up-to-date NHS reference cost price list. Some cost data could not be obtained from published sources or from NHS reference costs and therefore consensus methods were used in the Guideline Development Group to obtain an indicative estimate of the likely costs. The range of sources of cost data are set out in the appendix that explains the methodology adopted to construct each of the economic models created for this guideline.

In some cases (i.e., for screening for asymptomatic bacteriuria and for haemoglobinopathies), the economic modelling work began and had to be abandoned due to lack of data of the effectiveness of the different screening options. Appendix 2 provides some discussion of these models that could not be completed in the guideline and areas for future research.

Limitations of the economic evidence in this guideline

Economic analyses have been undertaken alongside a wide range of antenatal screening procedures. A systematic review of antenatal screening was undertaken in 2001.[7] This review found that many of the studies identified were of poor quality, since they did not consider the effects of screening on future health (of mother and baby) but only costs averted by a screening programme.

In this guideline, the costs of screening and the costs of the benefits or harm of screening have been considered simultaneously where possible (i.e. where the data exist). It has not been possible to include many of the consequences of a screening programme because the data do not exist on these less straightforward or measurable outcomes (such as the benefit foregone from ending pregnancy).

The economic analysis of screening methods in the guideline has not been able to consider the following:

- the value to the woman of being given information about the health of her future child
- the value of being able to plan appropriate services for children who are born with disabilities

- the value of a life of a child born with disability, to the child, to the family and to society in general
- the value to a woman of being able to choose whether to end a pregnancy
- the value of a life foregone as a consequence of screening.

The cost-effectiveness studies reviewed for this guideline had narrowly defined endpoints; for example, a case of birth defect detected and subsequently averted as a result of a screening test. Some of the studies have considered the cost consequences of avoiding the birth of an infant with severe disabilities and their long-term care costs. The value of future life foregone (of a healthy or a disabled infant's life) due to screening has not been explicitly considered in any of the economic evidence of antenatal screening. Since economic evaluation should always consider the costs and benefits of an intervention in the widest possible sense, this could be seen as a limitation of the analysis presented in this guideline. The consequences of this are discussed in Appendix 2.

Forming and grading the recommendations

The Guideline Development Group was presented with the summaries (text and evidence tables) of the best available research evidence to answer their questions. Recommendations were based on, and explicitly linked to, the evidence that supported them. A recommendation's grade may not necessarily reflect the importance attached to the recommendation. For example the Guideline Development Group felt that the principles of woman-centred care that underpin this guideline (Chapter 3) are particularly important but some of these recommendations receive only a D grade or good practice point (GPP).

The Group worked where possible on an informal consensus basis. Formal consensus methods (modified Delphi techniques or nominal group technique) were employed if required (e.g. grading recommendations or agreeing audit criteria).

The recommendations were then graded according to the level of evidence upon which they were based. The strength of the evidence on which each recommendation is based is shown in Table 1.2. The grading of recommendations will follow that outlined in the Health Technology Assessment (HTA) review *How to develop cost conscious guidelines*.

Limited results or data are presented in the text. More comprehensive results and data are available in the relevant evidence tables.

External review

The guideline has been developed in accordance with the NICE guideline development process.[6] This has included the opportunity for registered stakeholders to comment on the scope of the guideline, the first draft of the full and summary guidelines and the second draft of all versions of the guideline. In addition, the first draft was reviewed by nominated individuals with an interest in antenatal care. All drafts, comments and responses were also reviewed by the independent Guideline Review Panel established by NICE.

The comments made by the stakeholders, peer reviewers and the NICE Guideline Review Panel were collated and presented anonymously for consideration by the Guideline Development Group. All comments were considered systematically by the Group and the resulting actions and responses were recorded.

Table 1.2 Strength of the evidence upon which each recommendation is based

Grade	Definition
A	Directly based on level I evidence
B	Directly based on level II evidence or extrapolated recommendation from level I evidence
C	Directly based on level III evidence or extrapolated recommendation from either level I or II evidence
D	Directly based on level IV evidence or extrapolated recommendation from either level I, II or III evidence
Good practice point (GPP)	The view of the Guideline Development Group
NICE Technology Appraisal	Recommendation taken from the NICE Technology Appraisal

2. Summary of recommendations and practice algorithm

2.1 Summary of recommendations

Chapter 3 Woman-centred care and informed decision making

3.2 Antenatal education

Pregnant women should be offered opportunities to attend antenatal classes and have written information about antenatal care. [A]

Pregnant women should be offered evidence-based information and support to enable them to make informed decisions regarding their care. Information should include details of where they will be seen and who will undertake their care. Addressing women's choices should be recognised as being integral to the decision-making process. [C]

At the first contact, pregnant women should be offered information about the pregnancy care services and options available, lifestyle considerations, including dietary information, and screening tests. [C]

Pregnant women should be informed about the purpose of any screening test before it is performed. The right of a woman to accept or decline a test should be made clear. [D]

At each antenatal appointment, midwives and doctors should offer consistent information and clear explanations and should provide pregnant women with an opportunity to discuss issues and ask questions. [D]

Communication and information should be provided in a form that is accessible to pregnant women who have additional needs, such as those with physical, cognitive or sensory disabilities and those who do not speak or read English. [Good practice point]

Chapter 4 Provision and organisation of care

4.1 Who provides care?

Midwife- and GP-led models of care should be offered for women with an uncomplicated pregnancy. Routine involvement of obstetricians in the care of women with an uncomplicated pregnancy at scheduled times does not appear to improve perinatal outcomes compared with involving obstetricians when complications arise. [A]

4.2 Continuity of care

Antenatal care should be provided by a small group of carers with whom the woman feels comfortable. There should be continuity of care throughout the antenatal period. [A]

A system of clear referral paths should be established so that pregnant women who require additional care are managed and treated by the appropriate specialist teams when problems are identified. [D]

4.3 Where should antenatal appointments take place?

Antenatal care should be readily and easily accessible to all women and should be sensitive to the needs of individual women and the local community. [C]

The environment in which antenatal appointments take place should enable women to discuss sensitive issues such as domestic violence, sexual abuse, psychiatric illness and illicit drug use. [Good practice point]

4.4 Documentation of care

Structured maternity records should be used for antenatal care. [A]

Maternity services should have a system in place whereby women carry their own case notes. [A]

A standardised, national maternity record with an agreed minimum data set should be developed and used. This will help carers to provide the recommended evidence-based care to pregnant women. [Good practice point]

4.5 Frequency of antenatal appointments

A schedule of antenatal appointments should be determined by the function of the appointments. For a woman who is nulliparous with an uncomplicated pregnancy, a schedule of ten appointments should be adequate. For a woman who is parous with an uncomplicated pregnancy, a schedule of seven appointments should be adequate. [B]

Early in pregnancy, all women should receive appropriate written information about the likely number, timing and content of antenatal appointments associated with different options of care and be given an opportunity to discuss this schedule with their midwife or doctor. [D]

Each antenatal appointment should be structured and have focused content. Longer appointments are needed early in pregnancy to allow comprehensive assessment and discussion. Wherever possible, appointments should incorporate routine tests and investigations to minimise inconvenience to women. [D]

4.6 Gestational age assessment: LMP and ultrasound

Pregnant women should be offered an early ultrasound scan to determine gestational age (in lieu of last menstrual period (LMP) for all cases) and to detect multiple pregnancies. This will ensure consistency of gestational age assessments, improve the performance of mid-trimester serum screening for Down's syndrome and reduce the need for induction of labour after 41 weeks. [A]

Ideally, scans should be performed between 10 and 13 weeks and use crown–rump length measurement to determine gestational age. Pregnant women who present at or beyond 14 weeks of gestation should be offered an ultrasound scan to estimate gestational age using head circumference or biparietal diameter. [Good practice point]

4.7 What should happen at antenatal appointments?

The assessment of women who may or may not need additional clinical care during pregnancy is based on identifying those in whom there are any maternal or fetal conditions associated with an excess of maternal or perinatal death or morbidity. While this approach may not identify many of the women who go on to require extra care and will also categorise many women who go on to have normal uneventful births as 'high risk',[58,59] ascertainment of risk in pregnancy remains important as it may facilitate early detection to allow time to plan for appropriate management.

The needs of each pregnant woman should be assessed at the first appointment and reassessed at each appointment throughout pregnancy because new problems can arise at any time. Additional appointments should be determined by the needs of the pregnant woman, as assessed by her and her care givers, and the environment in which appointments take place should enable women to discuss sensitive issues Reducing the number of routine appointments will enable more time per appointment for care, information giving and support for pregnant women.

The schedule below, which has been determined by the purpose of each appointment, presents the recommended number of antenatal care appointments for women who are healthy and whose pregnancies remain uncomplicated in the antenatal period; ten appointments for nulliparous women and seven for parous women.

First appointment

The first appointment needs to be earlier in pregnancy (prior to 12 weeks) than may have traditionally occurred and, because of the large volume of information needs in early pregnancy, two appointments may be required. At the first (and second) antenatal appointment:

- give information, with an opportunity to discuss issues and ask questions; offer verbal information supported by written information (on topics such as diet and lifestyle considerations, pregnancy care services available, maternity benefits and sufficient information to enable informed decision making about screening tests)
- identify women who may need additional care (see Algorithm and Section 1.2) and plan pattern of care for the pregnancy
- check blood group and rhesus D (RhD) status
- offer screening for anaemia, red-cell alloantibodies, Hepatitis B virus, HIV, rubella susceptibility and syphilis
- offer screening for asymptomatic bacteriuria (ASB)
- offering screening for Down's syndrome
- offer early ultrasound scan for gestational age assessment
- offer ultrasound screening for structural anomalies (20 weeks)
- measure BMI and blood pressure (BP) and test urine for proteinuria.

After the first (and possibly second) appointment, for women who choose to have screening, the following test should be arranged before 16 weeks of gestation (except serum screening for Down's syndrome, which may occur up to 20 weeks of gestation):

- blood tests (for checking blood group and RhD status and screening for anaemia, red-cell alloantibodies, hepatitis B virus, HIV, rubella susceptibility and syphilis)
- urine tests (to check for proteinuria and screen for ASB)
- ultrasound scan to determine gestational age using:
  - crown–rump measurement if performed at 10 to 13 weeks
  - biparietal diameter or head circumference at or beyond 14 weeks
- Down's syndrome screening using:
- nuchal translucency at 11 to 14 weeks
- serum screening at 14 to 20 weeks.

16 weeks

The next appointment should be scheduled at 16 weeks to:

- review, discuss and record the results of all screening tests undertaken; reassess planned pattern of care for the pregnancy and identify women who need additional care (see Algorithm and Section 1.2)
- investigate a haemoglobin level of less than 11g/dl and consider iron supplementation if indicated
- measure BP and test urine for proteinuria
- give information, with an opportunity to discuss issues and ask questions; offer verbal information supported by antenatal classes and written information.

18–20 weeks

At 18–20 weeks, if the woman chooses, an ultrasound scan should be performed for the detection of structural anomalies. For a woman whose placenta is found to extend across the internal cervical os at this time, another scan at 36 weeks should be offered and the results of this scan reviewed at the 36-week appointment.

25 weeks

At 25 weeks of gestation, another appointment should be scheduled for nulliparous women. At this appointment:

- measure and plot symphysis–fundal height
- measure BP and test urine for proteinuria
- give information, with an opportunity to discuss issues and ask questions; offer verbal information supported by antenatal classes and written information.

28 weeks

The next appointment for all pregnant women should occur at 28 weeks. At this appointment:

- offer a second screening for anaemia and atypical red-cell alloantibodies
- investigate a haemoglobin level of less than 10.5 g/dl and consider iron supplementation, if indicated
- offer anti-D to rhesus-negative women
- measure BP and test urine for proteinuria
- measure and plot symphysis–fundal height
- give information, with an opportunity to discuss issues and ask questions; offer verbal information supported by antenatal classes and written information.

31 weeks

Nulliparous women should have an appointment scheduled at 31 weeks to:

- measure BP and test urine for proteinuria
- measure and plot symphysis–fundal height
- give information, with an opportunity to discuss issues and ask questions; offer verbal information supported by antenatal classes and written information
- review, discuss and record the results of screening tests undertaken at 28 weeks; reassess planned pattern of care for the pregnancy and identify women who need additional care (see Algorithm and Section 1.2).

34 weeks

At 34 weeks, all pregnant women should be seen in order to:

- offer a second dose of anti-D to rhesus-negative women
- measure BP and test urine for proteinuria
- measure and plot symphysis–fundal height
- give information, with an opportunity to discuss issues and ask questions; offer verbal information supported by antenatal classes and written information
- review, discuss and record the results of screening tests undertaken at 28 weeks; reassess planned pattern of care for the pregnancy and identify women who need additional care (see Algorithm and Section 1.2).

36 weeks

At 36 weeks, all pregnant women should be seen again to:

- measure BP and test urine for proteinuria
- measure and plot symphysis–fundal height
- check position of baby
- for women whose babies are in the breech presentation, offer external cephalic version (ECV)
- review ultrasound scan report if placenta extended over the internal cervical os at previous scan
- give information, with an opportunity to discuss issues and ask questions; offer verbal information supported by antenatal classes and written information.

38 weeks

Another appointment at 38 weeks will allow for:

- measurement BP and urine testing for proteinuria
- measurement and plotting of symphysis–fundal height
- information giving, with an opportunity to discuss issues and ask questions; verbal information supported by antenatal classes and written information.

40 weeks

For nulliparous women, an appointment at 40 weeks should be scheduled to:

- measure BP and test urine for proteinuria
- measure and plot symphysis–fundal height
- give information, with an opportunity to discuss issues and ask questions; offer verbal information supported by antenatal classes and written information.

41 weeks

For women who have not given birth by 41 weeks:

- a membrane sweep should be offered
- induction of labour should be offered
- BP should be measured and urine tested for proteinuria
- symphysis–fundal height should be measured and plotted
- information should be given, with an opportunity to discuss issues and ask questions; verbal information supported by written information.

General

Throughout the entire antenatal period, healthcare providers should remain alert to signs or symptoms of conditions which affect the health of the mother and fetus, such as domestic violence, pre-eclampsia and diabetes.

For an outline of care at each appointment see the Algorithm (Section 2.3).

Chapter 5 Lifestyle considerations

5.3 Working during pregnancy

Pregnant women should be informed of their maternity rights and benefits. [C]

The majority of women can be reassured that it is safe to continue working during pregnancy. Further information about possible occupational hazards during pregnancy is available from the Health and Safety Executive. [D]

A woman's occupation during pregnancy should be ascertained to identify those at increased risk through occupational exposure. [Good practice point]

5.5 Nutritional supplements

Pregnant women (and those intending to become pregnant) should be informed that dietary supplementation with folic acid, before conception and up to 12 weeks of gestation, reduces the risk of having a baby with neural tube defects (anencephaly, spina bifida). The recommended dose is 400 micrograms per day. [A]

Iron supplementation should not be offered routinely to all pregnant women. It does not benefit the mother's or the fetus's health and may have unpleasant maternal side effects. [A]

Pregnant women should be informed that vitamin A supplementation (intake greater than 700 micrograms) might be teratogenic and therefore it should be avoided. Pregnant women should be informed that as liver and liver products may also contain high levels of vitamin A, consumption of these products should also be avoided. [C]

There is insufficient evidence to evaluate the effectiveness of vitamin D in pregnancy. In the absence of evidence of benefit, vitamin D supplementation should not be offered routinely to all pregnant women. [A]

5.6 Food-acquired infections

Pregnant women should be offered information on how to reduce the risk of listeriosis by:

- drinking only pasteurised or UHT milk
- not eating ripened soft cheese such as Camembert, Brie and blue-veined cheese (there is no risk with hard cheeses, such as Cheddar, or cottage cheese and processed cheese)
- not eating pâté (of any sort, including vegetable)
- not eating uncooked or undercooked ready-prepared meals. [D]

Pregnant women should be offered information on how to reduce the risk of salmonella infection by:

- avoiding raw or partially cooked eggs or food that may contain them (such as mayonnaise)
- avoiding raw or partially cooked meat, especially poultry. [D]

5.7 Prescribed medicines

Few medicines have been established as safe to use in pregnancy. Prescription medicines should be used as little as possible during pregnancy and should be limited to circumstances where the benefit outweighs the risk. [D]

5.8 Over-the-counter medicines

Pregnant women should be informed that few over-the-counter (OTC) medicines have been established as being safe to take in pregnancy. OTC medicines should be used as little as possible during pregnancy. [D]

5.9 Complementary therapies

Pregnant women should be informed that few complementary therapies have been established as being safe and effective during pregnancy. Women should not assume that such therapies are safe and they should be used as little as possible during pregnancy. [D]

5.10 Exercise in pregnancy

Pregnant women should be informed that beginning or continuing a moderate course of exercise during pregnancy is not associated with adverse outcomes. [A]

Pregnant women should be informed of the potential dangers of certain activities during pregnancy, for example, contact sports, high-impact sports and vigorous racquet sports that may involve the risk of abdominal trauma, falls or excessive joint stress, and scuba diving, which may result in fetal birth defects and fetal decompression disease. [D]

5.11 Sexual intercourse in pregnancy

Pregnant woman should be informed that sexual intercourse in pregnancy is not known to be associated with any adverse outcomes. [B]

5.12 Alcohol and smoking in pregnancy

Excess alcohol has an adverse effect on the fetus. Therefore it is suggested that women limit alcohol consumption to no more than one standard unit per day. Each of the following constitutes one 'unit' of alcohol: a single measure of spirits, one small glass of wine, and a half pint of ordinary strength beer, lager or cider. [C]

Pregnant women should be informed about the specific risks of smoking during pregnancy (such as the risk of having a baby with low birthweight and preterm). The benefits of quitting at any stage should be emphasised. [A]

Women who smoke or who have recently stopped should be offered smoking cessation interventions. Interventions that appear to be effective in reducing smoking include advice by physician, group sessions and behavioural therapy (based on self-help manuals). [A]

Women who are unable to quit smoking during pregnancy should be encouraged to reduce smoking. [B]

5.13 Cannabis use in pregnancy

The direct effects of cannabis on the fetus are uncertain but may be harmful. Cannabis use is associated with smoking, which is known to be harmful; therefore women should be discouraged from using cannabis during pregnancy. [C]

5.14 Air travel during pregnancy

Pregnant women should be informed that long-haul air travel is associated with an increased risk of venous thrombosis, although whether or not there is additional risk during pregnancy is unclear. In the general population, wearing correctly fitted compression stockings is effective at reducing the risk. [B]

5.15 Car travel during pregnancy

Pregnant women should be informed about the correct use of seatbelts (that is, three-point seatbelts "above and below the bump, not over it"). [B]

5.16 Travelling abroad during pregnancy
Pregnant women should be informed that, if they are planning to travel abroad, they should discuss considerations such as flying, vaccinations and travel insurance with their midwife or doctor. [Good practice point]

Chapter 6 Management of common symptoms of pregnancy

6.1 Nausea and vomiting in early pregnancy
Women should be informed that most cases of nausea and vomiting in pregnancy will resolve spontaneously within 16 to 20 weeks of gestation and that nausea and vomiting are not usually associated with a poor pregnancy outcome. If a woman requests or would like to consider treatment, the following interventions appear to be effective in reducing symptoms [A]:

- nonpharmacological:
  - ginger
  - P6 acupressure
- pharmacological:
  - antihistamines.

Information about all forms of self-help and nonpharmacological treatments should be made available for pregnant women who have nausea and vomiting. [Good practice point]

6.2 Heartburn
Women who present with symptoms of heartburn in pregnancy should be offered information regarding lifestyle and diet modification. [Good practice point]

Antacids may be offered to women whose heartburn remains troublesome despite lifestyle and diet modification. [A]

6.3 Constipation
Women who present with constipation in pregnancy should be offered information regarding diet modification, such as bran or wheat fibre supplementation. [A]

6.4 Haemorrhoids
In the absence of evidence of the effectiveness of treatments for haemorrhoids in pregnancy, women should be offered information concerning diet modification. If clinical symptoms remain troublesome, standard haemorrhoid creams should be considered. [Good practice point]

6.5 Varicose veins
Women should be informed that varicose veins are a common symptom of pregnancy that will not cause harm and that compression stockings can improve the symptoms but will not prevent varicose veins from emerging. [A]

6.6 Vaginal discharge
Women should be informed that an increase in vaginal discharge is a common physiological change that occurs during pregnancy. If this is associated with itch, soreness, offensive smell or pain on passing urine there maybe an infective cause and investigation should be considered. [Good practice point]

A 1-week course of a topical imidazole is an effective treatment and should be considered for vaginal candidiasis infections in pregnant women. [A]

The effectiveness and safety of oral treatments for vaginal candidiasis in pregnancy is uncertain and these should not be offered. [Good practice point]

6.7 Backache
Women should be informed that exercising in water, massage therapy and group or individual back care classes might help to ease backache during pregnancy. [A]

Chapter 7 Clinical examination of pregnant women

7.1 Measurement of weight and body mass index

Maternal weight and height should be measured at the first antenatal appointment, and the woman's body mass index (BMI) calculated (weight [kg]/height[m]^2). [B]

Repeated weighing during pregnancy should be confined to circumstances where clinical management is likely to be influenced. [C]

7.2 Breast examination

Routine breast examination during antenatal care is not recommended for the promotion of postnatal breastfeeding. [A]

7.3 Pelvic examination

Routine antenatal pelvic examination does not accurately assess gestational age, nor does it accurately predict preterm birth or cephalopelvic disproportion. It is not recommended. [B]

7.4 Female genital mutilation

Pregnant women who have had female genital mutilation should be identified early in antenatal care through sensitive enquiry. Antenatal examination will then allow planning of intrapartum care. [C]

7.5 Domestic violence

Health care professionals need to be alert to the symptoms or signs of domestic violence and women should be given the opportunity to disclose domestic violence in an environment in which they feel secure. [D]

7.6 Psychiatric screening

Women should be asked early in pregnancy if they have had any previous psychiatric illnesses. Women who have had a past history of serious psychiatric disorder should be referred for a psychiatric assessment during the antenatal period. [B]

Pregnant women should not be offered routine screening, such as with the Edinburgh Postnatal Depression Scale, in the antenatal period to predict the development of postnatal depression. [A]

Pregnant women should not be offered antenatal education interventions to reduce perinatal or postnatal depression, as these interventions have not been shown to be effective. [A]

Chapter 8 Screening for haematological conditions

8.1 Anaemia

Pregnant women should be offered screening for anaemia. Screening should take place early in pregnancy (at the first appointment) and at 28 weeks when other blood screening tests are being performed. This allows enough time for treatment if anaemia is detected. [B]

Haemoglobin levels outside the normal UK range for pregnancy (that is, 11 g/dl at first contact and 10.5 g/dl at 28 weeks) should be investigated and iron supplementation considered if indicated. [A]

8.3 Blood grouping and red cell alloantibodies

Women should be offered testing for blood group and RhD status in early pregnancy. [B]

It is recommended that routine antenatal anti-D prophylaxis is offered to all non-sensitised pregnant women who are RhD negative. [NICE 2002]

Women should be screened for atypical red cell alloantibodies in early pregnancy and again at 28 weeks regardless of their RhD status. [B]

Pregnant women with clinically significant atypical red cell alloantibodies should be offered referral to a specialist centre for further investigation and advice on subsequent antenatal management.[D]

If a pregnant woman is RhD-negative, consideration should be given to offering partner testing to determine whether the administration of anti-D prophylaxis is necessary. [Good practice point]

Chapter 9 Screening for fetal anomalies

9.1 Screening for structural anomalies

Pregnant women should be offered an ultrasound scan to screen for structural anomalies, ideally between 18 and 20 weeks of gestation, by an appropriately trained sonographer and with equipment of an appropriate standard as outlined by the National Screening Committee. [A]

9.2 Screening for Down's syndrome

Pregnant women should be offered screening for Down's syndrome with a test that provides the current standard of a detection rate above 60% and a false positive rate of less than 5%. The following tests meet this standard:

- From 11 to 14 weeks:
  ○ nuchal translucency (NT)
  ○ the combined test (NT, hCG and PAPP-A)
- From 14 to 20 weeks:
  ○ the triple test (hCG, AFP and uE_3)
  ○ the quadruple test (hCG, AFP, uE_3, inhibin A)
- From 11 to 14 weeks AND 14 to 20 weeks:
  ○ the integrated test (NT, PAPP-A + hCG, AFP, uE_3, inhibin A)
  ○ the serum integrated test (PAPP-A + hCG, AFP, uE_3, inhibin A). [B]

By April 2007, pregnant women should be offered screening for Down's syndrome with a test which provides a detection rate above 75% and a false positive rate of less than 3%. These performance measures should be age standardised and based on a cutoff of 1/250 at term. The following tests currently meet this standard:

- From 11 to 14 weeks:
  ○ the combined test (NT, hCG and PAPP-A)
- From 14 to 20 weeks:
  ○ the quadruple test (hCG, AFP, uE_3, inhibin A)
- From 11 to 14 weeks AND 14 to 20 weeks:
  ○ the integrated test (NT, PAPP-A + hCG, AFP, uE_3, inhibin A)
  ○ the serum integrated test (PAPP-A + hCG, AFP, uE_3, inhibin A). [B]

Pregnant women should be given information about the detection rates and false positive rates of any Down's syndrome screening test being offered and about further diagnostic tests that may be offered. The woman's right to accept or decline the test should be made clear. [D]

Chapter 10 Screening for infections

10.1 Asymptomatic bacteriuria

Pregnant women should be offered routine screening for asymptomatic bacteriuria by midstream urine culture early in pregnancy. Identification and treatment of asymptomatic bacteriuria reduces the risk of preterm birth. [A]

10.2 Asymptomatic bacterial vaginosis

Pregnant women should not be offered routine screening for bacterial vaginosis because the evidence suggests that the identification and treatment of asymptomatic bacterial vaginosis does not lower the risk for preterm birth and other adverse reproductive outcomes. [A]

10.3 Chlamydia trachomatis

Pregnant women should not be offered routine screening for asymptomatic chlamydia because there is insufficient evidence on its effectiveness and cost effectiveness. However, this policy is likely to change with the implementation of the national opportunistic chlamydia screening programme. [C]

10.4 Cytomegalovirus

The available evidence does not support routine cytomegalovirus screening in pregnant women and it should not be offered. [B]

10.5 Hepatitis B virus

Serological screening for hepatitis B virus should be offered to pregnant women so that effective postnatal intervention can be offered to infected women to decrease the risk of mother-to-child transmission. [A]

10.6 Hepatitis C virus

Pregnant women should not be offered routine screening for hepatitis C virus because there is insufficient evidence on its effectiveness and cost effectiveness. [C]

10.7 HIV

Pregnant women should be offered screening for HIV infection early in antenatal care because appropriate antenatal interventions can reduce mother-to-child transmission of HIV infection. [A]

A system of clear referral paths should be established in each unit or department so that pregnant women who are diagnosed with an HIV infection are managed and treated by the appropriate specialist teams. [D]

10.8 Rubella

Rubella susceptibility screening should be offered early in antenatal care to identify women at risk of contracting rubella infection and to enable vaccination in the postnatal period for the protection of future pregnancies. [B]

10.9 Streptococcus Group B

Pregnant women should not be offered routine antenatal screening for group B streptococcus (GBS) because evidence of its clinical effectiveness and cost effectiveness remains uncertain. [C]

10.10 Syphilis

Screening for syphilis should be offered to all pregnant women at an early stage in antenatal care because treatment of syphilis is beneficial to the mother and fetus. [B]

Because syphilis is a rare condition in the UK and a positive result does not necessarily mean that a woman has syphilis, clear paths of referral for the management of women testing positive for syphilis should be established. [Good practice point]

10.11 Toxoplasmosis

Routine antenatal serological screening for toxoplasmosis should not be offered because the harms of screening may outweigh the potential benefits. [B]

Pregnant women should be informed of primary prevention measures to avoid toxoplasmosis infection such as:

- washing hands before handling food
- thoroughly washing all fruit and vegetables, including ready-prepared salads, before eating
- thoroughly cooking raw meats and ready-prepared chilled meals
- wearing gloves and thoroughly washing hands after handling soil and gardening
- avoiding cat faeces in cat litter or in soil. [C]

Chapter 11 Screening for clinical conditions

11.1 Gestational diabetes mellitus

The evidence does not support routine screening for gestational diabetes mellitus (GDM) and therefore it should not be offered. [B]

11.2 Pre-eclampsia

At first contact a woman's level of risk for pre-eclampsia should be evaluated so that a plan for her subsequent schedule of antenatal appointments can be formulated. The likelihood of developing pre-eclampsia during a pregnancy is increased in women who:

- are nulliparous
- are age 40 or older
- have a family history of pre-eclampsia (e.g., pre-eclampsia in a mother or sister)
- have a prior history of pre-eclampsia
- have a body mass index (BMI) at or above 35 at first contact
- have a multiple pregnancy or pre-existing vascular disease (for example, hypertension or diabetes). [C]

Whenever blood pressure is measured in pregnancy, a urine sample should be tested at the same time for proteinuria. [C]

Standardised equipment, techniques and conditions for blood-pressure measurement should be used by all personnel whenever blood pressure is measured in the antenatal period so that valid comparisons can be made. [C]

Pregnant women should be informed of the symptoms of advanced pre-eclampsia because these may be associated with poorer pregnancy outcomes for the mother or baby. Symptoms include headache, problems with vision, such as blurring or flashing before the eyes, bad pain just below the ribs, vomiting and sudden swelling of face, hands or feet. [D]

11.3 Preterm birth

Routine vaginal examination to assess the cervix is not an effective method of predicting preterm birth and should not be offered. [A]

Although cervical shortening identified by transvaginal ultrasound examination and increased levels of fetal fibronectin are associated with an increased risk for preterm birth, the evidence does not indicate that this information improves outcomes; therefore, neither routine antenatal cervical assessment by transvaginal ultrasound nor the measurement of fetal fibronectin should be used to predict preterm birth in healthy pregnant women. [B]

11.4 Placenta praevia

Because most low-lying placentas detected at a 20-week anomaly scan will resolve by the time the baby is born, only a woman whose placenta extends over the internal cervical os should be offered another transabdominal scan at 36 weeks. If the transabdominal scan is unclear, a transvaginal scan should be offered. [C]

Chapter 12 Fetal growth and wellbeing

12.1 Abdominal palpation for fetal presentation

Fetal presentation should be assessed by abdominal palpation at 36 weeks or later, when presentation is likely to influence the plans for the birth. Routine assessment of presentation by abdominal palpation should not be offered before 36 weeks because it is not always accurate and may be uncomfortable. [C]

Suspected fetal malpresentation should be confirmed by an ultrasound assessment. [Good practice point]

12.2 Measurement of symphysis–fundal distance

Pregnant women should be offered estimation of fetal size at each antenatal appointment to detect small- or large-for-gestational-age infants. [A]

Symphysis–fundal height should be measured and plotted at each antenatal appointment. [Good practice point]

12.3 Routine monitoring of fetal movements

Routine formal fetal-movement counting should not be offered. [A]

12.4 Auscultation of fetal heart

Auscultation of the fetal heart may confirm that the fetus is alive but is unlikely to have any predictive value and routine listening is therefore not recommended. However, when requested by the mother, auscultation of the fetal heart may provide reassurance. [D]

12.5 Cardiotocography

The evidence does not support the routine use of antenatal electronic fetal heart rate monitoring (cardiotocography) for fetal assessment in women with an uncomplicated pregnancy and therefore it should not be offered. [A]

12.6 Ultrasound assessment in the third trimester

The evidence does not support the routine use of ultrasound scanning after 24 weeks of gestation and therefore it should not be offered. [A]

12.7 Umbilical and uterine artery Doppler ultrasound

The use of umbilical artery Doppler ultrasound for the prediction of fetal growth restriction should not be offered routinely. [A]

The use of uterine artery Doppler ultrasound for the prediction of pre-eclampsia should not be offered routinely. [B]

Chapter 13 Management of specific clinical conditions

13.1 Pregnancy after 41 weeks (see also Chapter 4.6 Gestational age assessment)

Prior to formal induction of labour, women should be offered a vaginal examination for membrane sweeping. [A]

Women with uncomplicated pregnancies should be offered induction of labour beyond 41 weeks. [A]

From 42 weeks, women who decline induction of labour should be offered increased antenatal monitoring consisting of at least twice-weekly cardiotocography and ultrasound estimation of maximum amniotic pool depth. [Good practice point]

13.2 Breech presentation at term

All women who have an uncomplicated singleton breech pregnancy at 36 weeks of gestation should be offered external cephalic version (ECV). Exceptions include women in labour and women with a uterine scar or abnormality, fetal compromise, ruptured membranes, vaginal bleeding and medical conditions. [A]

Where it is not possible to schedule an appointment for ECV at 37 weeks of gestation, it should be scheduled at 36 weeks. [Good practice point]

2.2 Future research recommendations

Antenatal care is fortunate to have some areas where research evidence can clearly underpin clinical practice. However, it is noticeable that there are key areas within care where the research evidence is limited. For some of these areas, such as screening for gestational diabetes and first-trimester screening for anomalies, research is under way and results are awaited but for others there is an urgent need to address the gaps in the evidence.

- Effective ways of helping health professionals to support pregnant women in making informed decisions should be investigated. (Chapter 3)
- There is a lack of qualitative research on women's views regarding who provides care during pregnancy. (4.1)
- Alternative methods of providing antenatal information and support, such as drop in services, should be explored. (4.5)
- Research that explores how to ensure women's satisfaction and low morbidity and mortality with a reduced schedule of appointments should be conducted. (4.5)
- Further research to quantify the risk of air travel and to assess the effectiveness of interventions to prevent venous thromboembolism in pregnancy is needed. (5.14)

- More information on maternal and fetal safety for all interventions for nausea and vomiting in pregnancy (except antihistamines) is needed. (6.1)
- Further research into other nonpharmacological treatments for nausea and vomiting in pregnancy is recommended. (6.1)
- Although many treatments exist for backache in pregnancy, there is a lack of research evaluating their safety and effectiveness. (6.7)
- More research on effective treatments for symphysis pubis dysfunction is needed. (6.8)
- There is a lack of research evaluating effective interventions for carpal tunnel syndrome. (6.9)
- Although there are effective screening tools and screening for domestic violence has been shown to be acceptable to women, there is insufficient evidence on the effectiveness of interventions in improving health outcomes for women who have been identified. Therefore evaluation of interventions for domestic violence is urgently needed. (7.5)
- The effectiveness and costs of an ethnic question for antenatal screening for sickle cell and thalassaemia is needed. (8.2)
- The effectiveness and costs of laboratory methods for antenatal screening for sickle cell and thalassaemia is needed. (8.2)
- Up-to-date randomised controlled trials are needed to confirm the beneficial effect of screening for asymptomatic bacteriuria. (10.1)
- Further investigation into the benefits of screening for chlamydia in pregnancy is needed. (10.3)
- Further research into the effectiveness and cost effectiveness of antenatal screening for streptococcus group B are needed. (10.9)
- Research is needed to determine the optimal frequency and timing of blood pressure measurement and on the role of screening for proteinuria. (11.2)
- Further research on more effective ways to detect and manage small- and large-for-gestational-age fetuses is needed. (12.2)
- Further research is necessary to determine if tocolysis improves the success rate of external cephalic version. (13.2)

2.3 Algorithm: Antenatal care: routine care for the healthy pregnant woman

Antenatal care: routine care

The needs of each pregnant woman should be reassessed at each appointment throughout pregnancy

At each appointment, women should be given information with an opportunity to discuss issues and ask questions.

Women should usually carry their own case notes.

Women should be informed of the results of all tests and systems in place to communicate results to women.

Verbal information should be supported by classes and written information that is evidence based.

Nulliparous (1st pregnancy)	**Parous**

Identify women who may need additional care.

Give information on diet and lifestyle considerations, pregnancy care services, maternity benefits and screening tests.

Inform women about the benefits of folic acid supplementation (400 micrograms per day for up to 12 weeks).

➲ Offer screening tests. The purpose of all tests should be understood before they are undertaken.

Measure body mass index and blood pressure and test urine for proteinuria.

Support women who smoke or who have recently quit by offering anti-smoking interventions.

Prior to 12 weeks (may be 2 appts)

Review, discuss and record results of all screening tests undertaken.
Measure BP and test urine for proteinuria.

16

Measure symphysis fundal height + BP.
Urinalysis for proteinuria.

25

Measure SFH + BP. Urinalysis for proteinuria.
➲ Offer repeat screening for anaemia and atypical red cell alloantibodies.
➲ Offer 1st dose anti-D if rhesus negative.

28

SFH + BP + proteinuria urinalysis.
Review, discuss and record results of all screening tests undertaken.

31

Measure SFH + BP. Urinalysis for proteinuria. Offer 2nd dose anti-D if rhesus negative.
For parous women, review, discuss and record results of all screening tests undertaken.

34

Measure SFH + BP. Urinalysis for proteinuria. Check presentation: ➲ Offer ECV if breech

36

SFH + BP + urinalysis for proteinuria.

38

SFH + BP + urinalysis for proteinuria.

40

Measure SFH + BP + urinalysis for proteinuria.
➲ Offer membrane sweep.
➲ Offer induction after 41 weeks.

41

GESTATIONAL AGE

Total appointments for nulliparous women: 10	Total appointments for parous women: 7

Key: ECV external cephalic version • EPDS Edinburgh Postnatal Depression Scale • HELLP haemolysis, elev
LGA large for gestational age • SFH symphysis–fundal height • SGA small for gestational age • USS ultrasou

the healthy pregnant woman

Antenatal care should be provided by a small group of carers with whom the woman feels comfortable. There should be continuity of care throughout the antenatal period.

Healthcare professionals should be alert to the symptoms or signs of domestic violence and women should be given the opportunity to disclose domestic violence.

Women who may need additional care

Pregnant women should be informed about the purpose of any screening test before it is performed. The right of a woman to accept or decline a test should be made clear.

To be arranged early in pregnancy (before 16 weeks of gestation)

Blood tests to screen for:
- blood group, rhesus status and red cell antibodies
- haemoglobin (to screen for anaemia)
- hepatitis B virus
- HIV
- rubella susceptibility
- syphilis serology.

Urine test to screen for asymptomatic bacteriuria.

Ultrasound scan to determine gestational age.

Down's syndrome screening:
- Nuchal translucency at 11–14 weeks
- Serum screening at 14–20 weeks.

To be arranged between 18 to 20 weeks of gestation

Ultrasound scan for detection of structural anomalies.

If the placenta is found to extend across the internal cervical os at this time, another scan at 36 weeks should be offered and the results of this scan reviewed at the 36-week appointment.

Planning care: assessment
Are any of the following present?

- Conditions such as hypertension, cardiac or renal disease, endocrine, psychiatric or haematological disorders, epilepsy, diabetes, autoimmune diseases, cancer, HIV
- Factors that make the woman vulnerable such as those who lack social support
- Age 40 years and older or 18 years and younger
- BMI greater than or equal to 35 or less than 18
- Previous caesarean section
- Severe pre-eclampsia, HELLP or eclampsia
- Previous pre-eclampsia or eclampsia
- 3 or more miscarriages
- Previous preterm birth or mid trimester loss
- Previous psychiatric illness or puerperal psychosis
- Previous neonatal death or stillbirth
- Previous baby with congenital abnormality
- Previous SGA or LGA infant
- Family history of genetic disorder

These women are likely to need additional care which is outside the scope of this guideline. The care outlined here is the '*baseline care*'.

The following interventions are *NOT* recommended components of routine antenatal care:
- Repeated maternal weighing
- Breast examination
- Pelvic examination
- Screening for post natal depression using EPDS
- Iron supplementation
- Vitamin D supplementation
- Screening for the following infections
  - *Chlamydia trachomatis*
  - cytomegalovirus
  - hepatitis C virus
  - group B streptococcus
  - toxoplasmosis
  - bacterial vaginosis
- Screening for gestational diabetes mellitus (including dipstick testing for glycosuria)
- Screening for preterm birth by assessment of cervical length (either by USS or VE) or using fetal fibronectin
- Formal fetal movement counting
- Antenatal electronic cardiotocography
- Ultrasound scanning after 24 weeks
- Umbilical artery Doppler USS
- Uterine artery Doppler USS to predict pre-eclampsia

This algorithm should, where necessary, be interpreted with reference to the full guideline.

ver enzymes and low platelet count •
n • VE vaginal examination

3. Woman-centred care and informed decision making

3.1 Provision of information

Informed decision making has been described as "a reasoned choice made by a reasonable individual using relevant information about the advantages and disadvantages of all the possible courses of action, in accord with the individual's beliefs".[8]

In 1993, the Expert Maternity Group from the Department of Health released the *Changing Childbirth* report, which made explicit the right of women to be involved in decisions regarding all aspects of their antenatal care.[9] One of the priorities of antenatal care is to enable women to be able to make informed decisions about their care, such as where they will be seen, who will undertake their care, which screening tests they will undertake and where they plan to give birth. To do so, women require access to evidence-based information to take part in discussions with caregivers about these decisions. In practice however, it is reported that women feel that they have less say over some aspects of care than others and a substantial number of women would like to have more information about their options for care and services.[10] [Evidence level 3]

In a survey of maternity services in the NHS, just over 30% of recent mothers reported that they felt they had the option to choose where they received their pregnancy care. With screening tests, however, 60% of mothers reported feeling that they had been offered a choice. Women's assessment of information and communication in antenatal care indicated that 32–40% felt that they had not received enough spoken or written information about the risks and benefits of having different screening tests during pregnancy.[10] [Evidence level 3] Before making a decision about whether or not to have a test a woman needs to have information about what the test is looking for, what the test involves and any risks of the test itself to herself and her pregnancy, the type of result that will be reported (such as a probability or risk, the false positive and false negative rate) and the decisions she might face as a result of the test. However, it is not clear how this information should be given and how much information is optimal, as this is likely to vary among individual women.

In one survey, 1188 pregnant women's point of view on information needs were explored by means of self-completed postal questionnaires.[3] Half of the women reported that they would have liked additional information to be provided at their first antenatal appointment, with first time mothers most likely to believe that they had been provided with too little information. Written sources of information were also highly valued. [Evidence level 3]

In order to meet individual women's needs, it is likely that a variety of ways of giving information will be required. Written information varies widely in quality. A study of 81 leaflets used in antenatal screening programmes in England and Wales found that only 11 (14%) included comprehensive information on all aspects of screening.[11] [Evidence level 3]

An RCT that compared three methods of giving information about antenatal screening tests randomised pregnant women into three groups. In the first group, extra information was delivered to women on an individual basis. In the second group, women received extra information in classes and the third group (the control group), received routine antenatal clinic information. The study reported no differences between the groups in the uptake of screening for Down's syndrome and other fetal anomalies, haemoglobinopathies or cystic fibrosis. Anxiety, however, was reported to be higher by 20 weeks of gestation among women who were not offered extra information compared with women who received individual information.[12] [Evidence level 1b]

Another RCT assessed the impact of evidence-based leaflets to promote informed decision making among pregnant women compared with no leaflets.[13] The leaflets were designed to be used in a conscious and controlled way (i.e., not left in a rack at an antenatal clinic or GP office) and the information provided in them was the result of systematic review of the best available evidence and they were peer reviewed. No differences were detected in the proportion of women who reported that they had exercised informed choice or among those who reported an 'active' decision making role during antenatal care between the groups. Satisfaction with the amount of information between the two groups, however, was higher in the group that received the leaflets. [Evidence level 1b] Qualitative assessment within the trial of the use of the leaflets found that their potential as decision aids was greatly reduced due to competing demands within the clinical environment.[14] Time pressures limited discussion and hierarchical power structures resulted in defined norms, which dictated which 'choices' were available. This meant that women complied with their carers' choice rather than making an informed decision. [Evidence level 3]

Much of the responsibility for providing information, which should be unbiased and evidence-based, falls upon the healthcare provider. Although users of antenatal care services report that they place high value on quality information that will allow them to make an informed decision about antenatal screening tests,[15,16] [Evidence level 3] a study that recorded consultations in the USA and UK found that the information provided on antenatal screening tests was insufficient for informed decision making and occasionally misleading or inaccurate.[17] This may be explained by a lack of knowledge on the part of the carer,[18] [Evidence level 3] a lack of training on how to present information in an understandable way[19] or a lack of time and resources to present the information.[20] A comparison of those who completed and those who did not complete training to improve information providing skills in an RCT[19] found that those who dropped out were the ones who had poorer communication skills at baseline, suggesting that those most likely to need training in effective communication are the ones least likely to avail themselves of it.[21] [Evidence level 3]

Beyond the issue of poor understanding of tests undergone or declined, additional issues reported to be associated with antenatal screening programmes include anxiety following false positive results and false negative reassurance in those receiving negative test results.[22] This highlights the importance of the need for information on the outcomes of testing in order to make informed decisions. Although more is known about antenatal screening than other aspects of antenatal care, more research is needed to help ascertain how best to help parents make informed decisions about choices around antenatal testing. In addition, although the provision of information is perhaps a necessary condition for informed decision making, it is not sufficient. Other factors are necessary to achieve informed decision making and this may be difficult in the context of health care as, historically, pregnant women are not expected to make decisions themselves.

Available information

All first time pregnant women in England and Wales should be offered *The pregnancy book* (published by health departments in England and Wales)[23] by their carer. This book provides information on many aspects of pregnancy including: how the fetus develops; deciding where to have a baby; feelings and relationships during pregnancy; antenatal care and classes; a section for expectant fathers; problems in pregnancy; when pregnancy goes wrong; rights and benefits information and a list of useful organisations.

The Cochrane Database of Systematic Reviews (www.update-software.com/clibng/cliblogon.htm) provides the best available evidence on safe and effective antenatal care.

The MIDIRS Informed Choice initiative has produced 15 leaflets to assist women in making informed objective decisions during pregnancy. Each leaflet has a corresponding leaflet for professionals, aiming to help them guide pregnant women through decisions. Access to this resource is available online at www.nelh.nhs.uk/maternity.

A leaflet entitled *Tests for you and your baby during pregnancy* provides information to assist women in making informed decisions about the screening tests that are offered in pregnancy. It is published by Bro Taf Health Authority and may be tailored for specific health authorities.[24]

3.2 Antenatal education

There are many different ways of providing antenatal classes and antenatal education. There is variation in the underlying aims of antenatal education, in the number of classes offered, whether classes are offered individually or in groups, when during the course of pregnancy the classes are offered and the content of the classes. These factors may impact on the effectiveness of antenatal education programmes.

Antenatal classes are often used to give information regarding a woman's pregnancy, childbirth and parenting to expectant parents. However, antenatal education can encompass a broader concept of educational and supportive measures that help parents and prospective parents to understand and explore their own social, emotional, psychological and physical needs during pregnancy, labour and parenthood and enable them to be confident in their abilities to give birth and to parent successfully. In a study of three groups of childbirth teachers working in different organisations in the UK who were asked to identify the aims of antenatal education, the need to build women's confidence in their ability to give birth and care for their babies was reported as the most important aim.[25]

The scope of this guideline covers antenatal education relating to pregnancy, and does not cover important aspects of antenatal education that relate to childbirth or parenthood, although it is recognised that antenatal education is often considered the first step in the pathway of becoming a parent. Although women who experience fear of childbirth are not necessarily more likely to have interventions during labour such as emergency caesarean section, it is possible that building up a woman's confidence during pregnancy in her ability to give birth has the potential to influence her choices for the birth of her baby and the interventions she receives during birth.[26]

A systematic review based on six RCTs involving 1443 women assessed the effects of antenatal education on knowledge acquisition, anxiety, sense of control, pain, support, breastfeeding, infant care abilities, and psychological and social adjustment. The largest study (n = 1275) examined an educational intervention to increase vaginal birth after caesarean section only. The remaining five trials (combined n = 168, range n = 10–67) included more general educational interventions; however, the methodological quality of these trials is uncertain, as they do not report randomisation procedures, allocation concealment or accrual and loss of participants. None of the trials included labour and birth outcomes, anxiety, breastfeeding success or general social support. The effects on knowledge acquisition and infant care competencies were measured but interpretation is difficult because of the size and methodological quality of the trials.[27] [Evidence level 1b] The findings of observational studies are also inconsistent.[28–30] [Evidence level 3] One survey found acquisition of knowledge was increased among all women who attended antenatal education classes compared with women who did not attend, although antenatal classes appear to have stronger effects on women from higher socio-economic classes.[28] [Evidence level 3] Women who attended antenatal classes were also less anxious than women who did not attend antenatal classes. The inconsistency across the observational studies may be explained by confounding factors for which it is not possible to control in an analysis.

A survey of what women would like to learn in antenatal classes found that information on physical and psychological changes during pregnancy, fetal development, what will happen during labour and childbirth, their options during labour and childbirth and how to care for themselves during this time, possible complications and how to care for the baby after birth were the main issues.[31] [Evidence level 3] Evidence for the best method to deliver antenatal education is lacking. Ideally, the aims of antenatal education might include facilitating pregnant women to make informed decisions and to communicate more effectively with their carers, thus enabling them to contribute to the design of future antenatal education, to convey the issues they feel are most important to learn about and to feel empowered by their pregnancy and birth experience.

RECOMMENDATIONS

Pregnant women should be offered opportunities to attend antenatal classes and have written information about antenatal care. [A]

Pregnant women should be offered evidence-based information and support to enable them to make informed decisions regarding their care. Information should include details of where they will be seen and who will undertake their care. Addressing women's choices should be recognised as being integral to the decision-making process. [C]

At the first contact, pregnant women should be offered information about the pregnancy care services and options available, lifestyle considerations, including dietary information, and screening tests. [C]

Pregnant women should be informed about the purpose of any screening test before it is performed. The right of a woman to accept or decline a test should be made clear. [D]

At each antenatal appointment, midwives and doctors should offer consistent information and clear explanations and should provide pregnant women with an opportunity to discuss issues and ask questions. [D]

Communication and information should be provided in a form that is accessible to pregnant women who have additional needs, such as those with physical, cognitive or sensory disabilities and those who do not speak or read English. [Good practice point]

Future research

Effective ways of helping health professionals to support pregnant women in making informed decisions should be investigated.

4. Provision and organisation of care

4.1 Who provides care?

One systematic review assessed the clinical effectiveness and perception of antenatal care by type of antenatal care provider, i.e. midwife and general practitioner-led managed care was compared with obstetrician and gynaecologist-led shared care.[32] Three trials were included in the study, randomising 3041 women who were considered to be low risk (i.e. no medical or obstetrical complications). The two largest trials were set in Scotland (n = 2952). Of these, one assessed midwifery-led care and the other assessed care led by midwives and GPs.

No differences were observed between the midwife and GP-managed care and the obstetrician and gynaecologist-led shared care for preterm birth, caesarean section, anaemia, urinary tract infections, antepartum haemorrhage and perinatal mortality. However, the midwife and GP-managed care group had a statistically significant lower rate of pregnancy-induced hypertension (Peto OR 0.56, 95% CI 0.45 to 0.70) and pre-eclampsia (Peto OR 0.37, 95% CI 0.22 to 0.64) than the standard care group. This could result from either a decreased incidence or decreased detection. [Evidence level 1a]

There was no significant difference in the levels of satisfaction with the types of care provided between the two groups.

Based on this meta-analysis of 3041 women from three trials, midwife-managed or midwife and GP-managed antenatal care programmes for women at 'low risk' did not increase the risk of adverse maternal or perinatal outcomes.

RECOMMENDATION

Midwife and GP-led models of care should be offered for women with an uncomplicated pregnancy. Routine involvement of obstetricians in the care of women with an uncomplicated pregnancy at scheduled times does not appear to improve perinatal outcomes compared with involving obstetricians when complications arise. [A]

Future research

There is a lack of qualitative research on women's views regarding who provides care during pregnancy.

4.2 Continuity of care

The care of women during pregnancy, labour, and the postnatal period is often provided by many caregivers. Women may have caregivers who work only in particular settings, such as the antenatal clinic or the labour ward, and who cannot provide them with continuity of care. For the purposes of this guideline, continuity of care is defined as the provision of care by the same small team of caregivers throughout pregnancy. However, no trials investigated continuity of care solely in the antenatal period and therefore it is not possible to separate the results associated with continuity of care in the antenatal and intrapartum periods.

Two systematic reviews analysed the effects of continuous care during pregnancy and childbirth.[33,34]

One systematic review assessed the clinical effectiveness of continuity of care during pregnancy and childbirth and the postnatal period with routine care by multiple caregivers.[33] [Evidence level 1a] Two trials, one set in the UK, the other in Australia, were included in the review. They randomised 1815 women to continuity of care by a small group of midwives as well as consultation with an obstetrician compared with routine care provided by physicians and midwives. Women who had continuity of care by a team of midwives were less likely to:

- experience clinic waiting times greater than 15 minutes (Peto OR 0.14, 95% CI 0.10 to 0.19)
- be admitted to hospital antenatally (Peto OR 0.79, 95% CI 0.64 to 0.97)
- fail to attend antenatal classes (Peto OR 0.58, 95% CI 0.41 to 0.81)
- be unable to discuss worries in pregnancy (Peto OR 0.72, 95% CI 0.56 to 0.92)
- not feel well-prepared for labour (Peto OR 0.64, 95% CI 0.48 to 0.86).

There was no significant difference in the rates of caesarean section, induction of labour, stillbirth and neonatal death, preterm birth, admission to the neonatal unit, or birthweight less than 2500 g. Further outcomes are reported in the corresponding evidence table.

One other systematic review compared continuity of midwifery care with standard maternity services.[34] This review included seven RCTs, which randomised 9148 women. The women randomised to continuous care had significantly lower rates of many outcomes related to the intrapartum period, such as induction of labour, augmentation of labour and electronic fetal monitoring. There were no significant differences in the rates of caesarean section, admission to the neonatal unit, postnatal haemorrhage, antenatal admission to hospital or duration of labour. No maternal deaths were reported. Satisfaction with care was reported by six of the seven trials but not included in the meta-analysis due to lack of consistency between measures. However, women with continuous care were more satisfied with care during all phases of pregnancy and differences were statistically significant for each study separately. Women in the continuous care group were more pleased with information giving and communication with the caregivers and felt more involved in the decision making and more in control. [Evidence level 1a]

Four more recent RCTs that were not included in either of the above reviews were also located.[35 38]

Another RCT in England which compared caseload midwifery care with traditional shared care.[35] Caseload midwifery care refers to a group of midwives caring for a specific number of women where a midwife has her own group of women, with back-up support provided by another midwife when needed. This study found that although there was a significant difference between caseload and traditional care groups in terms of level of 'known carer at delivery', there were no significant differences in terms of rates of normal vaginal deliveries, operative deliveries or neonatal outcome. [Evidence level 1b]

An Australian RCT compared continuity of midwifery care in a community-based setting with standard care in a hospital-based antenatal clinic.[36] The latter was characterised by a lack of continuity of care as a large number of clinicians provided care. No differences in any clinical outcomes were reported except a significantly lower caesarean section rate in the midwife-led community-based care group (OR 0.6, 95% CI 0.4 to 0.9). [Evidence level 1b] The women in the community-based continuity of care group also reported significantly less waiting time and easier access to care and a higher perceived quality of care than the hospital-based control group.[37] [Evidence level 1b]

Another Australian RCT compared continuity of care provided by midwives with standard care provided by a variety of midwives and obstetric staff.[38] The women assigned to the intervention group experienced less augmentation of labour, less use of epidural analgesia and fewer episiotomies; no differences in perinatal mortality between the two groups was observed. [Evidence level 1b]

An RCT on satisfaction with continuity of care found that continuity of care provided by team midwifery was associated with increased satisfaction compared with standard care attended by various doctors.[39] A woman from the intervention group was twice as likely to agree with the statement, "Overall, care during pregnancy was very good" (OR 2.22, 95% CI 1.66 to 2.95). The intervention appeared to have greatest impact on satisfaction with care during the antenatal period compared with the intrapartum and postnatal period. [Evidence level 1b]

In most cases, the evidence demonstrates an association between continuity of care and lower intervention rates compared with standard maternity or hospital-based care as well as beneficial effects upon various psychosocial outcomes.

RECOMMENDATION

Antenatal care should be provided by a small group of carers with whom the woman feels comfortable. There should be continuity of care throughout the antenatal period. [A]

A system of clear referral paths should be established so that pregnant women who require additional care are managed and treated by the appropriate specialist teams when problems are identified. [D]

4.3 Where should antenatal appointments take place?

A meta-analysis of three RCTs examined whether a policy of home visits for antenatal care reduced the amount of antenatal care provided by nine hospital maternity units in France; 1410 women with pregnancy complications were assessed.[40] In the control group, women received the usual care provided by the maternity units with visits to the outpatient clinics as necessary. In the intervention group, the women received one or two home visits a week by a midwife in addition to the usual care. No difference in the rate of hospital admissions was found (pooled OR 0.9, 95% CI 0.7 to 1.2) but the average number of visits to the outpatient clinic was significantly lower in the two trials in which it was measured. [Evidence level 1a] Maternity care must be readily and easily accessible to all women. They should be sensitive to the needs of the local population and based primarily in the community.[9] [Evidence level 4]

RECOMMENDATION

Antenatal care should be readily and easily accessible to all women and should be sensitive to the needs of individual women and the local community. [C]

The environment in which antenatal appointments take place should enable women to discuss sensitive issues such as domestic violence, sexual abuse, psychiatric illness and illicit drug use. [Good practice point]

4.4 Documentation of care

The information in antenatal records is collected for two main purposes:

* administration
* identification of maternal risk, fetal risk, and special requirements so that further management can be planned.

Beyond the management of patient care, however, antenatal records also serve as vehicles for quality assurance, legal documentation, communication and epidemiological research for deciding future public health measures.

In an RCT of three methods of taking an antenatal history, unstructured histories taken on paper by midwives, structured paper histories (incorporating a checklist) and an interactive computerised questionnaire in an antenatal clinic in England were compared.[41] The number of clinical responses to factors arising from the antenatal histories were measured and each response was weighted for clinical importance. The structured questionnaires were reported to provide more and better information and their use improved clinical response to risk factors compared with unstructured paper histories. Computerised systems offered no further advantage over structured paper histories. [Evidence level 1b]

Women carrying their own case notes

Three RCTs have examined the effect of giving women their own maternity case notes to carry during pregnancy.[42–44] The impact on quality of care and maternal and perinatal outcomes was assessed. In all three trials, women were randomised either to carry their own antenatal case notes or to the usual system of case notes remaining in the hospital. In the latter case, women usually carried a cooperation card.

The first study (n = 246) found that both the women and health professionals involved considered that giving a woman her own maternity case notes during pregnancy was a good idea and was a positive step towards improving the quality of care.[44] [Evidence level 1b] No reasons were found during the study to deny women carrying their own notes and no insurmountable problems arose.

In the second study (n = 290) specific outcomes and hypotheses were proposed.[42] [Evidence level 1b] The two groups of women were comparable in terms of sociodemographic characteristics. Results from the questionnaires showed that:

- women carrying their own notes were nearly 50% more likely to say they felt in control of their pregnancy (rate ratio 1.45, 95% CI 1.08 to 1.95)
- more than 70% were more likely to say they found it easier to talk to the doctors and midwives during pregnancy (rate ratio 1.73, 95% CI 1.16 to 2.59).
- there were no other significant differences between the groups in terms of any of the other outcomes predicted
- there was no difference in the availability of notes for clinic appointments but approximately 1 hour of hospital clerical time was saved per week because of not having to retrieve and refile notes.

The third study (n = 150) was conducted among English-speaking women in an Australian metropolitan area, using open-ended questions.[43] [Evidence level 1b] Parous women who carried their own notes were significantly more likely to report that the doctors and midwives explained everything in their records to them than parous women with cooperation cards or nulliparous women from either group.

- 89% of women carrying their own notes responded positively. They felt more in control, felt more informed, liked having access to their results and felt it gave them an opportunity to share information particularly with other family members and partners.
- 11% of women carrying their own notes responded negatively, as they thought the record was too bulky, the system inconvenient or were worried they would forget notes.
- No differences were noted in numbers of lost records in each group.
- 89% of women in the hand-held notes group wanted to carry their notes in a future pregnancy as well as 52% of the cooperation-card group.

Women like to carry their own maternity care records. This can lead to an increased feeling of control during pregnancy. It may facilitate communication between the pregnant woman and the health professionals involved with her care.

RECOMMENDATIONS

Structured maternity records should be used for antenatal care. [A]

Maternity services should have a system in place whereby women carry their own case notes. [A]

A standardised, national maternity record with an agreed minimum data set should be developed and used. This will help carers to provide the recommended evidence-based care to pregnant women. [Good practice point]

4.5   Frequency of antenatal appointments

Antenatal care programmes as currently practised originate from models developed in 1929. As advances in medicine and technology have occurred, new components have been added to antenatal care, mostly for screening purposes. However, the significance of the frequency of antenatal care appointments and the interval between appointments has not been tested scientifically.

An observational study explored the relationship between the number of antenatal visits made by 17,765 British women and adverse perinatal outcomes.[45] [Evidence level 3] No consistent relationship between admission to the neonatal unit or perinatal mortality and number of antenatal visits was found. A significant positive relationship between number of antenatal visits and caesarean section was found and low birthweight (less than 2500 g) was positively associated with number of visits for nulliparous but not for parous women.

Two systematic reviews of RCTs have evaluated the evidence of the effectiveness of different models of care based on a reduced number of antenatal care visits compared with the standard number of antenatal care visits.[32,46] [Evidence level 1a] Both reviews included the same seven trials.

Both systematic reviews assessed the clinical effectiveness and perception of care (by women) of different antenatal care programmes. Frequency of antenatal care visits was one of the components of care assessed by the reviews. Four of the trials were conducted in developed countries and three in less developed countries, with a total of 57,418 women randomised to receive either a reduced number of antenatal care visits (with or without 'goal-oriented' components) or the standard number of antenatal care visits.

Between the two reviews, outcomes assessed were: preterm delivery (less than 37 weeks), pre-eclampsia, caesarean section, induction of labour, antenatal haemorrhage, postnatal haemorrhage, low birthweight, small-for-gestational-age at birth, postpartum anaemia, admission to neonatal intensive care unit, perinatal mortality, maternal mortality, urinary tract infection and satisfaction of care. The results did not demonstrate a difference in any of the biological outcomes. Women from the developed-country trials reported less satisfaction with the frequency of visits in the reduced number group (3 RCTs, n = 3393, Peto OR 0.61, 95% CI 0.52 to 0.72). However, the women in these trials were being told that they had fewer visits and were therefore aware that other women had more visits than they did. It should also be noted that there was clinical and statistical heterogeneity among the three trials that looked at this outcome.

The objective of both these systematic reviews was to demonstrate equivalent efficacy of the intervention. A problem with equivalence trials is that when the two interventions are similar the outcomes are also likely to be similar. A limitation common to both of these reviews, highlighted by the authors, was protocol deviations that resulted in nonsignificant reductions in the number of visits in the intervention group. The average difference in number of visits between the two arms in the trials was approximately two in both reviews. In the context of routine antenatal care in developed countries (10–14 visits), a difference of two visits would be unlikely to demonstrate a measurable impact upon pregnancy outcomes. However, when analysing the two largest trials, which took place in less developed countries, the reduction in the number of visits is proportionately much larger (from six to four visits). Within these trials, no adverse impact on maternal or perinatal outcomes was associated with reduced visits.

A moderate reduction in the traditional number of antenatal visits is not associated with an increase in adverse maternal or perinatal outcomes. However, a reduced number of appointments may be associated with a reduction in women's satisfaction with their antenatal care. It is likely that routine antenatal care for women without risk or complications can be provided with fewer appointments. It is possible that the key issue is not more or less antenatal care, but the implementation of procedures that have been shown to be effective and which may increase women's satisfaction with care. The frequency of appointments can then be planned accordingly.

In a secondary analysis of data from an RCT comparing a traditional and a reduced schedule of antenatal appointments in London, England, women who were satisfied with reduced schedules were more likely to have a caregiver who both listened and encouraged them to ask questions than women who were not satisfied with reduced schedules.[47] [Evidence level 3] A survey of women's expectations on number of antenatal care appointments in Sweden found that preference for more or fewer appointments was associated with parity, marital status, age, education, obstetric history, previous birth experience and timing of pregnancy.[48] [Evidence level 3] Older women (over 35 years), parous women, less educated women and women with more than two children preferred fewer appointments, whereas younger women (under 25 years), single women and women with a prior adverse pregnancy history indicated a preference for more appointments than the standard schedule.

Economic considerations

The cost of antenatal appointments is determined by the number of appointments overall, and the type and grade of health care provider. The cost effectiveness of the antenatal appointment schedule is determined by the primary outcomes of the antenatal care (preterm birth, low birthweight babies, maternal or infant mortality, birth complications and intensive care) and also secondary outcomes such as maternal and professional satisfaction with the package of care provided.

The evidence to date on the optimum number of antenatal appointments is inconclusive. The majority of studies have not focused on the cost effectiveness or cost benefit of the number of antenatal appointments. The World Health Organization (WHO) Antenatal Care Trial included an assessment of quality of care and an economic evaluation. The authors concluded that the provision of routine antenatal care by the new model did not affect maternal and perinatal outcomes and therefore was more cost effective. However, the study setting of the trial was developing countries.

Most of the existing research in industrialised countries is based on low-risk women as diagnosed at first contact. One UK based study compared a traditional antenatal appointment schedule with a reduced schedule of appointments.[49] The estimated total cost to the NHS of the traditional schedule (around 13 appointments) was £544, of which around £250 occurred antenatally. The estimated total costs for the reduced appointment schedule (six or seven appointments) were around £560, of which £255 occurred antenatally. The authors found that any reduced costs of fewer appointments were offset by the greater number of babies requiring special or intensive care, so that the total costs were not different. Sensitivity analyses varied the unit costs of care and length of postnatal stay and found substantial overlap between schedules, leading to inconclusive results. No difference was detected in the primary outcome (caesarean section) between the two groups. The authors reported differences in the secondary outcome (maternal satisfaction and psychological outcomes) that were significantly poorer for women receiving fewer appointments than for women receiving traditional care.

A study comparing pregnancy outcomes between England and Wales and France[50] demonstrated that, although the number of appointments is lower in France, there were no differences detected in pregnancy outcomes. This suggests that fewer appointments would be more cost effective if only these outcomes were considered.

Clearly, fewer routine antenatal appointments for low-risk pregnant women could release antenatal care resources for women who need additional support. The issue of 'satisfaction' is complex, since the long-term effects (and costs) of lower satisfaction and poorer psychosocial outcomes is not addressed in any of the studies.

Willingness-to-pay studies are one way of exploring whether one form of care is more highly valued by users of services (what they would be willing to sacrifice to have a particular form of care). This approach can incorporate the value of different forms of care and not only the final outcome. The value of information and reassurance to pregnant women is usually not included in economic evaluation.

Only one economic study has been undertaken to estimate women's valuation of antenatal care. This study did not address the number of appointments but did address the value of different providers of antenatal care. It suggested there was no significant difference in the monetary value women placed on alternatives forms of provision.[51]

RECOMMENDATIONS

A schedule of antenatal appointments should be determined by the function of the appointments. For a woman who is nulliparous with an uncomplicated pregnancy, a schedule of ten appointments should be adequate. For a woman who is parous with an uncomplicated pregnancy, a schedule of seven appointments should be adequate. [B]

Early in pregnancy, all women should receive appropriate written information about the likely number, timing and content of antenatal appointments associated with different options of care and be given an opportunity to discuss this schedule with their midwife or doctor. [D]

Each antenatal appointment should be structured and have focused content. Longer appointments are needed early in pregnancy to allow comprehensive assessment and discussion. Wherever possible, appointments should incorporate routine tests and investigations to minimise inconvenience to women. [D]

Future research

Alternative methods of providing antenatal information and support, such as drop in services, should be explored.

Research that explores how to ensure women's satisfaction and low morbidity and mortality with a reduced schedule of appointments should be conducted.

4.6 Gestational age assessment: LMP and ultrasound

Estimates of gestational duration based on the timing of the last normal menstrual period (LMP) are dependent upon a woman's ability to recall the dates accurately, the regularity or irregularity of her menstrual cycles and variations in the interval between bleeding and anovulation. Between 11% and 42% of gestational age estimates from LMP are reported as inaccurate.[52] However, there is thought to be little variation in fetal growth rate up to mid-pregnancy and therefore, estimates of fetal size by ultrasound scan provides estimates of gestational age which are not subject to the same human error as LMP.

Ultrasound assessment of gestational age at 10–13 weeks is usually calculated by measurement of the crown–rump length. For pregnant women who present in the second trimester, gestational age can be assessed with ultrasound measurement of biparietal diameter or head circumference. Ultrasound measurement of biparietal diameter is reported to provide a better estimate of date of delivery for term births than first day of the LMP.[53–55] [Evidence level 2a] Gestational age assessment with ultrasound occurs routinely prior to 24 weeks and where discrepancies between ultrasound and LMP exist, choosing to use the ultrasound dating reduces the number of births considered to be post-term.[53–56] [Evidence level 2a]

Routine ultrasound before 24 weeks is also associated with a reduction in rates of intervention for post-term pregnancies. One systematic review of nine RCTs found ultrasound scanning before 24 weeks to be associated with a reduction in the rate of induced labour for post-term pregnancy when compared to selective use of ultrasound (Peto OR 0.61, 95% CI 0.52 to 0.72). This may have consequences when pregnancies are misclassified as pre- or post-term and inappropriate action is taken. Earlier detection of multiple pregnancy was also reported, although this did not have a significant affect on perinatal mortality (twins undiagnosed at 26 weeks: Peto OR 0.08, 95% CI 0.04 to 0.16). No adverse influence on school performance or neurobehavioural function as a consequence of antenatal exposure to ultrasound was observed.[57] [Evidence level 1a]

Accurate assessment of gestational age also permits optimal timing of antenatal screening for Down's syndrome and fetal structural anomalies. Reliable dating is important when interpreting Down's syndrome serum results as it may reduce the number of false positives for a given detection rate. An RCT evaluating ultrasound assessment at the first antenatal appointment at less than 17 weeks of gestation compared with no ultrasound found that fewer women needed adjustment of the date of delivery in mid-gestation (9% versus 18%; RR 0.52, 95% CI 0.34 to 0.79) and that women who had an ultrasound at their first appointment reported more positive feelings about their pregnancy.[52] [Evidence level 1b]

RECOMMENDATIONS

Pregnant women should be offered an early ultrasound scan to determine gestational age (in lieu of LMP for all cases) and to detect multiple pregnancies. This will ensure consistency of gestational age assessments, improve the performance of mid-trimester serum screening for Down's syndrome and reduce the need for induction of labour after 41 weeks. [A]

Ideally, scans should be performed between 10 and 13 weeks and use crown – rump length measurement to determine gestational age. Pregnant women who present at or beyond 14 weeks of gestation should be offered an ultrasound scan to estimate gestational age using head circumference or biparietal diameter. [Good practice point]

4.7 What should happen at antenatal appointments?

The assessment of women who may or may not need additional clinical care during pregnancy is based on identifying those in whom there are any maternal or fetal conditions associated with an excess of maternal or perinatal death or morbidity. While this approach may not identify many of the women who go on to require extra care and will also categorise many women who go on to have normal uneventful births as 'high risk',[58,59] ascertainment of risk in pregnancy remains important as it may facilitate early detection to allow time to plan for appropriate management.

The needs of each pregnant woman should be assessed at the first appointment and reassessed at each appointment throughout pregnancy because new problems can arise at any time. Additional appointments should be determined by the needs of each pregnant woman, as assessed by her and her care givers, and the environment in which appointments take place should enable women to discuss sensitive issues Reducing the number of routine appointments will enable more time per appointment for care, information giving and support for pregnant women.

The schedule below, which has been determined by the purpose of each appointment, presents the recommended number of antenatal care appointments for women who are healthy and whose pregnancies remain uncomplicated in the antenatal period; ten appointments for nulliparous women and seven for parous women.

First appointment

The first appointment needs to be earlier in pregnancy (prior to 12 weeks) than may have traditionally occurred and, because of the large volume of information needs in early pregnancy, two appointments may be required. At the first (and second) antenatal appointment:

- give information, with an opportunity to discuss issues and ask questions; offer verbal information supported by written information (on topics such as diet and lifestyle considerations, pregnancy care services available, maternity benefits and sufficient information to enable informed decision making about screening tests)
- identify women who may need additional care (see Algorithm and Section 1.2) and plan pattern of care for the pregnancy
- check blood group and RhD status
- offer screening for anaemia, red-cell alloantibodies, Hepatitis B virus, HIV, rubella susceptibility and syphilis
- offer screening for asymptomatic bacteriuria (ASB)
- offering screening for Down's syndrome
- offer early ultrasound scan for gestational age assessment
- offer ultrasound screening for structural anomalies (20 weeks)
- measure BMI, blood pressure (BP) and test urine for proteinuria.

After the first (and possibly second) appointment, for women who choose to have screening, the following test should be arranged before 16 weeks of gestation (except serum screening for Down's syndrome, which may occur up to 20 weeks of gestation):

- blood tests (for checking blood group and RhD status and screening for anaemia, red-cell alloantibodies, hepatitis B virus, HIV, rubella susceptibility and syphilis)
- urine tests (to check for proteinuria and screen for ASB)
- ultrasound scan to determine gestational age using:
  - crown–rump measurement if performed at 10 to 13 weeks
  - biparietal diameter or head circumference at or beyond 14 weeks
- Down's syndrome screening using:
  - nuchal translucency at 11 to 14 weeks
  - serum screening at 14 to 20 weeks.

16 weeks

The next appointment should be scheduled at 16 weeks to:

- review, discuss and record the results of all screening tests undertaken; reassess planned pattern of care for the pregnancy and identify women who need additional care (see Algorithm and Section 1.2)
- investigate a haemoglobin level of less than 11g/dl and consider iron supplementation if indicated
- measure BP and test urine for proteinuria
- give information, with an opportunity to discuss issues and ask questions; offer verbal information supported by antenatal classes and written information.

18–20 weeks

At 18–20 weeks, if the woman chooses, an ultrasound scan should be performed for the detection of structural anomalies. For a woman whose placenta is found to extend across the internal cervical os at this time, another scan at 36 weeks should be offered and the results of this scan reviewed at the 36-week appointment.

25 weeks

At 25 weeks of gestation, another appointment should be scheduled for nulliparous women. At this appointment:

- measure and plot symphysis–fundal height
- measure BP and test urine for proteinuria
- give information, with an opportunity to discuss issues and ask questions; offer verbal information supported by antenatal classes and written information.

28 weeks

The next appointment for all pregnant women should occur at 28 weeks. At this appointment:

- offer a second screening for anaemia and atypical red-cell alloantibodies
- investigate a haemoglobin level of less than 10.5 g/dl and consider iron supplementation, if indicated
- offer anti-D to rhesus-negative women
- measure BP and test urine for proteinuria
- measure and plot symphysis–fundal height
- give information, with an opportunity to discuss issues and ask questions; offer verbal information supported by antenatal classes and written information.

31 weeks

Nulliparous women should have an appointment scheduled at 31 weeks to:

- measure BP and test urine for proteinuria
- measure and plot symphysis–fundal height
- give information, with an opportunity to discuss issues and ask questions; offer verbal information supported by antenatal classes and written information
- review, discuss and record the results of screening tests undertaken at 28 weeks; reassess planned pattern of care for the pregnancy and identify women who need additional care (see Algorithm and Section 1.2).

34 weeks

At 34 weeks, all pregnant women should be seen in order to:
- offer a second dose of anti-D to rhesus-negative women
- measure BP and test urine for proteinuria
- measure and plot symphysis–fundal height
- give information, with an opportunity to discuss issues and ask questions; offer verbal information supported by antenatal classes and written information
- review, discuss and record the results of screening tests undertaken at 28 weeks; reassess planned pattern of care for the pregnancy and identify women who need additional care (see Algorithm and Section 1.2).

36 weeks

At 36 weeks, all pregnant women should be seen again to:

- measure BP and test urine for proteinuria
- measure and plot symphysis–fundal height
- check position of baby
- for women whose babies are in the breech presentation, offer external cephalic version (ECV)
- review ultrasound scan report if placenta extended over the internal cervical os at previous scan
- give information, with an opportunity to discuss issues and ask questions; offer verbal information supported by antenatal classes and written information.

38 weeks

Another appointment at 38 weeks will allow for:

- measurement of BP and urine testing for proteinuria
- measurement and plotting of symphysis–fundal height
- information giving, with an opportunity to discuss issues and ask questions; verbal information supported by antenatal classes and written information.

40 weeks

For nulliparous women, an appointment at 40 weeks should be scheduled to:

- measure BP and test urine for proteinuria
- measure and plot symphysis–fundal height
- give information, with an opportunity to discuss issues and ask questions; offer verbal information supported by antenatal classes and written information.

41 weeks

For women who have not given birth by 41 weeks:

- a membrane sweep should be offered
- induction of labour should be offered
- BP should be measured and urine tested for proteinuria
- symphysis–fundal height should be measured and plotted
- information should be given, with an opportunity to discuss issues and ask questions; verbal information supported by written information.

General

Throughout the entire antenatal period, healthcare providers should remain alert to signs or symptoms of conditions which affect the health of the mother and fetus, such as domestic violence, pre-eclampsia and diabetes.

For an outline of care at each appointment see the Algorithm (Section 2.3).

5. Lifestyle considerations

5.1   Physiological, psychosocial and emotional changes in pregnancy

Many common physiological, psychosocial and emotional changes occur during pregnancy. Many of these changes may be due to the normal hormonal changes that are taking place in a pregnant woman's body or due to worries associated with pregnancy, such as concerns about the birth or the baby's wellbeing. *The pregnancy book*[23] has a chapter on feelings and relationships in pregnancy as well as a chapter on feelings that the father of the child may be encountering.

Some of the common changes that pregnant women might encounter include:

- bleeding gums or gingivitis (note that dental treatment is free during pregnancy and for a year after the birth of the baby) – see Section 5.2
- heartburn (indigestion) – see Section 6.2
- constipation – see Section 6.3
- vaginal discharge (thrush) – see Section 6.6
- varicose veins – see Section 6.5
- haemorrhoids (piles) – see Section 6.4
- backache – see Section 6.7
- swelling of the ankles, fingers, face and hands due to the body holding more fluid in pregnancy – a certain amount of swelling, or oedema, is normal later in pregnancy; however, more severe cases may indicate pre-eclampsia if present with other symptoms and signs (see Section 11.2).

Chapter 9 in *The Pregnancy Book*[23] addresses other common physiological problems encountered in pregnancy such as itching, feeling hot and skin and hair changes.

Not all women will experience all of the above symptoms but it is important for pregnant women to be aware that some of these changes are normal in pregnancy and to be alert to symptoms of potentially harmful complications. It is also important for pregnant women to be reassured that most symptoms of pregnancy are not putting them or their fetus in danger and to be made to feel comfortable about asking their healthcare provider about these changes.

5.2   Maternity health benefits

Prescriptions and dental treatment are free during pregnancy and for a year after the birth.

5.3   Working during pregnancy

Pregnant women want information about maternity benefits and rights. Healthcare professionals need to be aware of current UK legislation regarding employment. From 6 April 2003, women who work for an employer will qualify for 26 weeks' ordinary maternity leave and those who have worked for their employer continuously for 26 weeks by the 15th week before the baby is due may be entitled to additional maternity leave. Additional maternity leave lasts 26 weeks from the end of ordinary maternity leave.

Pregnant employees also have special employment rights; for example, the right to take time off work for antenatal care. Further rights are being introduced from 2003, such as the right to paid paternity leave and the right to apply for flexible working hours. Under current UK legislation:

- a woman in employment is not allowed to continue working beyond 33 weeks of gestation, unless the woman's GP informs her employer that she may continue to do so
- it is unlawful for an employer to require or allow a woman in their employment to return to work in the two weeks following childbirth
- employers are required to assess risks which might be posed to the health and safety of pregnant women, those who are breastfeeding or who have given birth in the past six months. If a significant risk is identified, steps to avoid the risk should be taken, such as:
  - use of preventative or protective behaviours
  - altering working conditions or hours
  - arranging alternative work.

As this information often changes with time, antenatal healthcare providers and pregnant women are encouraged to visit the Maternity Alliance website (www.maternityalliance.org.uk/) for more comprehensive and up-to-date information. Fact sheets on maternity benefits for students, single parents and young mothers can also be downloaded from this website. Further information may also be obtained from the Department of Trade and Industry (DTI) website (www.dti.gov.uk/er/workingparents.htm or telephone 0870 1502 500 for information leaflets) or the Government's interactive guidance site (www.tiger.gov.uk). Up-to-date information on maternity benefits can also be accessed at the Department for Work and Pensions (www.dwp.gov.uk).

In December 2002, a guide for employers, entitled *New and expectant mothers at work, a guide for employers* was published to assist employers in ensuring that pregnant women have a safe and healthy experience at work. These may be ordered from the Health and Safety Executive website at www.hsebooks.co.uk (Tel: 01787 881 165).

Exposure to radiation and chemicals

Some workers are occupationally exposed to potentially teratogenic or toxic substances or environments. For some of these, there is evidence to support an association between exposure and adverse maternal or neonatal outcomes, e.g. exposure to x-rays for healthcare workers. For other exposures, data are inconclusive, e.g. there are inconsistent data to support an association with miscarriage in workers exposed to vapours in the dry-cleaning and painting industries.[60-62] Further information on occupational hazards can be obtained from the Health and Safety Executive website: www.hse.gov.uk/mothers/index.htm.

Physical aspects of work

One meta-analysis of 29 observational studies analysed data on 160,988 women who worked during pregnancy.[63] The outcomes it considered were preterm birth, hypertension or pre-eclampsia and small-for-gestational-age babies. Physically demanding work and prolonged standing may be associated with poor outcomes but the evidence on prolonged hours and shift working is inconclusive. Employment per se has not been associated with increased risks in pregnancy.

One further cohort study from Poland that was not included in this review was located.[64] Although heavy physical work, as reported by the woman, was shown to be significantly associated with the birth of a small-for-gestational-age baby, no significant differences were reported when heavy physical work load was evaluated by level of energy expenditure. [Evidence level 2b]

RECOMMENDATIONS

Pregnant women should be informed of their maternity rights and benefits. [C]

The majority of women can be reassured that it is safe to continue working during pregnancy. Further information about possible occupational hazards during pregnancy is available from the Health and Safety Executive. [D]

A woman's occupation during pregnancy should be ascertained to identify those at increased risk through occupational exposure. [Good practice point]

5.4 Dietary information and education

In addition to the information contained in this guideline on what women should and should not eat during pregnancy, good sources of dietary information during pregnancy include *The Pregnancy Book*[23] and the publication *Eating While You Are Pregnant* from the Food Standards Agency, which may also be accessed online at: www.foodstandards.gov.uk/healthiereating/pregnancy/advice-for-you/pregnancy/.

In general, women should be given information about the benefits of eating a variety of foods during pregnancy including:

- plenty of fruit and vegetables
- starchy foods such as bread, pasta, rice and potatoes
- protein, such as lean meat, fish, beans and lentils
- plenty of fibre, which can be found in wholegrain breads and fruits and vegetables
- dairy foods, such as milk, yoghurt and cheese.

Pregnant women should be informed of foods that may put them or their fetus at risk including:

- soft mould ripened cheeses, such as Camembert, Brie and blue-veined cheese
- pâté (including vegetable pâté)
- liver and liver products
- uncooked or undercooked ready-prepared meals
- uncooked or cured meat, such as salami
- raw shellfish, such as oysters
- fish containing relatively high levels of methylmercury, such as shark, swordfish and marlin, which might affect the nervous system of the fetus.

The Food Standards Agency has also recently announced that pregnant women should limit their consumption of:

- tuna to no more than two medium size cans or one fresh tuna steak per week
- caffeine to 300 milligrams a day. Caffeine is present in coffee, tea and colas.

One systematic review of RCTs was located that assessed whether or not the provision of dietary information leads to improved maternal and perinatal outcomes compared with no dietary information.[65] The review was last updated in 1996, however, and although there was evidence that dietary information increased energy and protein intake, data concerning the outcome of pregnancy were available from only one trial, which was not of high quality.

5.5 Nutritional supplements

Folic acid

Neural tube defects, which comprise open spina bifida, anencephaly and encephalocele, affect 1.5/1000 pregnancies in the UK.[66] These congenital malformations, which arise from neural tube defects, are preventable through public health measures.

The effect of increased consumption of multivitamins or folic acid consumption before conception on the prevalence of neural tube defects was assessed in a systematic review of four RCTs of 6425 women.[67] In all the RCTs, folic acid was taken before conception and up to 6–12 weeks of gestation. This periconceptional folate supplementation was found to substantially reduce the prevalence of neural tube defects (relative risk 0.28, 95% CI 0.13 to 0.58). There was a reduction both where the mother had not had a previously affected fetus or infant (relative risk 0.07, 95% CI 0.00 to 1.32) and when the mother had given birth to a previously affected infant (OR 0.31, 95% CI 0.14 to 0.66). There were no significant differences found in the rates of miscarriage, ectopic pregnancy or stillbirth with folate supplementation compared with no folate supplementation. [Evidence level 1a] The effect of starting folic in early pregnancy has not been evaluated.

A concern raised in this review was the possible adverse effect of folate supplementation on causing an increase in the rate of twin pregnancies, with an associated increase in the rate of perinatal mortality. However, results from a large cohort study in China (n = 242,015 women) found no association between consumption of folic acid supplements in pregnancy (400 micrograms per day) and multiple births (rate ratio 0.91, 95% CI 0.82 to 1.0).[68] [Evidence level 2a]

It is estimated that only one-third of women take folic acid supplements before conception. As folic acid is needed at the time of embryogenesis and many women do not plan a pregnancy, folic acid-fortified foods have been advocated in the UK.[69] Folic acid-fortified foods have been found to be effective in achieving beneficial levels of red-cell folate. However, increasing intake through foods naturally containing folates has not been found to be effective.[70] While other countries, such as the USA, Canada and Chile, have put the fortification of wheat flour into practice and observed resultant decreases in the birth prevalence of neural tube defects, in May 2002, the UK Foods Standards Agency decided against recommending mandatory folic acid fortification.[69]

Current advice from an Expert Advisory Group report issued by the Department of Health[71] is that women who do not have a prior history of neural tube defects should take folic acid prior to conception and daily during the first 12 weeks of pregnancy. The recommended amount is 400 micrograms/day for women who have not had a previous baby with a neural tube defect. This report was largely based on evidence from a large multicentre RCT.[72] Although the size of effect for a given dose of folic acid has been quantified and modelling has indicated that a reduced risk is associated with higher doses (i.e., 500 micrograms in lieu of 400 micrograms), the practical application of an increased dose of folic acid has not yet been investigated in studies or trials and therefore cannot be recommended.[73]

RECOMMENDATION

Pregnant women (and those intending to become pregnant) should be informed that dietary supplementation with folic acid, before conception and up to 12 weeks of gestation, reduces the risk of having a baby with neural tube defects (anencephaly, spina bifida). The recommended dose is 400 micrograms/day. [A]

Iron supplementation

A systematic review of 20 randomised controlled trials compared iron supplementation with either placebo or no iron in pregnant women (n = 5552) with normal haemoglobin levels (greater than 10 g/dl) at less than 28 weeks of gestation.[74] Routine iron supplementation raised or maintained the serum ferritin level above 10 micrograms/litre and resulted in a substantial reduction in women with a haemoglobin level below 10 or 10.5g/dl in late pregnancy. There was no evidence of any beneficial or harmful effects on maternal or fetal outcomes. [Evidence level 1a]

The largest trial (n = 2682) of selective versus routine iron supplementation showed an increased likelihood of caesarean section and postpartum blood transfusion among those receiving selective supplementation, but fewer perinatal deaths.[75] [Evidence level 1b]

Another systematic review looked at the effects of routine iron and folate supplements on pregnant women with normal levels of haemoglobin.[76] Eight trials involving 5449 women were included. Routine supplementation with iron and folate raised or maintained the serum iron and ferritin levels and serum and red-cell folate levels. It also resulted in a substantial reduction of women with a haemoglobin level below 10 or 10.5 g/dl in late pregnancy. However, routine supplementation with iron and folate had no detectable effects, either beneficial or harmful, on any measures of maternal or fetal outcome. [Evidence level 1a]

Oral iron has also been associated with gastric irritation and altered bowel habit (i.e. constipation or diarrhoea).[77]

See also Section 8.1 on anaemia.

RECOMMENDATION

Iron supplementation should not be offered routinely to all pregnant women. It does not benefit the mother's or fetus's health and may have unpleasant maternal side effects. [A]

Vitamin A

In areas of the world where vitamin A deficiency is prevalent, supplementation may be beneficial for pregnant women.[78] [Evidence level 1a] Vitamin A deficiency is not prevalent among pregnant women in England and Wales and therefore the results of this review were not considered relevant to this guideline.

High levels of preformed vitamin A during pregnancy are considered to be teratogenic.[79–81] From the epidemiological evidence, it is not possible to establish a clear dose–response curve or threshold above which vitamin A intake may be harmful during the first trimester (considered to be the critical period for susceptibility). A dose between 10,000 and 25,000 iu of vitamin A may pose a teratogenic risk.

The intake of vitamin A during pregnancy should be limited to the recommended daily amount, which, in Europe, is 2310 iu, equivalent to 700 micrograms. As liver and liver products contain variable and sometimes very high amounts of vitamin A (10,000–38,000 mg per typical portion size of 100g), these foodstuffs should be avoided in pregnancy.

The consumption of liver and liver products by pregnant women (and moreover the intake of greater than 700 micrograms) is associated with an increase in the risk of certain congenital malformations.[81]

RECOMMENDATION

Pregnant women should be informed that vitamin A supplementation (intake greater than 700 micrograms) might be teratogenic and therefore it should be avoided. Pregnant women should be informed that, as liver and liver products may also contain high levels of vitamin A, consumption of these products should also be avoided. [C]

Vitamin D

Vitamin D requirements are thought to increase during pregnancy to aid calcium absorption. The main sources of vitamin D are sunlight and oily fish. Daily exposure to sunlight should avoid vitamin D deficiency. Maternal deficiency in Vitamin D is purported to be associated with neonatal rickets although this is a theoretical risk as we were unable to find evidence to quantify it.

Women from the Indian subcontinent living in England and Wales are thought to be particularly vulnerable to vitamin D deficiency. Those women who remain indoors, whose clothing leaves little exposed skin, who live in a sunless climate and who are vegetarian are also thought to be at higher risk of vitamin D deficiency.

One systematic review assessed the effects of vitamin D supplementation on pregnancy outcome.[82] Only two small RCTs were included (n = 232). Neonatal hypocalcaemia was less common in the supplemented group (OR 0.13, 95% CI 0.02 to 0.65). However, there were no other significant findings and there was not enough evidence to evaluate the effects of vitamin D supplementation during pregnancy. [Evidence level 1a]

Although the Food Standards Agency recommends vitamin D supplementation during pregnancy, there is no indication of what evidence this recommendation is based on.

RECOMMENDATION

There is insufficient evidence to evaluate the effectiveness of vitamin D in pregnancy. In the absence of evidence of benefit, vitamin D supplementation should not be offered routinely to pregnant women. [A]

5.6 Food-acquired infections

Listeriosis

Listeriosis is an illness caused by a bacterium called *Listeria monocytogenes*, which may present with mild, flu-like symptoms. It is also associated with miscarriage, stillbirth and

Hypnosis and aromatherapy

Although studies on hypnosis and aromatherapy during childbirth were located, no studies on their effectiveness or safety for use during pregnancy were found.

RECOMMENDATION

Pregnant women should be informed that few complementary therapies have been established as being safe and effective during pregnancy. Women should not assume that such therapies are safe and they should be used as little as possible during pregnancy. [D]

5.10 Exercise in pregnancy

Exercise includes a range of physical activities and not all sports have the same impact on pregnancy. The physiological and morphological changes that occur during pregnancy may interfere with a woman's ability to engage in some forms of physical activity safely. In the absence of any obstetric or medical complications, however, most women can begin or maintain a regular exercise regimen during pregnancy without causing harm to their fetus.

In an RCT that compared babies born to women who continued regular exercise during pregnancy with women who did not exercise regularly during pregnancy, no differences in neurodevelopmental outcomes at one year of age were reported.[100] [Evidence level 1b]

One systematic review assessed the effects of advising healthy pregnant women to engage in regular (at least two to three times per week) aerobic exercise on physical fitness, ease or difficulty of childbirth and delivery, and on the course and outcome of pregnancy.[101]. Ten trials randomising 688 women were included, all of which had methodological shortcomings. Five of the ten trials reported significant improvement in physical fitness in the exercise group; however, the measures used to assess fitness varied across the trials and were therefore not subject to meta-analysis. A conflicting result with no mean difference in gestational age (three RCTs, n = 416; WMD 0.02, 95% CI – 0.4 to 0.4) and an increased risk of preterm birth in the exercise group was found (three RCTs, n = 421; RR 2.29, 95% CI 1.02 to 5.13). No other adverse outcomes were reported and one trial (n = 15) found improvement among exercising women in several aspects of self-reported body image, including muscle strength, energy level and body build.[101] [Evidence level 1a]

Pregnant women should avoid exercise that involves the risk of abdominal trauma, falls or excessive joint stress, as in high impact sports, contact sports and vigorous racquet sports. They are also recommended not to scuba dive, because the risk of birth defects seems to be greater among those who do, and there is a serious risk of fetal decompression disease.[102] [Evidence level 3]

Maternal exercise during pregnancy does not appear to have a negative effect on the fetus or on birth outcomes.

RECOMMENDATION

Pregnant women should be informed that beginning or continuing a moderate course of exercise during pregnancy is not associated with adverse outcomes. [A]

Pregnant women should be informed of the potential dangers of certain activities during pregnancy, for example, contact sports, high-impact sports and vigorous racquet sports that may involve the risk of abdominal trauma, falls or excessive joint stress, and scuba diving, which may result in fetal birth defects and fetal decompression disease. [D]

5.11 Sexual intercourse in pregnancy

Two American cohort studies of over 52,000 pregnant women reported an inverse association between the frequency of sexual intercourse at various times during pregnancy and the risk of preterm delivery.[103,104] [Evidence level 2a] No association between frequency of sexual intercourse and perinatal mortality was observed.[104] A study among women identified with bacterial vaginosis (BV) or *Trichomonas vaginalis* in the USA reported a similar decreased risk for preterm birth among women who reported more frequent intercourse than women who reported less frequent intercourse, but this finding applied only to women with BV and not to those with *T. vaginalis*.[105]

RECOMMENDATION

Pregnant woman should be informed that sexual intercourse in pregnancy is not known to be associated with any adverse outcomes. [B]

5.12   Alcohol and smoking in pregnancy

Alcohol consumption in pregnancy

Alcohol passes freely across the placenta to the fetus and, while there is general agreement that women should not drink excessively during pregnancy, it remains unclear what level of drinking is harmful to a pregnant woman and her fetus. Investigating the effects of maternal drinking on fetal development is difficult, due to confounding factors such as socio-economic status and smoking.

Research evidence is consistent in finding no evidence of fetal harm among women who drink one or two units of alcohol per week.[106] There is also little or no evidence of harm in women who drink up to ten units per week. However, binge drinking or otherwise heavy consumption of alcohol is associated with adverse baby outcomes such as low birthweight[107,108] and behavioural and intellectual difficulties later in life.[109] [Evidence level 3] Binge drinking is also associated with fetal alcohol syndrome and the incidence in Europe is reported to be 0.4 cases/1000.[110]

As a safe low level of alcohol consumption has yet to be ascertained and associations with fetal alcohol syndrome exist only with binge or heavy drinking, guidance from professional bodies is slightly inconsistent. One guideline recommends that while there is no conclusive evidence that consumption levels below 15 units/week have an adverse effect on fetal growth or childhood IQ levels, pregnant women should be careful about the amount of alcohol they consume and limit it to no more than one standard unit of alcohol per day.[111] [Evidence level 4] Other guidance (e.g. MIDIRS Informed Choice and Foods Standards Agency) recommends one to two units once or twice a week. [Evidence level 4]

RECOMMENDATION

Excess alcohol has an adverse effect on the fetus. Therefore it is suggested that women limit alcohol consumption to no more than one standard unit per day. Each of the following constitutes one 'unit' of alcohol: a single measure of spirits, one small glass of wine, and a half pint of ordinary strength beer, lager or cider. [C]

Smoking in pregnancy

Although it is estimated that up to 25% of women who smoke stop before their first antenatal appointment,[112] 27% of pregnant women in the UK report that they are current smokers at the time of the birth of the baby.[113]

Smoking is a significant modifiable cause of adverse pregnancy outcome in women and its dangers have been widely established. Meta-analyses have shown significant associations between maternal cigarette smoking in pregnancy and increased risks of perinatal mortality,[114] sudden infant death syndrome,[114] placental abruption,[115,116] preterm premature rupture of membranes,[116] ectopic pregnancies,[116] placenta praevia,[116] preterm delivery,[117] miscarriage,[114] low birthweight[114] and the development of cleft lip and cleft palate in children.[118] [all studies: Evidence levels 2 and 3] Smoking during pregnancy has also been reported to reduce the incidence of pre-eclampsia;[116,119] however, this association should be considered in context with the many negative risks associated with smoking during pregnancy. [Evidence levels 2 and 3]

Cohort studies have shown significant associations between maternal cigarette smoking in pregnancy and increased risks of small-for-gestational-age infant,[120] stillbirth[121] and fetal and infant mortality.[122] [Evidence level 2]

In addition, the link between maternal cigarette smoking and reduced birthweight has been established in over 100 publications based on studies of more than 500,000 births published between 1957 and 1986, with babies born to smokers being a consistent 175–200 g smaller than those born to similar non-smokers.[123] It has been estimated that if all pregnant women stopped smoking, a 10% reduction in infant and fetal deaths would be seen.[122] As smoking is a potentially preventable activity, it is an important public health issue in pregnancy.

Long-term effects on children born to mothers who smoked during pregnancy have been studied but report conflicting results.[124–126] [Evidence level 3] It is possible that effects of smoking in pregnancy resolve later in childhood.

One review of systematic reviews of RCTs found two systematic reviews and three additional RCTs that assessed the effects of smoking cessation programmes implemented during pregnancy.[127]

The first review (44 trials, n = 16,916 women) found a significant reduction in smoking in late pregnancy among women who attended smoking cessation programmes compared with no programme (Peto OR 0.53, 95% CI 0.47 to 0.60)[112] [Evidence level 1a] The trials in this review showed substantial clinical heterogeneity; however, the effect was still present when analysis was restricted to trials in which abstinence from smoking was confirmed by means other than self-report (Peto OR 0.53, 95% CI 0.44 to 0.63). A subset of ten trials that included information on fetal outcome showed a reduction in low birthweight (Peto OR 0.8, 95% CI 0.67 to 0.95), a reduction in preterm birth (Peto OR 0.83, 95% CI 0.69 to 0.99) and an increase in mean birthweight of 28 g (95% CI 9 g to 49 g) among women who attended anti-smoking programmes. However, no differences in very low birthweight or perinatal mortality were observed.

The second review (10 RCTs, n = 4815 pregnant women) included a trial of physician advice, a trial of advice from a health educator, a trial of group sessions, and seven trials on behavioural therapy based on self-help manuals.[128] Cessation rates ranged from 1.9% to 16.7% among those who did not receive an intervention and from 7.1% to 36.1% among those who participated in an intervention. The review found that cessation programmes significantly increased the rate of quitting (absolute risk increase with intervention versus no intervention 7.6%, 95% CI 4.3 to 10.8). [Evidence level 1a]

Three additional RCTs compared nicotine patches with placebo, a brief (10–15 minutes) smoking intervention delivered by a midwife compared with usual care (n = 1120 pregnant women), and motivational interviewing with usual care (n = 269 women in their 28th week of pregnancy). Nicotine patches were not significantly associated with a difference in quit rates.[129] [Evidence level 1b] Furthermore, the safety of nicotine replacement therapy in pregnancy has not been established. The intervention delivered by midwives was based on a 10–15 minute session in which verbal counselling was backed up with written information and arrangements for continuing self-help support were made, if necessary. This intervention found no difference in smoking behaviour when compared with the women who received usual care.[130] [Evidence level 1b] The motivational interviewing trial was based on intensified, late pregnancy counselling of 3 to 5 minutes plus the distribution of self-help booklets mailed weekly, and follow-up letters and telephone calls. This trial also reported no difference in cessation rates when compared with women in their 34th week of pregnancy or at 6 months postpartum.[131] [Evidence level 1b]

An RCT was conducted in three NHS trusts in England.[132] The intervention consisted of giving self-help booklets on quitting smoking to pregnant women at the first opportunity, together with a booklet for partners, family members and friends. Four more booklets were sent to the woman at weekly intervals. The intervention was reported to be ineffective at increasing smoking cessation. [Evidence level 1b]

Pregnant women who are unable to quit during pregnancy often reduce the number of cigarettes that they smoke. Data indicate this can significantly reduce nicotine concentrations and can offer some measure of protection for the fetus, with a 50% reduction being associated with a 92 g increase in birthweight.[133,134]

The NHS pregnancy smoking telephone help line is available at 0800 169 9 169.

RECOMMENDATIONS

Pregnant women should be informed about the specific risks of smoking during pregnancy (such as the risk of having a baby with low birthweight and preterm). The benefits of quitting at any stage should be emphasised. [A]

Women who smoke or who have recently stopped should be offered smoking cessation interventions. Interventions that appear to be effective in reducing smoking include advice by physician, group sessions, and behavioural therapy (based on self-help manuals). [A]

Women who are unable to quit smoking during pregnancy should be encouraged to reduce smoking. [B]

5.13 Cannabis use in pregnancy

There is limited evidence on the impact of maternal cannabis consumption during pregnancy. Cannabis is often smoked as a mix with tobacco. One of the problems with research into cannabis consumption during pregnancy is accurately measuring the amount of cannabis consumed. Research can also be confounded by factors such as socio-economic status, alcohol use, smoking and the use of other drugs.

An estimated 5% of mothers reported smoking cannabis before and during pregnancy in England.[135] [Evidence level 3]

A meta-analysis of ten observational studies that were adjusted for cigarette smoking presented data on 32,483 live births.[136] Studies were examined where possible according to an arbitrarily defined dose response. Infrequent use was defined as no greater than once a week, and frequent use was defined as at least four times a week. Where possible, results were presented by gestational age at time of consumption. In the five studies that reported mean birthweight:

- any cannabis use during the first trimester of pregnancy reduced the mean birthweight by 48 g (95% CI –83 g to –14 g)
- any cannabis use during the second trimester of pregnancy reduced the mean birthweight by 39 g (95% CI –75 g to –3 g)
- any cannabis use during the third trimester of pregnancy reduced the mean birthweight by 35 g (95% CI –71 g to 1 g)
- infrequent use of cannabis resulted in an increase in mean birthweight of 62 g (95% CI 8 g to 132 g)
- frequent use of cannabis resulted in a reduction in mean birthweight of 131 g (95% CI –209 g to –52 g).

In the five studies that reported the odds ratio for low birthweight (less than 2500 g), the pooled OR was 1.09 (95% CI 0.94 to 1.27) for any cannabis use during pregnancy.

A study of over 12,000 women in England found no association between any level of cannabis use (weekly, less than weekly, or no cannabis and before, during or after the first trimester) and perinatal death, preterm delivery and admission to the neonatal unit.[135] [Evidence level 3] After adjustment for confounding (youth, caffeine, alcohol and illicit drug use), no statistically significant association between cannabis use and birthweight was found.

There is insufficient evidence to conclude that maternal cannabis use at the levels reported causes low birthweight. However, a study on behavioural outcomes of children at three years of age found increased fearfulness and poorer motor skills among those who were born to mothers who used cannabis during pregnancy.[126] [Evidence level 3] Taking the precautionary principle based on the positive associations between cannabis use and cigarette smoking, it is recommended that women should be discouraged from using cannabis in pregnancy.

Note

As women who use heroin, cocaine (including crack cocaine), ecstasy, ketamine, amphetamines or other drugs during pregnancy are likely to require additional care due to more adverse effects, these topics were deemed to be outside the remit of this guideline which is intended for healthy women with uncomplicated singleton pregnancies.

RECOMMENDATION

The direct effects of cannabis on the fetus are uncertain but may be harmful. Cannabis use is associated with smoking, which is known to be harmful; therefore women should be discouraged from using cannabis during pregnancy. [C]

5.14 Air travel during pregnancy

No direct estimates of the risk of travel-related venous thromboembolism in pregnancy were located. The overall incidence of symptomatic venous thrombosis after a long-haul flight has been estimated to be around 1/400 to 1/10,000. Asymptomatic venous thrombosis is estimated to be about ten times this figure.[137] [Evidence level 4] Venous thromboembolism is reported to complicate 0.13/1000 to 1/1000 pregnancies,[137–140] [Evidence level 3] and it has been suggested that this risk is increased in pregnant women during air travel.[137] [Evidence level 4]

The risk of venous thromboembolism is attributed predominantly to immobility during air travel. In a trial of 231 passengers randomised to wearing below-knee elastic stockings on both legs compared with passengers who did not wear such stockings, a decreased risk of deep vein thrombosis was observed in the intervention group (OR 0.07, 95% CI 0 to 0.46).[141] [Evidence level 1b] No evidence on the effectiveness of compression stockings specifically in pregnant women was located. Other precautionary measures for all travellers that pregnant women should be informed about include isometric calf exercises, walking around the aircraft cabin when possible and avoiding dehydration by drinking plenty of water and by minimising alcohol and caffeine intake.[137] [Evidence level 4]

Commercial flights are normally safe for a pregnant woman and her fetus. However, most airlines restrict the acceptance of pregnant women. In general, uncomplicated singleton pregnancies may fly long distances until the 36th week of gestation and a letter from a doctor or midwife confirming good health, normal pregnancy and the expected date of delivery should be carried after the 28th week of pregnancy.[142] Medical clearance is required by some airlines for pregnant women if delivery is expected less than 4 weeks after the departure date or if any complications in delivery may be expected. As different airlines may have different restrictions, specific airlines should be contacted directly for more information.

RECOMMENDATION

Pregnant women should be informed that long-haul air travel is associated with an increased risk of venous thrombosis, although whether or not there is additional risk during pregnancy is unclear. In the general population, wearing correctly fitted compression stockings is effective at reducing the risk. [B]

Future research

Further research to quantify the risk of air travel and to assess the effectiveness of interventions to prevent venous thromboembolism in pregnancy is needed.

5.15 Car travel during pregnancy

From 1997 to 1999, seven pregnant women were killed in road traffic accidents.[143] [Evidence level 3] Irrespective of where one is sitting in the car, it has been a legal requirement in the UK to wear a seatbelt since 1991 and this law applies to pregnant women.

A 1998 survey on pregnant women's knowledge and use of seatbelts showed that, while 98% of pregnant front-seat passengers wore a seatbelt, only 68% wore one in the back of the car.[144] The survey also found that only 48% of women correctly identified the correct way to use a seatbelt, with only 37% reporting that they had received information on the correct use of seatbelts while pregnant. The women who had received information while pregnant were more likely to correctly position their seatbelts than women who had received no information (OR 0.35, 95% CI 0.17 to 0.70). [Evidence level 3]

An American study investigating the education of pregnant women on the correct use of seatbelts found that, even with minimal information on wearing a seatbelt, seatbelt use increased from 19.4% to 28.6%.[145] [Evidence level 2a]

The correct use of seatbelts is particularly important in pregnant women, as incorrect use may cause harm to the fetus and fail to protect the woman in the case of an accident. A retrospective study of 43 pregnant women involved in road traffic accidents showed an increase in adverse fetal outcome, including fetal loss, with improper maternal restraint use compared with women who used seatbelts properly: in minor crashes 33% (2/6) versus 11% (2/18); moderate crashes 100% (1/1) versus 30% (3/10); severe crashes 100% (5/5) versus 100% (3/3).[146] [Evidence level 3]

In an older study comparing lap-belt restraint with no seatbelt use among 208 pregnant women who were involved in severe rural car accidents, maternal mortality was 3.6% among those wearing a lap belt compared with 7.8% among those not wearing a seatbelt.[147] Total maternal injuries, including death, was 10.7% among women wearing a lap belt compared with 21.1% among those not wearing a seatbelt. Fetal mortality was 16.7% among women wearing a lap belt compared with 14.4% among women not wearing a seatbelt. [Evidence level 3]

No human studies on the comparison of lap belts compared with three-point seatbelts in pregnant women were located; however, a study in pregnant baboons investigating the use of three-point restraints versus lap belts found a fetal death rate of 8.3 % among animals wearing with a three-point restraint on impact compared with a 50% fetal death rate among animals impacted with lap belts only.[148] [Evidence level 2a]

A study on pregnancy outcomes in pregnant women drivers found that women who were not wearing seatbelts were 1.9 times more likely to have a low birthweight baby (95% CI 1.2 to 2.9) and 2.3 times more likely to give birth within 48 hours after a motor vehicle crash (95% CI 1.1 to 4.9) when compared with women drivers who were wearing seatbelts (adjusted for age and gestational age at crash).[149] Fetal death was 0.5% (7/1349) in women who did not use seatbelts and 0.2% (2/1243) in women who did use seatbelts. [Evidence level 3]

The Confidential Enquiry into Maternal Deaths in the United Kingdom provides information on the correct use of seatbelts in pregnancy:[143]

- Above and below the bump, not over it.
- Use three-point seatbelts with the lap strap placed as low as possible beneath the 'bump', lying across the thighs with the diagonal shoulder strap above the bump lying between the breasts.
- Adjust the fit to be as snug as comfortably possible.

RECOMMENDATIONS

Pregnant women should be informed about the correct use of seatbelts (that is, three-point seatbelts "above and below the bump, not over it"). [B]

5.16 Travelling abroad during pregnancy

Vaccinations

In the event that a pregnant woman is travelling abroad, care must be taken to ensure that any vaccines that are received are not contraindicated in pregnancy. In general, killed or inactivated vaccines, toxoids and polysaccharides can be given during pregnancy, as can oral polio vaccine.

Live vaccines are generally contraindicated because of largely theoretical risks to the fetus. Measles, mumps, rubella, BCG and yellow fever vaccines should be avoided in pregnancy.[150]

The risks and benefits of specific vaccines should be examined in each individual case and the advice of a travel medicine doctor should be sought for women considering travel in pregnancy. Table 5.1 summarises the WHO-compiled information on the use of various vaccines in pregnancy.

Yellow fever

Vaccination against yellow fever may be considered after the sixth month of pregnancy when the risk from exposure is deemed greater than the risk to the fetus and pregnant women. Yellow fever is transmitted by mosquitoes and fatality from yellow fever in unimmunised adults is 50%.[151] Women should be informed about the risks of yellow fever and about areas where the risk of exposure to yellow fever is high.[150]

Malaria

Malaria in a pregnant woman increases the risk of maternal death, miscarriage, stillbirth and low birthweight with associated risk of neonatal death and preterm birth.[154,155] [Evidence level 2a] The risks associated with malaria infection in nonimmune pregnant women include miscarriage in up to 60% of cases and maternal mortality of up to 10%.[156]

As with all travellers, taking precautions against insect bites is an important preventive measure. This includes minimising skin exposure and the use of bed nets. As pregnant women appear to attract twice as many malaria-carrying mosquitoes as women who are not pregnant,[157] [Evidence level 3] pregnant women should be extra diligent in using measures to protect against mosquito bites, but should take care not to exceed the recommended dosage of insect repellents as the safety of DEET (N,N-diethyl-m-toluamide, now called N,N-diethyl-3-methylbenzamide) has not been established in pregnancy.[154] [Evidence level 3] One case report was found of a child who was born with mental disability, impaired sensorimotor coordination and craniofacial dysmorphology to a woman who had applied DEET on a daily basis throughout pregnancy in addition to using chloroquine.[158] [Evidence level 3] One study on the use of permethrin bed nets

Table 5.1 Vaccination in pregnancy[150]

Vaccine	Use in pregnancy	Comments
BCG*	No	
Cholera	No[151]	Safety not determined
Hepatitis A	Yes, administer if indicated	Safety not determined
Hepatitis B	Yes, administer if indicated	
Influenza	Yes, administer if indicated	In some circumstances; consult a physician
Japanese encephalitis**	No	Safety not determined
Measles*	No***	
Meningococcal disease	Yes, administer if indicated	Only if significant risk of infection[151]
Mumps*	No***	
Oral poliomyelitis vaccine	Yes, administer if indicated	
Inactivated poliomyelitis vaccine	Yes, administer if indicated	Normally avoided
Rabies	Yes, administer if indicated	
Rubella*	No***	
Tetanus/diphtheria	Yes, administer if indicated	
Typhoid Ty21a		Safety not determined
Smallpox	No[152]	
Varicella*	No	
Yellow fever*	Yes, administer if indicated	Avoid unless at high risk

*   live vaccine, to be avoided in pregnancy
**   Contrary to the WHO, other reports indicate that the vaccine is both contraindicated in pregnancy and may be administered in pregnancy[152,153]
*** Pregnancy should be delayed for 3 months after vaccine given

in pregnancy on the Thai–Burmese border reported no adverse effects on pregnancy or infant outcome but also reported a marginal effect of bed nets on the reduction of malaria compared with no bed nets (reduction seen in one of three test sites, RR 1.67, 95% CI 1.07 to 2.61).[159] [Evidence level 1b]

The antimalarials chloroquine and proguanil may be given in usual doses in areas where *Plasmodium falciparum* strains of malaria are not resistant. In the case of proguanil, 5 mg of folic acid/day should be given. The manufacturer of mefloquine advises avoidance as a matter of principle but studies of mefloquine in pregnancy (including during the first trimester) have revealed no evidence of harm; it may therefore be considered for travel to chloroquine-resistant areas. Pyrimethamine with dapsone (Maloprim®, GSK) should not be used in pregnancy; the preparation has been discontinued in the UK. Doxycycline is contraindicated during pregnancy. Proguanil hydrochloride with atovaquone (Malarone®, GSK) should be avoided during pregnancy unless there is no suitable alternative.[77]

Travel insurance

Women who will be travelling while pregnant should obtain adequate medical and travel insurance, ensuring in advanced that complications relating to pregnancy are covered, as well as medical care in the case of birth overseas for both the mother and baby. Most insurance companies will cover up to 28 weeks and there are a few that cover to 32 weeks.[160] Insurance companies will generally cover pregnant women, providing that:

- the pregnant woman returns to this country by the time stated
- the pregnant woman has had no antenatal problems that have required treatment, especially if this has entailed a stay in hospital
- the pregnant woman is travelling with the consent of her doctor.[160]

Travel insurance agencies should be contacted directly for more comprehensive information. Pregnant women should compare various policies and read the exclusion clauses carefully before choosing. In some cases, insurance policies will terminate benefit if medical care is sought from medical facilities that are not approved[161] and some policies will cover the mother but will not extend to coverage of the baby if it is born while the woman is travelling.[162] Other policies will not cover medical expenses after a certain gestation date or for specific outcomes of pregnancy, such as miscarriage.[163]

If the pregnant woman is travelling within the European Economic Area (EEA), then she will need an E111 form. This will cover the cost of care in a hospital but it does not cover the cost of transport to get to the hospital or to bring the baby home. If the pregnant women is more than 36 weeks' pregnant or intends to have the baby within the EEA but outside the UK, she needs form E112. The Department of Health International Relations Unit can be contacted to obtain the leaflet *Health Advice for Travellers*, which gives more information. This leaflet may also be available from the local post office or health centre.[160]

RECOMMENDATION

Pregnant women should be informed that, if they are planning to travel abroad, they should discuss considerations such as flying, vaccinations and travel insurance with their midwife or doctor. [Good practice point]

6. Management of common symptoms of pregnancy

6.1   Nausea and vomiting in early pregnancy

The causes of nausea and vomiting in pregnancy are not known and, although the rise in human chorionic gonadotrophin (hCG) during pregnancy has been implicated, data about its association are conflicting.[164] Nausea and vomiting occurs more commonly in multiple pregnancies and molar pregnancies.[165] Nausea is the most common gastrointestinal symptom of pregnancy, occurring in 80–85% of all pregnancies during the first trimester, with vomiting an associated complaint in approximately 52% of women.[166,167] [Evidence level 3] Hyperemesis gravidarum refers to pregnant women in whom fluid and electrolyte disturbances or nutritional deficiency from intractable vomiting develops early in pregnancy. This condition is much less common with an average incidence of 3.5/1000 deliveries[168] and usually requires hospital admission.

The severity of nausea and vomiting varies greatly among pregnant women. The majority of women with nausea and vomiting report symptoms within 8 weeks of their last menstrual period (94%), with over one-third of women (34%) reporting symptoms within 4 weeks of their last menstrual period.[166,167] [Evidence level 3] Most women (87–91%) report cessation of symptoms by 16–20 weeks of gestation and only 11–18% of women report having nausea and vomiting confined to the mornings.[166,167] [Evidence level 3]

One systematic review of observational studies found a reduced risk associated with nausea and vomiting and miscarriage (OR 0.36, 95% CI 0.32 to 0.42) and conflicting data regarding reduced risk for perinatal mortality.[165] [Evidence level 3] No association with nausea and vomiting and teratogenicity has been reported.[169] [Evidence level 3]

Despite reassurance that nausea and vomiting does not have harmful effects on pregnancy outcomes, nausea and vomiting can severely impact on a pregnant woman's quality of life. Two observational studies have reported on the detrimental impact that nausea and vomiting may have on day-to-day activities, including interfering with household activities, restricting interaction with children, greater use of healthcare resources and time lost off work.[170,171] [Evidence level 3]

Interventions for nausea and vomiting that do not require prescription include ginger, acupressure and vitamin B. Prescribed treatments for nausea and vomiting include antihistamines and phenothiazines.

Ginger

One RCT of ginger treatment (250 mg four times daily) compared with placebo reported a significant reduction in the severity of nausea and vomiting (p = 0.014) and a reduction in episodes of vomiting (p = 0.021) after four days in the treatment group.[172] [Evidence level 1b] No difference in the rates of miscarriage, caesarean section or congenital anomalies was observed between the two groups.

Two systematic reviews on various treatments for nausea and vomiting in pregnancy reported on the results of one RCT of ginger which was a double-blind, placebo-controlled crossover trial of 27 women who were hospitalised for hyperemesis and used ginger (250 mg four times daily).[173,174] [Evidence level 1b] Both the degree of nausea and number of attacks of vomiting were reduced with the ginger treatment (p = 0.035).[174] [Evidence level 1b]

Another RCT assessed ginger syrup to alleviate nausea and vomiting in pregnancy.[175] The intervention included 1 tablespoon of ginger syrup or placebo in 4 to 8 fluid ounces of water four times daily. Higher improvement on a nausea scale was observed by women in the ginger group and vomiting resolved in 67% of the women in this group by day 6 compared with only 20% in the control group. [Evidence level 1b]

P6 acupressure

The P6 point (Neiguan) point is located on the volar surface of the forearm approximately three fingerbreadths proximal to the wrist.

Three systematic reviews of RCTs on P6 acupressure for the relief of nausea and vomiting were found.[173,174,176] [Evidence level 1a] The reviews used different inclusion criteria and each included four or more of seven RCTs. Six out of the seven trials showed a positive effect for stimulation of the P6 pressure point. The seventh trial (n = 161) showed no difference between acupressure and sham acupressure or no treatment.[174,176] [Evidence level 1a] This trial did not present its data in a form that could be included in a meta-analysis.[173] [Evidence level 1a]

The review that excluded three of the seven trials did so because they were of crossover design without separate results from the first crossover period being available. A meta-analysis of dichotomised data from two of the trials reported evidence of benefit (Peto OR 0.35, 95% CI 0.23 to 0.54) but the continuous data from a third trial did not (in contrast to the finding in the reviews above).

More recent RCTs have also reported a reduction in symptoms of nausea and vomiting among women with acupressure wristbands compared with women with dummy bands or no treatment at all.[177–180] [Evidence level 1b] A possible placebo effect with sham acupressure was also reported in two of the studies.[178,180]

The risk of adverse effects of acupressure on pregnancy outcome was assessed in one RCT.[181] No differences in perinatal outcome, congenital abnormalities, pregnancy complications and other infant outcomes were found between the acupressure, sham acupressure or no treatment. [Evidence level 1b]

Antihistamines (promethazine, prochlorperazine, metoclopramide)

In a meta-analysis of 12 RCTs that included a comparison of antiemetics (antihistamines ± pyridoxine) with placebo or no treatment, there was a significant reduction in nausea in the treated group (Peto OR 0.17, 95% CI 0.13 to 0.21).[173] [Evidence level 1a] Although the results suggest an increase in drowsiness associated with antihistamines (Peto OR 2.19, 95% CI 1.09 to 4.37),[173] a review of the safety of antihistamines in relation to teratogenicity found no significant increased risk (24 studies, n > 200,000; OR 0.76, 95% CI 0.60 to 0.94).[182] [Evidence level 2a] Metoclopramide, however, has insufficient data on safety to be recommended as a first-line agent, though no evidence of association with malformations has been reported.[183]

Phenothiazines

One systematic review of three RCTs (n = 389 women) found that phenothiazines reduced nausea or vomiting when compared with placebo (RR 0.31, 95% CI 0.24 to 0.42).[182] [Evidence level 1a] However, this analysis included different phenothiazines as a group and one of the RCTs recruited women after the first trimester. The bulk of evidence demonstrates no association between teratogenicity and phenothiazines (nine studies, n = 2948; RR 1.03, 95% CI 0.88 to 1.22).[171,182] [Evidence level 2a & 3]

Pyridoxine (vitamin B6)

RCTs in the two reviews that studied pyridoxine considered doses of 25–75 mg up to three times daily.[173,174] [Evidence level 1a] Although the review suggests a reduction in nausea, it was not effective in reducing vomiting (Peto OR 0.91, 95% CI 0.60 to 1.38). Although concerns about possible toxicity at high doses have not yet been resolved and it is not recommended for use, one cohort study found no association between pyridoxine and major malformations (n = 1369, RR 1.05, 95% CI 0.60 to 1.84).[182] [Evidence level 2a] The Committee on Toxicity of Foods has recommended a safe upper limit of 10 milligrams a day for pyridoxine in the UK.

Cyanocobalamin (vitamin B12)

Two RCTs assessed the effect of cyanocobalamin (one trial gave multivitamins containing cyanocobalamin) compared with placebo and found a significant reduction in nausea and vomiting (pooled RR 0.49, 95% CI 0.28 to 0.86).[182] [Evidence level 1a] No studies assessing the safety of cyanocobalamin were located but this vitamin is thought to play a role in inhibiting malformations associated with neural tube defects.

Summary

Ginger, P6 acupressure and medication with antihistamines reduce the frequency of nausea in early pregnancy. Pyridoxine (vitamin B6) also appears to be effective, although concerns about the toxicity of vitamin B6 remain. Cyanocobalamin (vitamin B12) is also effective in reducing nausea and vomiting, although no data on its safety were located.

Most cases of nausea and vomiting resolve within 16 to 20 weeks with no harm to the pregnancy, prescribed treatment in the first trimester is usually not indicated unless the symptoms are severe and debilitating.[77]

RECOMMENDATIONS

Women should be informed that most cases of nausea and vomiting in pregnancy will resolve spontaneously within 16 to 20 weeks of gestation and that nausea and vomiting are not usually associated with a poor pregnancy outcome. If a woman requests or would like to consider treatment, the following interventions appear to be effective in reducing symptoms [A]:

- nonpharmacological:
  - ginger
  - P6 acupressure
- pharmacological:
  - antihistamines

Information about all forms of self-help and nonpharmacological treatments should be made available for pregnant women who have nausea and vomiting. [Good practice point]

Future research

More information on maternal and fetal safety for all interventions for nausea and vomiting in pregnancy (except antihistamines) is needed.

Further research into other nonpharmacological treatments for nausea and vomiting in pregnancy is recommended.

6.2   Heartburn

Heartburn is described as a burning sensation or discomfort felt behind the sternum or throat or both. It may be accompanied by acid regurgitation reaching the throat or the mouth, causing a bitter or sour taste in the mouth. The pathogenesis of heartburn during pregnancy is unclear but may be the consequence of the altered hormonal status interfering with gastric motility, resulting in gastro-oesophageal reflux. It is not associated with adverse outcomes of pregnancy and therefore its treatment is intended to provide relief of symptoms rather than to prevent harm to the fetus or mother. Heartburn should be distinguished from epigastric pain associated with pre-eclampsia. This may be done by checking the woman's blood pressure and urine for proteinuria.

Heartburn is a frequent complaint during pregnancy. One large study involving 607 pregnant women reported an increased frequency of heartburn with gestation, with 22% of women reporting heartburn in the first trimester, 39% in second and 72% in third trimester.[184] [Evidence level 3] Another study reported a weekly prevalence of 60% from the 31st week of gestation until delivery.[185] [Evidence level 3] An English study that separated white Europeans from Asian women reported a slightly higher prevalence of 76–87% for white Europeans and 78–81% for Asians.[186] [Evidence level 3]

Treatment options for heartburn include lifestyle modification, use of antacids or alkali mixtures, H_2 receptor antagonists and proton pump inhibitors, which aim to alleviate symptoms by reducing the acid reflux.

Information on lifestyle modification includes awareness of posture, maintaining upright positions, especially after meals, sleeping in a propped up position and dietary modifications such as small frequent meals, reduction of high-fat foods and gastric irritants such as caffeine. Antacids, which neutralise and bind bile acids, may also be considered for the relief of heartburn. An RCT of antacid treatment compared with placebo found that 80% of women reported relief of heartburn pain within one hour compared with 13% from the placebo group.[187] [Evidence level 1b]

Alginate preparations, such as Gaviscon® (Reckitt & Coleman), reduce reflux by inhibiting the regurgitation of gastric contents. One RCT compared alginate with magnesium trisilicate and both were found to relieve symptoms of heartburn and no differences in the effects of each treatment were reported.[188] [Evidence level 1b] The manufacturers of Gaviscon® state that it may be taken during pregnancy.[189]

Another RCT compared acid and alkali mixtures with placebo and reported that there was no difference in relief of heartburn symptoms when women were given either the acid or alkali mixtures but better relief was achieved using these rather than using a placebo.[190] [Evidence level 1b]

H_2 receptor antagonists or blockers, which reduce acid secretion and volume, have also been reported to treat heartburn effectively and safely in pregnant women. Two trials that investigated the effect of ranitidine, an H^2 receptor blocker, given once and twice daily, compared with a placebo found that there was a significant improvement in heartburn symptoms, especially when ranitidine was taken twice daily, morning and afternoon.[191,192] [Evidence level 1b] H_2 blockers in the first trimester have also been assessed for safety in a cohort of 178 women and no association with fetal malformations was found.[193] [Evidence level 2a] Nevertheless, the manufacturers of ranitidine and cimetidine advise the avoidance of these products unless essential.[77]

A meta-analysis (five cohort studies, n = 593 infants) of the safety of proton pump inhibitors such as omeprazole, which suppress gastric acid secretion also reported no association between exposure to proton pump inhibitors and fetal malformations.[194] [Evidence level 2a] However, the manufacturer of omeprazole advises caution with its use in pregnancy due to toxicity shown in animal studies and does not advise its use unless there is no alternative.[77,189]

RECOMMENDATIONS

Women who present with symptoms of heartburn in pregnancy should be offered information regarding lifestyle and diet modification. [Good practice point]

Antacids may be offered to women whose heartburn remains troublesome despite lifestyle and diet modification. [A]

6.3 Constipation

Constipation is the delay in the passage of food residue, associated with painful defecation and abdominal discomfort. Constipation during pregnancy may not only be associated with poor dietary fibre intake but also with rising levels of progesterone causing a reduction in gastric motility and increased gastric transit time.

It is a commonly reported condition during pregnancy that appears to decrease with gestation. One study found that 39% of pregnant women reported symptoms of constipation at 14 weeks of gestation, 30% at 28 weeks and 20% at 36 weeks.[195] [Evidence level 3] The results of this study, however, may be over-estimates, as routine iron supplementation was recommended for all pregnant women in the UK at the time the study was conducted and iron consumption is associated with constipation.

One systematic review of two RCTs (n = 215) randomised women to fibre supplements or nothing.[196] Wheat or bran fibre supplements were significantly more effective in increasing stool frequency (Peto OR 0.18, 95% CI 0.05 to 0.67). When discomfort was not alleviated by fibre supplementation, stimulant laxatives were more effective than bulk-forming laxatives (Peto OR 0.30, 95% CI 0.14 to 0.61). However, significantly more abdominal pain and diarrhoea was observed when stimulants were used and no differences in nausea were reported. [Evidence level 1a]

No evidence was found for the effectiveness or safety of osmotic laxatives (e.g. lactulose) or softeners for use in pregnancy.

RECOMMENDATION

Women who present with constipation in pregnancy should be offered information regarding diet modification, such as bran or wheat fibre supplementation. [A]

6.4 Haemorrhoids

Haemorrhoids are swollen veins around the anus that are characterised by anorectal bleeding, anal pain and anal itching. This is thought to be a result of the prolapse of the anal canal cushions, which play a role in maintaining continence. A low-fibre diet and pregnancy are both precipitating factors for haemorrhoids.

One recent observational study found that 8% of pregnant women experienced haemorrhoidal disease in the last three months of pregnancy.[197] [Evidence level 3]

Treatment for haemorrhoids includes diet modification, creams (such as Anusol-HC®, Kestrel, Anacal®, Sankyo Pharma) oral medication and surgical intervention.

No evidence for the effectiveness or safety of creams used in pregnancy was found. However, the manufacturers of Anusol-HC® and Anacal® state that, "no epidemiological evidence of adverse effects to the pregnant mother or fetus" has been reported.[189]

One RCT of oral medication or placebo for pregnant women with haemorrhoids found that 84% of women in the treatment group reported an improvement in symptoms compared with 12% in the placebo group, after two weeks. No significant differences in side effects or fetal outcome were reported.[198] [Evidence level 1b]

In another study of oral flavonoid therapy, 50 pregnant women were treated over three phases.[199] The majority of women reported an improvement in symptoms (bleeding, pain, rectal exudation and rectal discomfort) after 7 days, the first phase of treatment. Six women complained of nausea and vomiting, which resolved over the course of treatment. [Evidence level 3]

In extreme circumstances, surgical removal of haemorrhoids has been used. In a study where closed haemorrhoidectomy, under local anaesthesia, was performed on 25 women with thrombosed or gangrenous haemorrhoids in the third trimester, 24 women reported immediate pain relief with no resultant fetal complications related to the surgery.[200] [Evidence level 3] Surgery is rarely considered an appropriate intervention for the pregnant woman since haemorrhoids may resolve after delivery.

RECOMMENDATION

In the absence of evidence for the effectiveness of treatments for haemorrhoids in pregnancy, women should be offered information concerning diet modification. If clinical symptoms remain troublesome, standard haemorrhoid creams should be considered. [Good practice point]

6.5 Varicose veins

Varicose veins are caused by the pooling of blood in the surface veins as a result of inefficient valves that would normally prevent blood draining back down the leg. They can occur as blue swollen veins on the calves and inside of the legs, and cause itching and general discomfort. Feet and ankles can also become swollen. They are a common complaint in pregnancy.

One systematic review addressed this issue.[119] Three RCTs of three different treatments in 115 women were included. One RCT investigated external pneumatic intermittent compression and another RCT investigated immersion in water and bed rest in pregnant women with leg oedema. The outcomes studied (leg volume, diuresis, blood pressure) did not appear to be important for the women themselves. In addition, only effects immediately after treatment were studied. The third trial administered rutoside capsules or placebo for 8 weeks in the third trimester, which led to a subjective improvement of symptoms at 36 weeks of gestation (Peto OR 0.30 95% CI 0.12 to 0.77). However, no data were provided on the safety or side effects of the administration of rutosides at this stage of pregnancy.

An RCT published after this review was also located.[201] The efficacy of compression stockings (compression class I and compression class II) in preventing emergent varicose veins during pregnancy was compared with no stockings among 42 women at less then 12 weeks of gestation. Both classes of compression stockings failed to prevent the emergence of varicose veins but more treated women reported improved leg symptoms (p = 0.045). [Evidence level 1b]

RECOMMENDATION

Women should be informed that varicose veins are a common symptom of pregnancy that will not cause harm and that compression stockings can improve the symptoms but will not prevent varicose veins from emerging. [A]

6.6 Vaginal discharge

The quality and quantity of vaginal discharge often changes in pregnancy. Women usually produce more discharge during pregnancy. If the discharge has a strong or unpleasant odour, is associated with itch or soreness or associated with pain on passing urine, the woman may have bacterial vaginosis (see Section 10.2), vaginal trichomoniasis or candidiasis. However, vaginal discharge may also be caused by a range of other physiological or pathological conditions such as vulval dermatoses or allergic reactions.

Trichomoniasis, infection with the parasitic protozoan *Trichomonas vaginalis*, is characterised by green-yellow frothy discharge from the vagina and pain upon urination and is one of the most commonly sexually transmitted infections. A systematic review of RCTs assessed the effects of trichomoniasis and its treatment during pregnancy.[202] Two RCTs were located. Both trials used metronidazole as the treatment intervention. However, the dose used in one trial (2 g, 48 hours apart and repeated after 2 weeks), conducted in the USA, was double the dose used in the other trial, which was conducted in South Africa. Both studies demonstrated high rates of cure (two RCTs, n = 703, RR 0.11, 95% CI 0.08 to 0.17) but a higher risk for preterm birth was observed in the treatment group in the US study when compared with the placebo group (RR 1.78, 95% CI 1.19 to 2.66). No significant differences in low birthweight were observed between the two groups in either trial and the South African study also reported no differences in mean birthweight or gestational age when compared with the control group, who received no treatment. Therefore, although trichomoniasis is associated with adverse pregnancy outcomes,[203] the effect of metronidazole for its treatment during pregnancy remains unclear. [Evidence level 1a]

There is no evidence that vaginal candidiasis (also called thrush), which is caused by the yeast *Candida albicans*, harms the unborn child. One systematic review of ten RCTs assessed the effectiveness of topical treatments for vaginal candidiasis in pregnant women.[204] Meta-analysis showed that imidazoles (miconazole cream and clotrimazole pessaries) were more effective than nystatin pessaries or placebo for symptomatic relief and resolution of persistent candidiasis (five RCTs, n = 793, Peto OR 0.21, 95%I 0.16 to 0.29 for nystatin pessaries; one RCT, n = 100, Peto OR 0.14, 95% CI 0.06 to 0.31 for placebo). Two RCTs (n = 91) also demonstrated that treatment with miconazole or econazole for 1 week was just as effective as treatment for 2 weeks (Peto OR 0.41, 95% CI 0.16 to 1.05). However, treatment for 4 days was not as effective as treatment for 1 week (two RCTs, n = 81, Peto OR 11.07, 95% CI 4.21 to 29.15). One RCT (n = 38) found that terconazole cream was as effective as clotrimazole cream for treatment of vaginal candidiasis (Peto OR 1.41, 95% CI 0.28 to 7.10). [Evidence level 1a]

Although one-dose oral treatments for the treatment of vaginal candidiasis are now available, their safety or efficacy in pregnancy has not yet been evaluated.

RECOMMENDATIONS

Women should be informed that an increase in vaginal discharge is a common physiological change that occurs during pregnancy. If this is associated with itch, soreness, offensive smell or pain on passing urine, there maybe an infective cause and investigation should be considered. [Good practice point]

A 1-week course of a topical imidazole is an effective treatment and should be considered for vaginal candidiasis in pregnant women. [A]

The effectiveness and safety of oral treatments for vaginal candidiasis in pregnancy is uncertain and these should not be offered. [Good practice point]

6.7 Backache

The definition of back pain or back discomfort during pregnancy is subjective, due to the nature of this discomfort. The estimated prevalence of backache during pregnancy ranges between 35% and 61%.[205–210] Among these women, 47–60% reported backache first developing during the 5th to 7th months of pregnancy. It was also reported that the symptoms of backache were worse in the evenings. [Evidence level 3]

Back pain during pregnancy has been attributed to an altered posture due to the increasing weight in the womb and increased laxity of supporting muscles, as a result of the hormone relaxin. Back pain during pregnancy is potentially debilitating, since it can interfere with a woman's daily activities and sleep patterns, particularly during the third trimester.

A systematic review assessed three RCTs to identify the most appropriate interventions for the prevention and treatment of back pain in pregnancy.[211] The three RCTs investigated three types of interventions: water gymnastics compared with no intervention, Ozzlo pillows compared with standard pillows, and acupuncture compared with physiotherapy. [Evidence level 1a] Women who participated in water gymnastics took less sick leave when compared with women who had no specific intervention (OR 0.38, 95% CI 0.16, 0.88). In the second trial, Ozzlo pillows, which are hollowed out nest-shaped pillows, were more effective in relieving back pain and improving sleep for women at more than 36 weeks of gestation compared with a standard pillow (OR 0.32, 95% CI 0.18 to 0.58 for backache relief; OR 0.35, 95% CI 0.20 to 0.62 for sleep). In the third RCT, ten acupuncture sessions were rated more helpful when compared with ten group physiotherapy sessions in pregnant women who developed back pain before 32 weeks of pregnancy (OR 6.58, 95% CI 1.00 to 43.16).

Two additional studies not included in the systematic review were identified. One RCT compared the effect of massage therapy with relaxation classes and found that back pain relief scores diminished significantly with the women who had received massage therapy when compared with the women in the relaxation group (n = 26 women, p < 0.01)[212] [Evidence level 1b]

The other study, which was excluded from the systematic review because it was quasi-randomised, was conducted in Sweden and compared three management options for backache. These were: group back-care classes, individual back-care classes and routine antenatal care (control).[213] Women who received either individual or group back-care classes reported an improvement in pelvic or back pain compared with the control group (n = 407, p < 0.05). Women who received individual classes also reported a significant improvement in pain relief while those in the control group and those receiving group sessions did not report any pain relief. The group receiving individual training also reported significantly less sick leave (p < 0.05) than those in the control group and those who had group training. [Evidence level 1b]

Another Swedish study compared the effects of a physiotherapy programme (five visits for teaching on anatomy, posture, vocational ergonomics, gymnastics and relaxation) and an exercise programme compared with no specific intervention on 135 pregnant women with backache.[214] This cohort study found a significantly reduced number of sick leave days taken during pregnancy by an average of 24 days per woman (p < 0.001). [Evidence level 2a]

Other interventions identified for the treatment of backache and reported to have a beneficial effect were autotraction, a chiropractic, mechanical treatment for back pain,[215] spinal manipulative therapy,[216] rotational mobilisation exercise[217] and manual joint mobilisation applied to symptomatic vertebral segments.[218] [Evidence level 3] However, all these studies had problems with study design or the data were derived from a small sample size.

RECOMMENDATION

Women should be informed that exercising in water, massage therapy and group or individual back care classes might help to ease backache during pregnancy. [A]

Future research

Although many treatments exist for backache in pregnancy, there is a lack of research evaluating their safety and effectiveness.

6.8 Symphysis pubis dysfunction

Symphysis pubis dysfunction has been described as a collection of signs and symptoms of discomfort and pain in the pelvic area, including pelvic pain radiating to the upper thighs and perineum. Complaints vary from mild discomfort to severe and debilitating pain that can impede mobility.

The reported incidence of symphysis pubis during pregnancy varies in the literature from 0.03% to 3%. In Leeds, a hospital survey of women (n = 248) in whom a diagnosis of symphysis pubis dysfunction had been made, estimated that 1/36 deliveries were associated with symphysis pubis dysfunction either during pregnancy or soon after delivery.[219] Among the respondents (57% response rate), 9% reported that symptoms first occurred in the first trimester, 44% reported symptoms in the second trimester, 45% in the third trimester and 2% during labour or the postnatal period. [Evidence level 3]

There is little evidence in the literature on which to base clinical practice. No higher levels of evidence than case reports were located on effective therapies for symphysis pubis dysfunction, although the use of elbow crutches, pelvic support and prescribed pain relief have been suggested.[220] [Evidence level 4] It is important to remember that many medications for pain relief for bones and joints may not be appropriate for use in pregnancy.

Future research

More research on effective treatments for symphysis pubis dysfunction is needed.

6.9 Carpal tunnel syndrome

Carpal tunnel syndrome results from compression of the median nerve within the carpal tunnel in the hand. It is characterised by tingling, burning pain, numbness and a swelling sensation in the hand that may impair sensory and motor function of the hand.

Carpal tunnel syndrome is not an uncommon complaint among pregnant women and estimates of incidence during pregnancy range from 21% to 62%.[221–223] [Evidence level 3]

Interventions to treat carpal tunnel syndrome include wrist splints[224,225] and wrist splints plus injections of corticosteroid and analgesia.[226] However, case series reports were the highest level of evidence identified that evaluated these therapies and the studies were not of good quality.

Future research

There is a lack of research evaluating effective interventions for carpal tunnel syndrome.

7. Clinical examination of pregnant women

7.1   Measurement of weight and body mass index

A retrospective study of 1092 pregnant women found that, after taking into account maternal gestation, age and smoking habit, weekly weight gain and maternal weight at booking were the only factors that had an association with infant birthweight.[227] Low maternal booking weight (< 51 kg) was the most effective for antenatal detection of small-for-gestational-age infants (positive predictive value 20%). Low average weekly maternal weight gain (< 0.20 kg) had a positive predictive value of 13% for detecting small-for-gestational-age infants (lower than the PPV of 16% for maternal smoking). Weight loss or failure to gain weight over a two-week interval in the third trimester was observed in 46% of all women studied.

The normal range of weight gain during pregnancy varies for each pregnant individual. Based on observational data, total weight gain ranges for healthy pregnant women giving birth to babies between three and four kilograms are between 7 and 18 kg.[228] A prospective observational study of 7589 women in their first pregnancy examined the differences in pattern of weight gain according to trimester for women who delivered at term versus preterm.[229] Women who delivered preterm had patterns of weight gain similar to women delivering at term. Underweight status (BMI < 19.8 kg/m^2) before pregnancy increased the likelihood of delivering preterm (adjusted OR 1.98, 95% CI 1.33 to 2.98). Inadequate weight gain in the third trimester (defined as < 0.34, 0.35, 0.30 and 0.30 kg/week for underweight, normal weight, overweight and obese women, respectively) increased the risk by a similar magnitude (adjusted OR 1.91, 95% CI 1.40 to 2.61).

Body mass index (BMI) is calculated by taking a person's weight in kilograms (1 kg = 2.2 lb) and dividing it by the square of their height (weight [kg]/height[m^2], 1 in = 2.5 cm). A longitudinal study of 156 healthy pregnant women investigated whether BMI was related to energy intake during pregnancy and whether BMI, energy intake and other factors were related to net weight gain.[230] Women at the highest level of BMI were significantly less often in the high-energy intake category than women at the medium or low level of BMI. Net weight gain during pregnancy was independently influenced by BMI status and energy intake. Women at the highest level of BMI gained significantly less weight from first to third trimester compared with women at the medium or low levels of BMI. The mean birth weight in the three BMI groups did not differ and was not influenced by age, marital status, education, parity or smoking.

Routine weighing to monitor the nutrition of all pregnant women was begun in antenatal clinics in London in 1941.[227] There is a correlation between maternal weight gain and infant birthweight but this is not effective for screening for small size (low birthweight) babies. It is still important to measure maternal weight and height at least once; for example, at first contact, in order to document weight and height distributions in various subgroups of the clinic population. However, measuring maternal weight (or height) routinely during pregnancy should be abandoned as it may produce unnecessary anxiety with no added benefit. The exception is pregnant women in whom nutrition is of concern.

RECOMMENDATIONS

Maternal weight and height should be measured at the first antenatal appointment, and the woman's BMI calculated (weight [kg]/height[m]^2). [B]

Repeated weighing during pregnancy should be confined to circumstances where clinical management is likely to be influenced. [C]

7.2 Breast examination

Breast examination at the first antenatal appointment was traditionally used to determine whether any problems with breastfeeding could be anticipated. In particular, women were examined for the presence of flat or inverted nipples as potential obstacles to breastfeeding so that breast shields or nipple exercises could be prescribed to remedy the situation. However, an RCT examining the effectiveness of breast shields versus no breast shields or nipple exercises (Hoffman's exercises) versus no exercises found that the presence of flat or inverted nipples did not mean that women could not successfully breastfeed.[231] In fact, breast shells reduced the chances of successful breastfeeding and no differences in breastfeeding were found between the two exercise groups. [Evidence level 1b]

RECOMMENDATION

Routine breast examination during antenatal care is not recommended for the promotion of postnatal breastfeeding. [A]

7.3 Pelvic examination

Pelvic examination during pregnancy is used to detect a number of clinical conditions such as anatomical abnormalities and sexually transmitted infections, to evaluate the size of a woman's pelvis (pelvimetry) and to assess the uterine cervix so as to be able to detect signs of cervical incompetence (associated with recurrent mid-trimester miscarriages) or to predict preterm labour (see Section 11.3).

Pelvimetry has been used to predict the need for caesarean section in pregnant women. A systematic review of four RCTs (n = 895) assessed the effects of pelvimetry (x-ray) on method of delivery.[232] Women on whom pelvimetry was performed were more likely to be delivered by caesarean section (Peto OR 2.17, 95% CI 1.63 to 2.88). No differences in the perinatal mortality were found, but the numbers were not large enough to assess this adequately. There were also no differences in asphyxia, admission to neonatal unit, scar dehiscence or blood transfusion reported between the two groups. Although the risk of caesarean section was increased, no increased benefit of pelvimetry to the pregnant woman, fetus or neonate was found.

In an RCT that assessed the relationship between antenatal pelvic examinations and premature rupture of the membranes (PROM), 175 women were assigned to no examinations and 174 women were assigned to routine digital pelvic examinations commencing at 37 weeks and continuing until delivery.[233] In the group of women who had no pelvic examination, ten women developed PROM (6%) compared with 32 women (18%) from the group of women who were examined weekly. This three-fold increase in the occurrence of PROM among women who had pelvic examinations was significant (p = 0.001). [Evidence level 1b]

With regard to ovarian cysts, the majority are benign and ovarian cancer is rare in pregnancy: 1/15,000 to 1/32,000 pregnancies.[234] [Evidence level 3] A study that retrospectively reviewed 11,622 antenatal records found 16 cysts, 14 of which were later detected also at ultrasound examination.[235] In total, 57 ovarian cysts were detected, but 40 were detected only by ultrasound scan. [Evidence level 3]

RECOMMENDATION

Routine antenatal pelvic examination does not accurately assess gestational age, nor does it accurately predict preterm birth or cephalopelvic disproportion. It is not recommended. [B]

7.4 Female genital mutilation

WHO defines female genital mutilation as, "all procedures that involve partial or total removal of the female external genitalia or other injury to the female genital organs whether for cultural, religious or other non-therapeutic reasons".[236] It is further classified as follows:

Type I   Excision of the prepuce with or without excision of part or all of the clitoris

Type II   Excision of the prepuce and clitoris, together with partial or total excision of the labia minora

Type III Excision of part or all of the external genitalia and stitching/narrowing of the vaginal opening (infibulation)

Type IV   Unclassified: pricking, piercing or incision of the clitoris or labia; stretching of the clitoris or labia; cauterisation by burning of the clitoris and surrounding tissues; scraping (angury cuts) of the vaginal orifice or cutting (gishiri cuts) of the vagina; introduction of corrosive substances into the vagina to cause bleeding or herbs into the vagina with the aim of tightening or narrowing the vagina; any other procedure that falls under the definition of female genital mutilation given above.

Most of the girls and women who have undergone female genital mutilation live in 28 African countries, although some live in Asia and the Middle East. Prevalence rates at or above 90% are found in Djibouti, Guinea and Somalia, Eritrea, Mali, Sierra Leone and Sudan.[237] They are also increasingly found in Europe, Australia, Canada and the USA, primarily among immigrants from the above countries.[236]

The total number of girls and women who have undergone female genital mutilation, which is also often referred to as 'female circumcision', is estimated to be between 100 and 140 million. Each year, an estimated additional 2 million girls are at risk of undergoing genital mutilation.[236] An estimated 10,000 to 20,000 girls in the UK are thought to have undergone genital mutilation[238] and information on its prevalence among pregnant women in the UK was not located.

Ninety-four percent of referral to specialist African well-woman clinics in the UK is through midwives.[238] Twenty percent of women attending an African well-woman clinic had previously informed their GP that they had undergone genital mutilation because of underlying medical problems. However, it was also reported that some women did not want their GP to know that they had undergone this procedure.[238] In a study of women attending an African well-woman clinic, among pregnant women who required defibulation and were offered it antenatally, 8% (3 out of 39) agreed to the procedure. The rest preferred to be defibulated during the second stage of labour because they would "rather go through a painful procedure once".[238]

The reduced vaginal opening affects not only delivery but appears to be the main factor responsible for other obstetric problems caused by genital mutilation, making antenatal assessment, intrapartum vaginal examination or catheterisation difficult or impossible. Inadequate assessments at these times as a result of genital mutilation may compromise mother and fetus physically.[239]

Female genital mutilation type III causes a direct mechanical barrier to delivery; types I, II and IV can produce severe, although perhaps unintentional vulval and vaginal scarring that can act as an obstruction to delivery.[239] In 20 studies (one from the UK and one from the USA), where 75 cases are described, with primary data on second-stage labour, obstruction is described relating to soft-tissue dystocia and many cases of such obstruction are described as being easily overcome by episiotomies.[239]

In a series of African women with genital mutilation in Middlesex, of the 14 primigravid patients, seven had a pinhole introitus or an introitus that would require defibulation for adequate intrapartum care. In all 23 parous women, the introitus was perceived to be adequate for vaginal examination in labour; 13/14 primigravid women had normal vaginal deliveries, although all 13 had episiotomies or perinatal lacerations; 1/14 primigravid women had a caesarean section for obstetric reasons unrelated to the fact that she was infibulated; 14/23 parous women had a normal vaginal delivery, 3/23 had instrumental deliveries and 6/23 were delivered by caesarean section.[240]

Episiotomies and perineal tears are the most common complications reported, with a statistically significant increased episiotomy seen in nulliparous women with female genital mutilation compared with women with no genital mutilation (89% versus 54%).[239] There is also evidence for increased fetal distress and higher Apgar scores among women with female genital mutilation compared with women with no genital mutilation.[239] Evidence that genital mutilation leads to a higher incidence of postpartum haemorrhage, maternal death, fetal death, postpartum genital wound infection and fistulae formulation has also been reported.[239]

In 1985, the UK Parliament passed the Prohibition of Female Circumcision Act, which made female genital mutilation an illegal act punishable by a fine or imprisonment. This includes the repair of the vulva of a woman who has delivered a baby vaginally; i.e., this Act makes it illegal to repair the labia in a way that makes intercourse difficult or impossible.[241]

The management of birth in women with female genital mutilation will be covered more comprehensively in the Intrapartum Care Guideline.

RECOMMENDATION

Pregnant women who have had female genital mutilation should be identified early in antenatal care through sensitive enquiry. Antenatal examination will then allow planning of intrapartum care. [C]

7.5   Domestic violence

Domestic violence has been defined as "Physical, sexual or emotional violence from an adult perpetrator directed towards an adult victim in the context of a close relationship".[242] Surveys suggest a lifetime prevalence of domestic violence against women of between 25% and 30%, with an annual prevalence of 2% to 12%.[243–246] [Evidence level 3] Variability in these estimates has been attributed in part to differences in the definitions used.

Pregnancy is a time when abuse may start or escalate.[242,247] In pregnancy, the prevalence of domestic violence has been shown to be as high as 17% in England.[248] [Evidence level 3]. In the last Confidential Enquiries into Maternal Deaths for the triennia 1997–1999, eight deaths were due to domestic violence.[143] [Evidence level 3]

Women who experience domestic violence are at increased risk of injury and death, as well as physical, emotional and social problems. During pregnancy, domestic violence can result in direct harm to the pregnancy, such as preterm birth,[249–251] antepartum haemorrhage,[252] and perinatal death,[252] [Evidence level 3] and also indirect harm through a woman's inability to access antenatal care. As such, domestic violence is a major public health problem and priority. Several professional and governmental bodies recommend 'routine enquiry' about domestic violence for all women; for example, the British Medical Association,[242] the Royal College of Midwives,[253] the Royal College of Obstetricians and Gynaecologists[247] and the Royal College of Psychiatrists[254].

Two systematic reviews have been published evaluating screening for domestic violence: the availability of screening tools, the acceptability of screening to women and healthcare professionals and the effectiveness of interventions in improving health outcomes for women.[255,256] [Evidence level 2] Both reviews identified valid screening tools for domestic violence. Screening with a single question was as effective as screening with multiple questions. Screening is likely to increase the number of women identified as experiencing domestic violence. Both reviews reported that screening was acceptable to the majority of women but that acceptance among health professionals was lower. A UK survey of the levels of detection, knowledge and attitudes of healthcare workers to domestic violence found that knowledge about domestic violence as a healthcare issue was poor and that this sometimes resulted in inappropriate referrals to agencies.[257]

Both reviews highlighted that there is insufficient evidence for the effectiveness of intervention in healthcare settings for women identified by screening programmes. Interventions evaluated in these studies included women staying at a shelter, counselling for women, and interventions for the male partner or couple such as counselling. Three of the studies included pregnant women. Both reviews identified the studies as of poorer quality and note that 'surrogate' outcomes rather than substantive health outcomes have been used.

There is a need for additional research to test the effectiveness of interventions on improving health outcomes before recommending routine screening. Healthcare professionals need to be alert to the possibility of domestic violence in women with symptoms or signs of domestic violence.

Further information on domestic violence is offered in the Department of Health publication, *Domestic violence: a resource manual for health care professionals.*[258]

RECOMMENDATION

Healthcare professionals need to be alert to the symptoms or signs of domestic violence and women should be given the opportunity to disclose domestic violence in an environment in which they feel secure. [D]

Future research

Although there are effective screening tools and screening for domestic violence has been shown to be acceptable to women, there is insufficient evidence on the effectiveness of interventions in improving health outcomes for women who have been identified. Therefore, evaluation of interventions for domestic violence is urgently needed.

7.6 Psychiatric screening

Depression in the childbearing years is a recognised problem, as are its associated effects on a child's behavioural and cognitive development. From 1997 to 1999, there were approximately 640,000 live births per year in England and Wales. In that same period, the Confidential Enquiries into Maternal Deaths in the UK[143] received reports of 11 deaths during pregnancy related to psychiatric causes. [Evidence level 3]

An association between antenatal and postnatal depression has been identified. In one systematic review,[259] a strong association between women experiencing antepartum depression and subsequently having postnatal depression was reported. [Evidence level 3] With regard to the effect of depression on obstetric complications, some investigators conclude that there is no relationship,[260] while others report an association between anxiety and depression with preterm labour (OR 2.1, 95% CI 1.1 to 4.1).[261] [Evidence level 3]

Babies of mothers who experience antenatal depression are also reported to have higher norepinephrine levels and demonstrate poorer performance on neonatal assessment tests (orientation, reflex, excitability) when compared with babies of mothers who do not experience antenatal depression.[262] [Evidence level 3]

While the Edinburgh Postnatal Depression Scale (EPDS) has been validated against a 30–60-minute semi-structured psychiatric interview as a tool for screening for antenatal depression.[263] No studies confirming the effective use of the EPDS as a screening tool in practice were located. [Evidence level 3] Using the EPDS to determine the incidence of antenatal depression, however, identified 24% of pregnant women in one survey as having clinically significant depression.[264] An association between depressive symptoms and socio-demographic status, e.g. no educational qualifications, unmarried, unemployed, was also reported. [Evidence level 3] In a cohort study that assessed mood during pregnancy and childbirth with the EPDS (n = 14,541 women), 13.5% of women scored for probable depression at 32 weeks of pregnancy while 9.1% scored for depression at 8 weeks postpartum.[265] [Evidence level 3]

An association between antenatal and postnatal depression has been reported in cohort and case–control studies[259] and numerous studies assessing antenatal prevention of postnatal depression have been conducted. Using antenatal screening as a predictor for postnatal depression, a systematic review of 16 studies found that the two largest studies predicted 16% and 52% of the women would develop postnatal depression but only 35% and 8% of women, respectively, actually developed depression after birth.[266] [Evidence level 3] In an RCT assessing the impact of an antenatal education programme on postnatal depression, no difference in reduction of depression scores was found between the intervention and control groups.[267] [Evidence level 1b]

In another RCT, the benefits of providing a 'preparing for parenthood' course versus routine antenatal care for the prevention of postnatal depression were investigated.[268] Among 209 women screened to be at risk of developing postnatal depression, no reduction in the rates of postnatal depression were observed when the intervention group was compared with the control group (OR 1.22, 95% CI 0.63 to 2.39). [Evidence level 1b] Thus, assessment of antenatal screening for the detection of postnatal depression has poor sensitivity and educational antenatal interventions do not appear to reduce postnatal depression.

However, while antenatal assessment for the detection of postnatal depression appears to have poor sensitivity in the general population, this is not the case among women with previous episodes of puerperal illness. Among these women, there is a 1/2 or 1/3 chance of recurrence and these are also the women who are at higher risk for suicide.[143] Therefore, sensitive questioning of pregnant women about previous or current mental illness is warranted for the identification of this subgroup of women. [Evidence level 3]

RECOMMENDATIONS

Women should be asked early in pregnancy if they have had any previous psychiatric illnesses. Women who have a past history of serious psychiatric disorder should be referred for a psychiatric assessment during the antenatal period. [B]

Pregnant women should not be offered routine screening, such as with the Edinburgh Postnatal Depression Scale, in the antenatal period to predict the development of postnatal depression. [A]

Pregnant women should not be offered antenatal education interventions to reduce perinatal or postnatal depression, as these interventions have not been shown to be effective. [A]

8 Screening for haematological conditions

8.1 Anaemia

The most common cause of anaemia in pregnancy worldwide is iron deficiency. Maternal iron requirements increase in pregnancy because of the requirements of the fetus and placenta and the increase in maternal red cell mass. Iron absorption increases to meet this increased demand. In normal pregnancy, maternal plasma volume increases by up to 50% and the red cell mass gradually increases by about 20%. Hence, the haemoglobin (Hb) concentration drops. This normal physiological response may resemble iron deficiency anaemia.[269]

The haemoglobin level, which defines anaemia, is controversial and lacks consistency across studies, although most studies report 11 g/dl to 12 g/dl to be the mean minimum haemoglobin concentration in pregnancy. Because haemoglobin levels vary depending upon the time of gestation, it is recommended that levels are checked against a gestation-sensitive threshold. In the UK, the normal range of haemoglobin in pregnant women up to 12 weeks should be at or above 11 g/dl and 10.5 g/dl at 28 to 30 weeks of gestation.[270]

Low haemoglobin values such as those between 8.5 g/dl and 10.5 g/dl may be associated with reduced risks of low birthweight and preterm labour.[271] [Evidence level 3] Increased risks of poor fetal outcome are associated with particularly low and very high levels of haemoglobin.[271,272] [Evidence level 3]

In order to correctly diagnose iron deficiency anaemia, the impact of gestational age on the change in plasma volume must be considered. Because of the diverse pathogenesis of anaemia (e.g., iron deficiency anaemia, thalassaemia, sickle cell anaemia) the use of haemoglobin as the sole means of diagnosing anaemia is not a sensitive test although this is often used as the first indicator in clinical practice. When there is a suspicion of iron deficiency, more sensitive and specific tests should be considered. Serum ferritin is the most sensitive single screening test to detect adequate iron stores. Using a cutoff of 30 micrograms/litre a sensitivity of 90% has been reported.[273]

Routine iron supplements for women with normal haemoglobin levels

A systematic review of 20 randomised controlled trials compared iron supplementation with either placebo or no iron in pregnant women with normal haemoglobin levels (> 10 g/dl) at less than 28 weeks of gestation.[76] [Evidence level 1a] Routine iron supplementation raised or maintained the serum ferritin level above 10 micrograms/litre (Peto OR 0.12, 95% CI 0.08 to 0.17) and resulted in a substantial reduction in women with a haemoglobin level below 10 g/dl or 10.5 g/dl in late pregnancy (Peto OR 0.15, 95% CI 0.11 to 0.20). There was no evidence of any beneficial or harmful effects on maternal or fetal outcomes. One trial of routine versus selective iron supplementation included in this review showed a reduced likelihood of caesarean section and postpartum blood transfusion, but there were more perinatal deaths in the routinely supplemented group.[76] [Evidence level 1b]

Another systematic review looked at the effects of routine iron and folate supplements on pregnant women with normal levels of haemoglobin.[74] [Evidence level 1a] Eight trials involving 5449 women were included. Routine supplementation with iron and folate raised or maintained the serum iron and ferritin levels and serum and red-cell folate levels. It also resulted in a substantial reduction of women with a haemoglobin level below 10 g/dl or 10.5 g/dl in late pregnancy (Peto OR 0.19, 95% CI 0.13 to 0.27). However, routine supplementation with iron and folate had no detectable effects, either beneficial or harmful, on rates of caesarean section, preterm delivery, low birthweight, admission to neonatal unit or stillbirth and neonatal deaths.

Effect of iron supplementation for iron deficiency in pregnancy

A third review assessed the effectiveness of different treatments (oral, intramuscular and intravenous) for iron deficiency anaemia in pregnancy (defined as haemoglobin less than 11 g/dl) on maternal and neonatal morbidity and mortality. Five trials randomising 1234 women were included. The author concluded that the evidence was inconclusive on the effects of treating iron deficiency anaemia in pregnancy because of the lack of good quality trials. There is an absence of evidence to indicate the timing of, and who should be receiving, iron supplementation during pregnancy.[274] [Evidence level 1a]

RECOMMENDATIONS

Pregnant women should be offered screening for anaemia. Screening should take place early in pregnancy (at the first appointment) and at 28 weeks, when other blood screening tests are being performed. This allows enough time for treatment if anaemia is detected. [B]

Haemoglobin levels outside the normal UK range for pregnancy (that is, 11 g/dl at first contact and 10.5 g/dl at 28 weeks) should be investigated and iron supplementation considered if indicated. [A]

8.2 Screening for sickle cell disorders and thalassaemia

Haemoglobin (Hb) disorders are autosomal recessive; however, it is possible to inherit more than one haemoglobin disorder. Sickle cell disorders include a variety of disorders, the most common of which are haemoglobins SS, Hb SC, Hb SD Punjab, HbS B thalassaemia and HbS O Arab. Hb SS causes anaemia, increased susceptibility to infection and infarction of various organs, including the brain. It is characterised by sickle-shaped red blood cells, resulting in their premature removal from the circulation. The prevalence of sickle cell trait in Northern European populations is 0.05% compared with 4% to 11% in black Caribbean populations, 20% (range 10% to 28%) in black African populations, 1% (range 0% to 1%) in Indians and 0.75% (range 0.5% to 10%) in Cypriot populations.[275] It is estimated 160 babies are born each year with sickle cell disorder in England. Implementation of the national universal screening of newborn babies for sickle cell disorders began in April 2003 in England and Wales.

Beta thalassaemia major causes severe anaemia from infancy, which is usually fatal within ten years if not treated. It is most common in people of Mediterranean origin and across the Middle and Far East. Prevalence estimates for thalassaemia trait are 0.9% among black Caribbean populations and black African populations, 3.5% (range 2.55 to 4.5%) among Indian populations, 4.5% (range 3.5% to 5.5%) among Pakistani populations, 3.0% among Bangladeshi populations (range 2.0% to 4.0%) and Chinese populations (range 1.0% to 4.0%) and 16% among Cypriot populations, compared with 0.1% among Northern Europeans.[275] Seventeen babies are born each year with thalassaemia, but there may be two to three times this number of pregnancies affected.[275] [Evidence level 3]

The aim of antenatal screening for sickle cell disorders and thalassaemia is to identify women at risk early in pregnancy, so that genetic counselling can be provided and women may make timely and informed reproductive choices. An audit of current practice in the UK indicated that about 50% of thalassaemia-affected pregnancies in England were not offered prenatal diagnosis, although a risk was recognised in 43–55% of pregnancies,[276] [Evidence level 3] while an audit of prenatal diagnosis found that only 50% and 13% of couples at risk for thalassaemia and sickle cell disorder, respectively, actually have a prenatal diagnosis.[277] [Evidence level 3]

Screening may be based on an ethnic question used to identify pregnant women at higher risk, who are then investigated for haemoglobin abnormalities, or on offering laboratory screening to all pregnant women. Irrespective of which method is used, information on ethnicity (ancestry) needs to be collected for interpretation of screening results.

In 1993, the UK Standing Medical Advisory Committee recommended screening using laboratory methods in districts where 15% or more of the antenatal population were from ethnic minorities.[278] [Evidence level 4] More recently, two Health Technology Assessment (HTA) reports have evaluated the effectiveness of screening in the antenatal, neonatal or preconceptual period and have addressed the question of screening using an ethnic question or using laboratory methods.[275,279]

Screening using an ethnic question is based on questions to identify ethnic origin of the pregnant woman. Ethnic origin is an important issue in screening, as sickle cell trait is found predominantly in people of African-Caribbean and sub-Saharan African origin, and thalassaemia trait is found predominantly in people of Arab, Mediterranean and Indian origin. The effectiveness and suitability of questions about ethnic origin is uncertain.[280] It is reported that data from the Department of Health showed that ethnic origin information was missing from 43% of records in London and 37% in England although the collection of this information is mandatory.[281] Substantial variability in practice and in the quality of data collected has also been reported, with up to 20% of high-risk ethnic origins being misclassified.[281] Further evaluation of using an ethnic question as the basis for screening is currently under way.

Screening antenatal women using laboratory methods involves both screening to detect haemoglobin variants and the interpretation of red cell indices with investigation of those identified as screen positive. If the pregnant woman has confirmed sickle cell or thalassaemia trait (or any other genetic mutation of haemoglobin), the father of the fetus should be offered testing. If both parents have the trait, counselling should be offered. Prenatal diagnosis usually involves chorionic villus sampling. Parents who would like to consider prenatal diagnosis of the fetus must be referred to a specialist centre.[282] More information on screening for thalassaemia and abnormal haemoglobins is available from the NHS sickle cell and thalassaemia website (www.kcl-phs.org.uk/haemscreening/).

Issues around the psychological impact of screening for haemoglobinopathies also exist as ending the pregnancy may be considered if the fetus is affected. For this reason, women at risk should be identified as soon as possible. Among couples counselled in the first trimester, one study reported that 85–95% of couples at risk request prenatal diagnosis for thalassaemias and 50–80% request prenatal diagnosis for sickle cell disorders.[282,283] A UK audit reported that the uptake of prenatal diagnosis for thalassaemia trait is sensitive to gestational age and that when offered, uptake ranged from 70% to 95% in the first trimester, depending upon ethnic origin with 11 of 12 affected pregnancies being terminated among British Pakistani women.[276] [Evidence level 3] In a study of the response of Muslim communities in Pakistan to antenatal diagnosis and termination of pregnancies due to thalassaemia, 89% of woman carrying an affected fetus chose to terminate their pregnancy.[284] [Evidence level 3]

Economic considerations

The search for economic papers on this topic found 13 studies including two HTA reports. The first HTA examined the total costs of screening programmes in high and low prevalence areas of people of specific ethnic origins.[279] The report indicated that the relative cost effectiveness of the strategies were highly sensitive to:

- the uptake of screening
- the presumed fetal prevalence of sickle cell disease
- the ethnic composition
- the inter-ethnic union rates.

The second HTA report included a systematic review of published studies.[275] No studies reporting the full benefits of screening and no good-quality UK-based cost data were found. A cost study based on one hospital estimated that the cost of identification of an at-risk fetus was £2455 per woman, including follow-up costs. The cost of treatment was estimated to be around £5000 per annum. The question of whether a universal or selective programme should be adopted was not directly addressed but it was suggested that a screening programme would be cost effective in areas with haemoglobinopathy traits at or above 2.5%.

It was first envisaged that a model could be constructed for this guideline, using census data to assess which areas of the UK might benefit from a more selective approach to screening.

However, despite efforts to obtain these data, it was not possible in the end to construct the model due to the inadequacy of the data that could be obtained.

The parameters that they suggest may be important in deciding whether to adopt a selective screening strategy are the ethnic composition of geographical area and the number of inter-ethnic unions resulting in a pregnancy. Since these rates may change quickly in any given population, this policy may not be effective or equitable to implement in practice.

Future research

The effectiveness and costs of an ethnic question for antenatal screening for sickle cell and thalassaemia is needed.

The effectiveness and costs of laboratory methods for antenatal screening for sickle cell and thalassaemia is needed.

8.3 Blood grouping and red cell alloantibodies

Identifying blood group, RhD status and red cell antibodies in pregnant women is important to prevent haemolytic disease of the newborn (HDN) and to identify possible transfusion problems. 15% of women are RhD negative. It is important to ascertain maternal RhD status so that RhD-negative women can be offered appropriate antenatal and postnatal immunoprophylaxis with the aim of preventing RhD alloimmunisation in subsequent pregnancies.

The reasons for identifying other red cell antibodies in pregnant women are the prevention of haemolytic disease of the newborn, which may cause jaundice, severe anaemia, heart failure and death, and for the identification of possible transfusion problems. These can occur in RhD-positive and -negative women. A significant number of women will have red cell antibodies.[285] The main antibodies that can cause severe alloimmune anaemia in the fetus are anti-D, anti-c and anti-Kell. Of lesser importance but still with the potential to cause HDN are anti-e, -Ce, -Fya, -Jka and-Cw. Anti-Lea, -Leb, -Lua, -P, -N, -Xga and high-titre low-avidity antibodies such as anti-Kna have not been associated with HDN.[286] There is no value in identifying group O pregnant women with high titres of anti-A or anti-B. Antenatal testing for these antibodies has been shown to have no value in predicting the incidence of HDN caused by ABO incompatibility.[287,288]

Antibody screening should be undertaken using an indirect antiglobulin test and a red cell panel conforming to current UK guidelines.[285]

Two Swedish surveys of red cell antibody screening in similar populations used different testing schedules and both concluded that their particular schedule detected all women at risk of HDN, yet one tested once only in early pregnancy[289] and the other tested RhD-positive women twice in pregnancy and RhD-negative women three times in pregnancy.[290]

Routine antenatal serological testing has been practised throughout the UK for about 30 years. There are currently recommendations that all women should be tested as early in pregnancy as possible, usually at 8 to 12 weeks of gestation.[291] This initial testing should include ABO and RhD typing as well as a screening test to detect any irregular red cell antibodies. Testing should be undertaken again at 28 weeks of gestation for all women with no antibodies on initial testing to ensure that no additional antibodies have developed.[291] No RCTs of different testing schedules were found.

When an antibody is detected, the clinician responsible for the woman's antenatal care must be informed of its likely significance, with respect to both the development of HDN and transfusion problems. Management of pregnancies in which red cell antibodies are detected varies depending upon the clinical significance and titre of the antibody detected.

Guidance on the routine administration of antenatal anti-D prophylaxis for RhD-negative women has been recently issued, which recommends that anti-D is offered to all pregnant women who are RhD negative.[292] However, in the case where a woman is RhD negative, consideration should also be given to offering partner testing because, if the biological father of the fetus is negative as well, anti-D prophylaxis, which is a blood product, will not need to be administered. Other situations where antenatal anti-D prophylaxis may not be necessary include cases where a woman has opted to be sterilised after the birth of the baby or when a woman is otherwise certain that she will not have another child after the current pregnancy.

RECOMMENDATIONS

Women should be offered testing for blood group and RhD status in early pregnancy. [B]

It is recommended that routine antenatal anti-D prophylaxis is offered to all non-sensitised pregnant women who are RhD negative. [NICE 2002]

Women should be screened for atypical red cell alloantibodies in early pregnancy and again at 28 weeks, regardless of their RhD status. [B]

Pregnant women with clinically significant atypical red cell alloantibodies should be offered referral to a specialist centre for further investigation and advice on subsequent antenatal management. [D]

If a pregnant woman is RhD-negative, consideration should be given to offering partner testing to determine whether the administration of anti-D prophylaxis is necessary. [Good practice point]

9 Screening for fetal anomalies

Screening tests that aim to detect structural and chromosomal anomalies include ultrasound scan assessment and maternal serum screening (for open neural tube defects and Down's syndrome) early in pregnancy. The objectives of fetal anomaly screening include the identification of:[293]

- anomalies that are not compatible with life
- anomalies associated with high morbidity and long-term disability
- fetal conditions with the potential for intrauterine therapy
- fetal conditions that will require postnatal investigation or treatment.

The scope of any screening test for fetal anomalies should be made clear to women when the screening is offered. Although results from RCTs have not yet demonstrated whether informed decision making in screening affects uptake,[294] the UK National Screening Committee has adopted the principle that screening programmes should offer choice to individuals and that each person should make an informed decision about screening based upon appreciation of the risks and benefits.[295] Although the amount of information needed to make choices about antenatal screening varies from person to person, a report from the RCOG outlines the topics that should be discussed with a woman before screening.[296] Written information should be provided on details of the nature and purpose of the screening (i.e. for ultrasound scans, explanation of the structures examined), the screening procedure, details of detection rates for defined common conditions, the meaning of a positive and negative screening result, and actions to be taken if a test is reported as 'normal' or 'abnormal'.

9.1 Screening for structural anomalies

The aim of screening for fetal anomalies is to identify specific structural malformations. This allows the parents to plan appropriate care during pregnancy and childbirth or for the parents to be offered other reproductive choices. The detection of fetal anomalies varies, depending upon the anatomical system being examined, the gestational age at assessment, the skill of the operator and the quality of the equipment.

Ultrasound scanning for structural anomalies

A systematic review, based on 11 studies (one RCT, six retrospective cohorts and four prospective cohorts) was undertaken to examine the use of routine ultrasound to detect fetal anomalies.[297] The studies, which included 96,633 babies, were performed in Europe, the USA and Korea between 1988 and 1996. The overall prevalence of fetal anomaly was 2.09%, ranging from 0.76% to 2.45% in individual studies and including major and minor anomalies. [Evidence level IIa]

None of the studies conducted screening for anomalies at less than 15 weeks of gestation. Detection rates at less than 24 weeks was 41.3%, and 18.6% at greater than 24 weeks. Overall, detection of fetal anomaly was 44.7%, with a range of 15.0% to 85.3%, as different anomalies are more or less likely to be correctly identified. For example, anomaly scanning at 14 to 22 weeks for anencephaly can detect nearly 100% of cases.[298] [Evidence level 3]

Detection rates of ultrasound in the studies from the review may be inflated, as some studies reported the number of anomalies detected rather than the number of babies with structural anomalies. However, the authors also only included studies that reported adequate methods of

Box 9.1. Minimum standards for the 20-week anomaly scan, derived from the RCOG[302]

Fetal normality:

- Head shape and size and internal structures (cavum pellucidum, cerebellum, ventricular size at atrium < 10 mm)

- Spine: longitudinal and transverse

- Abdominal shape and content at level of stomach

- Abdominal shape and content at level of kidneys and umbilicus

- Renal pelvis < 5 mm anterior–posterior measurement

- Longitudinal axis abdominal–thoracic appearance (diaphragm and bladder)

- Thorax at level of a four-chamber cardiac view

- Arms: three bones and hand (not counting fingers)

- Legs: three bones and foot (not counting toes)

Optimal standard for a 20-week anomaly scan:

- Cardiac outflow tracts

- Face and lips

postnatal ascertainment of anomalies to verify their presence and allow a more accurate calculation of test performance. Variation in detection rate occurs with:

- the type of anomaly being screened (see Table 9.1)
- the gestational age at scanning
- the skill of the operator
- the quality of the equipment being used
- the time allocated for the scan.

The use of ultrasound to detect fetal anomalies reduces perinatal mortality only if the parents choose to end the pregnancy following the detection of those anomalies.[297] [Evidence level 1b & 2a]

Another RCT that was not included in the above review compared routine ultrasound scanning with selective ultrasound.[299] [Evidence level 1b] A better detection rate for major malformations was reported for routine ultrasound than for selective ultrasound (40% versus 28%). A significantly lower perinatal mortality rate in the routine ultrasound group was also reported and was mainly attributed to differences in termination of pregnancy after detection. There was more than a two-fold difference in the detection rates between the two hospitals that participated in this trial (75% versus 35%), which reinforces the need to ensure a high skill level among those performing the scan.

As detection rates vary, those providing ultrasound scanning need to monitor the quality of their service. This requires the collection of follow-up information on all babies scanned during

Table 9.1 Percentage of fetal anomalies detected by routine ultrasound screening in the second trimester according to anatomical system.[297] [Evidence level IIa]

Anatomical systems	Detected (%)
Central nervous system	76
Urinary tract	67
Pulmonary	50
Gastrointestinal	42
Skeletal	24
Cardiac	17

pregnancy. As detection rates are influenced both by the skill of the operator and the quality of the ultrasound scanning equipment, the RCOG working party report outlined standards for training and equipment (Appendix 3).

The detection rate of fetal structural anomalies also varies with gestational age at the time of ultrasound. An observational study on the detection of major structural anomalies with a scan at 12 to 13 weeks reported an 84% detection rate for anencephaly.[300] [Evidence level 3] The potential benefit of scanning for structural anomalies in the first trimester is that gestational age assessment (see Section 4.6) and Down's syndrome screening (i.e. nuchal translucency) could be performed concurrently.

In Wales, 100% of maternity units currently offer a routine 18- to 20-week anomaly scan.[301] A UK recommended minimum standard for the 20-week anomaly scan is provided by the RCOG (Box 9.1). The standards for an 'optimal scan' include additional features to improve the detection of cardiac anomalies and facial cleft defects.[302] [Evidence level 4] Although many maternity units may not currently be able to afford the additional scanning time or scans required, these have been included as a standard that maternity units may aspire to achieve.

When a screening result for structural anomalies suggests a malformation, all women should be offered a more detailed ultrasound scan, if necessary at a regional centre, for a definitive diagnosis.

RECOMMENDATION

Pregnant women should be offered an ultrasound scan to screen for structural anomalies, ideally between 18 to 20 weeks of gestation, by an appropriately trained sonographer and with equipment of an appropriate standard as outlined by the National Screening Committee. [A]

9.2 Screening for Down's syndrome

Down's syndrome, also termed Trisomy 21, is a congenital syndrome that arises when the affected baby has an extra copy of chromosome 21. The birth incidence of Down's syndrome in England and Wales was 6.2/10,000 live and still births in 1998.[303] [Evidence level 3] The main clinical feature of this disorder is intellectual impairment, although it is also associated with excess mortality due to congenital malformations (of which cardiac anomalies are the most common), leukaemia and increased incidence of thyroid disorders, epilepsy and Alzheimer's disease. An estimated 80% of children affected with Down's syndrome will have profound or severe intellectual disability and 20% will have mild or no intellectual disability. About 46% of children with Down's syndrome are born with a congenital heart defect that may require surgery.[304]

Principles of screening for Down's syndrome

The first step of any screening for congenital anomalies should include the provision of unbiased, evidence-based information so that the pregnant woman will be able to make autonomous informed decisions. This should include information on Down's syndrome, the characteristics of the screening test the woman is being offered and the implications of the test results.[305] The results of a cross-sectional study have shown, however, that although many women understand practical aspects of the test (e.g. that serum screening occurs at 16 to 18 weeks of gestation and that blood would be needed for the test), they lack knowledge about the likelihood and implications of possible results.[306] Women were surveyed after consultation with a midwife or obstetrician during which serum screening for Down's syndrome was offered and only 36% of women answered correctly the question, "Negative results do not guarantee that everything is all right with the baby". [Evidence level 3] Women should be made aware that they could opt out of the screening process at any time. However, knowing about a problem that the baby may have will allow for reproductive choice and also the opportunity for doctors and midwives to provide optimal care during pregnancy and childbirth.

Antenatal screening for Down's syndrome can take place during the first or second trimester of pregnancy and a variety of screening tests can be used. In the first trimester, nuchal translucency

(NT), which is the measurement of the normal subcutaneous space between the skin and the cervical spine in the fetus early in pregnancy, can be used to identify women at increased risk of carrying a Down's syndrome baby at around 10 to 14 weeks. Nuchal translucency may be used with or without two first-trimester maternal serum markers, human chorionic gonadotrophin (hCG) and pregnancy-associated plasma protein A (PAPP-A): i.e., the combined test, or as part of the integrated test. In the early second trimester, screening techniques include biochemical marker screening at around 15 to 16 weeks.

Once a screening test is performed, the risk of Down's syndrome is calculated, taking into account maternal age, gestational age and the levels of biochemical markers. Results are 'positive' or classified as 'high risk' if the risk is equal to or greater than a locally agreed cutoff level. This is often expressed numerically to indicate the likelihood that a woman has a baby with Down's syndrome when a positive screening result is returned; e.g., a 1/250 chance that a pregnant woman is carrying an affected baby. When a high-risk screening result is returned, a woman will usually be offered a diagnostic test, such as amniocentesis, which has an excess fetal loss rate of 1%.[307] [Evidence level 1b]

It should be made clear to the woman that the nature of screening tests is such that a number of 'false positives' and 'false negatives' will result from a screening programme. The effectiveness of Down's syndrome screening tests are often reported with a 'false positive rate', which indicates the proportion of positive screening tests that indicate there may be a problem when there is not.

Differences in the performance of screening tests between studies may occur for a number of reasons:

- variation in statistical models of both prior age-related maternal risk and risk calculation from biochemical markers
- variation in biochemical assays used
- variation in the test thresholds, i.e. cutoff levels
- methodological quality of studies leading to both under- or over-ascertainment of cases in cohort studies or the use of case–control designs leading to biased estimates of test performance.[308,309]
- chance variation.

An associated increase in miscarriage throughout pregnancy has been reported among pregnant women known to have a fetus affected by Down's syndrome compared with pregnant women with unaffected fetuses.[310] [Evidence level 3] Therefore the prevalence of Down's syndrome is likely to be higher early in pregnancy than at birth. Down's syndrome screening tests performed early in pregnancy will identify fetuses that may be lost spontaneously later in pregnancy. This affects the accuracy of cutoff rates in the determination of women who are 'high risk' or will be offered a diagnostic test and becomes relevant when the 'detection rate' of an earlier screening test is compared with that of a later screening test. A later screening test may not identify as high a proportion of Down's syndrome fetuses as an earlier test. However, it should not necessarily be interpreted that the later test is less efficient than the earlier test. Adjustment for the loss of Down's syndrome fetuses that have been terminated or spontaneously aborted needs to be made in order to provide accurate estimates of risk and screening performance.

Methods of screening for Down's syndrome

The risk of Down's syndrome increases with maternal age. The odds of having a baby affected by Down's syndrome at age 20 years are approximately 1:1,440 rising to 1:338 at 35 years and 1:32 at 45 years.[311] [Evidence level 3] Therefore, before the development of biochemical and ultrasound screening methods, screening for Down's syndrome was based on maternal age only and all women over the age of 35 to 37 years were offered amniocentesis as a screening test. In 2000, in England and Wales, 16.5% of mothers were older than 35 years at the birth of their baby[312] and would have been offered invasive diagnostic testing, based on a policy of screening by maternal age alone.

Invasive diagnostic testing and karyotyping is the gold standard test for confirming the diagnosis but it is associated with an excess risk for fetal loss of 1% compared with women with no invasive diagnostic testing.[307] In 1998, a survey found that 8% of UK health authorities screened on the basis of maternal age alone.[313] One study estimated that screening by maternal age alone detected 53% of Down's syndrome cases antenatally over a three-year period, though this was thought to be an overestimate, as the total number of liveborn Down's syndrome babies was not obtainable.[314]

In the 1980s, a number of biochemical markers were found to be associated with Down's syndrome and this marked the advent of screening being offered to women younger than 35 years. This was important because, although the risk of Down's syndrome increases with age, younger women have the majority of pregnancies and therefore give birth to the majority of children with Down's syndrome. First-trimester biochemical markers now include hCG (total and free beta) and PAPP-A. hCG may also be measured in the second trimester. Other second-trimester biochemical markers include alphafetoprotein (AFP), unconjugated oestriol (uE$_3$) and dimeric inhibin A.

The associations between specific ultrasonographic markers and Down's syndrome have also been identified. One meta-analysis assessed which second-trimester ultrasound markers were effective for the detection of fetuses with Down's syndrome. The findings suggested that a thickened nuchal fold was the most accurate ultrasound marker in the second trimester. The six other markers that were assessed were reported to be of little value in screening for Down's syndrome, as they would result in more fetal losses than cases of Down's syndrome detected.[315] [Evidence level 2a & 3] However, the review concluded that the sensitivity of a thickened nuchal fold in the second trimester was not high enough to be used as a practical screening test for Down's syndrome on its own. NT measurement for Down's syndrome screening commonly occurs between 11 and 14 weeks of gestation and detection rates for this are reported below. The presence or absence of fetal nasal bone, another possible ultrasound marker, is currently being researched.

Current screening for Down's syndrome

There is an extensive body of literature on Down's syndrome screening that investigates the numerous combinations of individual and multimarker screening in the first or second trimester, ultrasound screening and the integrated approach, which includes screening tests in the both the first and second trimester. If PAPP-A, hCG and NT are used as a first-trimester screening test (at 10 to 12 weeks), this is commonly referred to as the 'combined test'. When hCG and AFP are used between 14 to 20 weeks as a screening test, this is often called the 'double test'. If uE$_3$ is added to the double test combination, it becomes known as the 'triple test'. The addition of inhibin A to the triple test comprises the 'quadruple test'. The 'integrated test' uses NT and PAPP-A at 10 to 12 weeks of gestation with hCG, AFP, uE$_3$ and inhibin A at 14 to 20 weeks of gestation, requiring women to be managed through the first and second trimester for screening. Although the efficacy of this test is known, the acceptability of this approach to testing to pregnant women is not known. The 'serum integrated test' is the same as the integrated test without NT.

A 2001 survey of all maternity centres and primary care trusts in England indicated that the majority of units offered some form of screening for Down's syndrome. However, a variety of screening tests are used including: first-trimester NT screening with or without biochemical markers or biochemical marker screening in the second trimester (personal communication, Helen Janecek, 2003). In addition, an HTA monograph presented results for the integrated test.[316] The detection rates for each of these screening test combinations are presented in Table 9.2.

Considerable discrepancy between reported detection and false positive rates between studies often exist, due to differences in study design, varying cutoff rates, skill of the ultrasound operator, and the times at which the screening was conducted. All these factors should be taken into account when planning which screening method will be used for a pregnant population. In addition, other factors, such as the practicality of managing women through two trimesters for screening or the introduction of NT for Down's syndrome screening in the context of extra time required for ultrasound (assuming that a unit already offers first trimester dating scans) should also be considered.

Diagnosis after a positive screening result

Diagnostic tests are offered to women identified as at high risk of having an affected pregnancy. Antenatal diagnosis of Down's syndrome is currently done by culture of fetal cells and fetal cells can currently only be acquired by invasive methods: amniocentesis, chorionic villus sampling (CVS) or fetal blood sampling. All of these methods carry a risk of miscarriage. The excess risk

Table 9.2 Detection and false positive rates for various combinations of markers used for Down's syndrome screening

Measurements (cutoff)	False positive rate (%)	Detection rate (%)
Nuchal translucency at 9 to 14 weeks* (13 cohort studies, n = 170,343)[317]	4.7	77
Combined test : NT plus serum screening (10 studies, range reported)[318]	5	85–89
Double test (6 cohort studies, n = 110,254)[319]	Not reported**	66
Triple test (20 cohort studies, n = 194,326, medians and ranges reported)[320]		
For a risk cutoff 1:190–200	4 (range 3–7)	67 (range 48–91)
For a risk cutoff 1:250–295	6 (range 4–7)	71 (range 48–80)
For a risk cutoff 1:350–380	8 (range 7–13)	73 (range 70–80)
Quadruple test (1 cohort study, n = 46,193)[321]	5	75 (95% CI 66–84)
Serum integrated test (1 nested case–control study, n = 28,434)[316]	2.7	85
Integrated test (1 nested case–control study, n = 28,434)[316]	1.3	85

* These data are from published cohort studies; data from the SURUSS report[316] have not been included as this was a nested case–control study and higher level evidence was available

** Due to variation in practice between screening programmes being compared

of miscarriage following amniocentesis is approximately 1%.[307] [Evidence level 1b] Among women who were screened in the first trimester and had a positive result, the reported rate of uptake for invasive testing for prenatal diagnosis was 77%.[322] [Evidence level 2a] Among women who were screened in the second trimester and had a positive result, reported uptake of invasive testing ranged from 43% to 74%, depending upon the magnitude of the risk.[321]

CVS is commonly performed between 11 and 13 weeks of gestation and amniocentesis after 15 weeks of gestation. However, first-trimester CVS is associated with a higher sampling failure rate (Peto OR 2.86, 95% CI 1.93 to 4.24) and also a higher pregnancy loss rate (Peto OR 1.33, 95% CI 1.17 to 1.52) than second-trimester amniocentesis.[323] [Evidence level 1a] Amniocentesis should not be carried out in the first trimester. When compared with CVS, early amniocentesis was associated with a higher failure rate (0.4% versus 2%, RR 0.23, 95% CI 0.08 to 0.65) though there was no significant difference in pregnancy loss between the two procedures (6.2% versus 5%, RR 1.24, 95% CI 0.85 to 1.81)[324] [Evidence level 1a] When early amniocentesis (before 14 weeks) was compared with amniocentesis at 15 weeks or later, however, a significantly higher rate of fetal loss (7.6% versus 5.9%, p = 0.012), fetal talipes (1.3% versus 0.1%, p = 0.0001) and sampling difficulty has been reported.[307] [Evidence level 1b] Therefore, associated risks are lowest for amniocentesis performed after fifteen weeks and highest for CVS at all times during pregnancy.

When a pregnant woman is offered a diagnostic test after a positive screening result, she should be informed of the risks associated with invasive testing and that other chromosomal anomalies, not just Down's syndrome, may be identified and that in some cases the prognosis for the fetus may not be clear. Although considerable anxiety is reported to be associated with diagnostic testing for Down's syndrome,[325,326] uptake of diagnostic testing after a high-risk screening result (1:250–300) in UK populations has been reported to range from 43% to 77%.[321,322]

A recent study examining the effect of prenatal diagnosis on infant mortality reported a decline in infant deaths due to congenital anomalies.[327] The authors suggested that the increased availability of reproductive choice upon diagnosis of congenital anomaly was related to the observed decrease in overall infant mortality. [Evidence level 3]

The future of Down's syndrome screening

The recommendations stated below accord with the current recommendations of the Antenatal Subcommittee of the UK National Screening Committee (NSC). However, as some screening tests for Down's syndrome are performed early in pregnancy, consideration should be given to ensuring that pregnant women who present late for antenatal care can also be offered screening for Down's syndrome.

Research surrounding the issue of screening for Down's syndrome is moving quickly and, while the NSC hopes that all units will achieve the standard of a 60% detection rate with a 5% false positive rate by April 2004, they also propose that a 75% detection rate with a less than 3% false positive rate should be achieved by April 2007 (www.nelh.nhs.uk/screening/dssp/home.htm). These performance meaures should be age standardised and based on a cutoff of 1/250 at term. A pilot programme in preparation for the introduction of inhibin A for Down's syndrome screening to address concerns about its reliability is currently under way. The feasibility and acceptability of the integrated and serum-integrated approach are also being explored.

RECOMMENDATIONS

Pregnant women should be offered screening for Down's syndrome with a test that provides the current standard of a detection rate above 60% and a false positive rate of less than 5%. The following tests meet this standard:

- From 11 to 14 weeks:
  - nuchal translucency (NT)
  - the combined test (NT, hCG and PAPP-A)
- From 14 to 20 weeks:
  - the triple test (hCG, AFP and uE_3)
  - the quadruple test (hCG, AFP, uE_3, inhibin A)
- From 11 to 14 weeks AND 14 to 20 weeks:
  - the integrated test (NT, PAPP-A + hCG, AFP, uE_3, inhibin A)
  - the serum integrated test (PAPP-A + hCG, AFP, uE_3, inhibin A). [B]

By April 2007, pregnant women should be offered screening for Down's syndrome with a test which provides a detection rate above 75% and a false positive rate of less than 3%. These performance measures should be age standardised and based on a cutoff of 1/250 at term. The following tests currently meet this standard:

- From 11 to 14 weeks:
  - the combined test (NT, hCG and PAPP-A)
- From 14 to 20 weeks:
  - the quadruple test (hCG, AFP, uE_3, inhibin A)
- From 11 to 14 weeks AND 14 to 20 weeks:
  - the integrated test (NT, PAPP-A + hCG, AFP, uE_3, inhibin A)
  - the serum integrated test (PAPP-A + hCG, AFP, uE_3, inhibin A). [B]

Pregnant women should be given information about the detection rates and false positive rates of any Down's syndrome screening test being offered and about further diagnostic tests that may be offered. The woman's right to accept or decline the test should be made clear. [D]

10. Screening for infections

10.1   Asymptomatic bacteriuria

Asymptomatic bacteriuria (ASB) is defined as persistent bacterial colonisation of the urinary tract without urinary tract symptoms. Its incidence has been quoted as being 2–10% in studies conducted in the USA, with the higher incidence among women of lower socio-economic status.[328] Studies in the UK have shown that it occurs in 2–5% of pregnant women.[329-331] [Evidence level 3]

Evidence from randomised controlled trials that were conducted to show the benefit of treatment among women with ASB indicate an increased risk between ASB and maternal and fetal outcomes, such as preterm birth and pyelonephritis, among untreated women compared with women without bacteriuria.[329,331-337] [Evidence level 1b] The reported increased risk of pyelonephritis among pregnant women with ASB ranges from a risk difference of 1.8% to 28%.[329,331-333,335,338] [Evidence levels 2a & 1b]

These trials also indicate an increased risk of preterm birth in women who have untreated ASB compared with women who do not have ASB. The risk difference ranges from 2.1% to 12.8%.[329,332,333,338] [Evidence level 1b] The large range in risk difference may be due to variation in effect size over time because earlier studies reported larger effects than more recent studies. Also, with regards to randomisation, many of the older studies did not specify the method of randomisation or were open to bias because of quasi-random allocation to treatment versus control groups.

Urine culture (midstream) has been used as the reference standard for diagnosis of ASB. In studies of ASB, a growth of 105 organisms of a single uropathogen per millilitre in a single midstream sample of urine is considered significant,[339,340] although some tests have used figures such as 104 and 108.[330] When urine culture is used in screening for ASB, the drawbacks include the time lag: results are not usually available for at least 24 hours,[341] and the cost: £1.40 in a 1993 UK study[342] compared with the maximum cost of a reagent strip test of £0.14. Its advantages are in being able to identify causative organisms and determine antibiotic sensitivities.

A number of rapid tests have been evaluated against urine culture in test evaluation studies. These include:

- reagent strip tests which test for one or more of the following:
  - nitrite
  - protein
  - blood
  - leucocyte esterase
- microscopic urinalysis
- Gram stain with or without centrifugation
- urinary interleukin
- rapid enzymatic screening test (detection of catalase activity)
- bioluminescence assay.

Reagent strip testing

This has the advantage of being rapid and inexpensive and requiring little technical expertise. Reagent strips have panels that have nitrites and leucocyte esterase,[343-346] and in which the presence of either nitrites or leucocyte esterase is considered positive.[345,347] Other strips have protein, blood, nitrite and leucocyte esterase.[348] In test evaluation studies with all four panels, a positive test result is defined as a strip showing any of the following:

- more than a trace of protein
- more than a trace of blood
- any positive result for nitrite
- any positive result for leucocyte esterase.[348]

The sensitivity of reagent strip testing, using two or four panels in combination (all tests positive) ranges from 8.18% to 50.0%.[342,343,345,347,348] [Evidence level 2a] With either test positive, in the case of the nitrite and leucocyte esterase test, two studies from the USA conducted in 2001 and 1993, respectively, showed sensitivities of 45% and 50%,[343,347] [Evidence level 2a] whereas a 1988 study, also from the USA, showed a sensitivity of 92%.[346] [Evidence level 2a] These findings are confirmed in another study, where the reported sensitivity of testing for protein alone for ASB was 57% with a specificity of 93.2%.[342] [Evidence level 2a] This implies that, at best, reagent strip testing will detect 50% of women with ASB.

Microscopic urinalysis

This test consists of microscopic analysis of urinary sediment and pyuria is deemed significant with ten cells per high-power field.[345,347] [Evidence level 2a] A study that examined a population of women attending an antenatal clinic found a sensitivity of 25%, which means that 75% of women with ASB will be missed using this test.[347] Two other studies report higher sensitivities but the population in one of the studies was a mixture of women attending an antenatal clinic and women in preterm labour and the second study used a wide range of pyuria of between one and eight per high-power field.[345,349]

Gram stain

Two American studies were identified in which Gram staining was compared with urine culture. In one study, a specificity of 7.7% was reported when urine was centrifuged and considered positive if the same morphotype of bacteria was seen in more than 6 of 12 high-power fields.[345] [Evidence level 2a] In the other study, urine was not centrifuged and a positive smear was defined as more than two organisms per high-power field. This yielded a specificity of 89.2%.[347] [Evidence level 2a] With the low specificity in the more rigorous estimation, more than 90% of women who do not have ASB will be incorrectly identified as cases.[345] [Evidence level 2a]

Other tests

Other tests identified include the urinary interleukin-8 test[343] and the rapid enzymatic test,[344] both of which have a sensitivity of 70% and will potentially miss 30% of women with ASB. [Evidence level 2a] A bioluminescence test has been described, with a sensitivity of 93% and a specificity of 78%.[350] [Evidence level 2a]

Treatment

A systematic review of 14 RCTs compared antibiotic treatment with no treatment or placebo. Antibiotic treatment reduced persistent bacteriuria during pregnancy (Peto OR 0.07, 95% CI 0.05 to 0.10), reduced risk of preterm delivery or low-birthweight babies (OR 0.60, 95% CI 0.45 to 0.80), and reduced the risk of development of pyelonephritis (OR 0.24, 95% CI 0.19 to 0.32, NNT 7).[351] [Evidence level 1a]

A systematic review that compared single-dose antibiotic treatment with a 4 to 7 day course of antibiotic treatment for asymptomatic bacteriuria showed no difference in the prevention of preterm birth (RR 0.81, 95% CI 0.26 to 2.57) or pyelonephritis (RR 3.09, 95% CI 0.54 to 17.55). Longer duration of treatment, however, was associated with increased reports of adverse effects (RR 0.53, 95% CI 0.31 to 9.91).[352] [Evidence level 1a]

Economic considerations (see Appendix 2)

Screening antenatally for asymptomatic bacteriuria can have important healthcare resource consequences associated with the reduction of maternal and infant morbidity. Using resources to screen women antenatally could save the future costs of treating pyelonephritis (which can have severe symptoms in pregnant women) and preterm birth and the consequent lifetime costs of disability associated with preterm birth. Screening and treating pregnant women can lead to healthier mothers and infants and does not lead to a choice to end a pregnancy. Therefore, screening and consequent treatment has only positive benefits for pregnant women and their children.

Implementing either of the screening strategies is more cost effective than a policy of no screening. There is controversy around whether to use a dipstick or a culture test for screening. The culture test is relatively more expensive but has a higher sensitivity and specificity. One economic study concluded that the urine culture, which is regarded as the gold standard, is not cost beneficial when compared with the dipstick strategy.[600] However, this study did not consider the cost consequences of preterm birth in their analysis. Since these costs may be quite high (considering the lifetime costs of an infant born with disability), it was decided to try and model the alternative screening programmes and include these costs.

For that reason, a decision analytic model was created to compare the two strategies:

1. screening with urine culture
2. screening with leukocyte esterase-nitrite dipstick.

The economic data used in the model were extracted from five papers that met the criteria for high-quality economic evaluation (see Appendix 2). The clinical effectiveness data were extrapolated from the evidence tables of the present guideline document.

The model indicated the difference in costs and benefits of adopting a dipstick method when compared with the culture method (the current gold standard). The unit of effectiveness was defined as cases of pyelonephritis averted and cases of preterm birth averted. The value and non-resource consequences of averting these cases could not be explored as data were not available.

The costs were expressed in three different ways:

1. the cost of screening only
2. the cost of screening and treatment (of ASB and pyelonephritis)
3. the cost of screening, treatment and the cost of preterm birth.

The model showed that the mean cost per case of pyelonephritis averted for the dipstick method was £4,300 when preterm birth was excluded and £115,000 when preterm birth was included. The mean cost per case averted for the culture method was £82,500 with and £36,500 without preterm birth. The results of the models indicate that it would cost an extra £32,400 for an extra case of preterm birth prevented if the dipstick method was followed instead of the culture.

The analysis supports the conclusion that the culture method is favourable, taking into account the wider cost consequences of ASB. The model indicated that if the policy of using a dipstick test led to only one additional case of preterm birth, then this is no longer the more favourable screening option, relative to the urine culture method.

Threshold analysis was also undertaken to explore the circumstances under which the screening options would have similar costs. The analysis indicated that for the two screening strategies to have equal overall costs (including the cost of preterm birth), the sensitivity of the dipstick method would have to be equal to or greater than 0.912, which is very high for this method of screening. Any sensitivity below this makes the culture method more cost effective in comparison to the dipstick method.

This result has not yet been fully explored in primary cost effectiveness studies and should be considered a priority for future research.

RECOMMENDATION

Pregnant women should be offered routine screening for asymptomatic bacteriuria by midstream urine culture early in pregnancy. Identification and treatment of asymptomatic bacteriuria reduces the risk of preterm birth. [A]

Future research

Up-to-date RCTs are needed to confirm the beneficial effect of screening for asymptomatic bacteriuria.

10.2   Asymptomatic bacterial vaginosis

Bacterial vaginosis results from the relative deficiency of normal *Lactobacillus* species in the vagina and relative overgrowth of anaerobic bacteria. These may include *Mobiluncus* species, *Gardnerella vaginalis*, *Prevotella* species and *Mycoplasma hominis*. This results in a reduction of the normal acidity of the vagina. It is the most common cause of vaginal discharge and malodour,[353] although 50% of women with bacterial vaginosis infection during pregnancy will be asymptomatic.[354] Why these organisms, many of which are present in small numbers in the vagina normally, multiply is not well understood. The condition is not sexually transmitted, although it is associated with sexual activity.

The presence of bacterial vaginosis during pregnancy varies according to ethnicity and how often a population is screened. In a cross-sectional study of 13,747 pregnant women in the USA, 8.8% of white women had bacterial vaginosis compared with 22.7% in black women (p < 0.05), 15.9% in Hispanic women (p < 0.05) and 6.1% in Asian-Pacific Islander women.[355] [Evidence level 3] In a northwest area of London, screening before 28 weeks of gestation found a prevalence of 12%.[356] [Evidence level 3]

Bacterial vaginosis is associated with preterm birth. In a review of case–control and cohort studies, women with bacterial vaginosis infection were found to be 1.85 times more likely (95% CI 1.62 to 2.11) to deliver preterm than women without bacterial vaginosis.[357] [Evidence levels 2 & 3] The higher risk of preterm birth remains in women diagnosed with bacterial vaginosis early in pregnancy even if the bacterial vaginosis spontaneously recovers later in pregnancy.[358] [Evidence level 3]

Bacterial vaginosis may be diagnosed by either Amsel's criteria (thin white-grey homogenous discharge, pH greater than 4.5, release of 'fishy odour' on adding alkali, clue cells present on direct microscopy)[359] or Nugent's criteria (Gram-stained vaginal smear to identify proportions of bacterial morphotypes with a score of less than 4 normal, 4–6 intermediate, and greater than 6 bacterial vaginosis).[360] Culture of *G. vaginalis* is not recommended as a diagnostic tool because it is not specific. Cervical Papanicolaou tests have limited clinical utility for the diagnosis of bacterial vaginosis because of low sensitivity.

One RCT was located which investigated the efficacy of yoghurt in treating bacterial vaginosis compared with vaginal metronidazole and vaginal placebo.[361] Although metronidazole was the most effective treatment against persistence of infection (relative risk reduction 62%, 95% CI 50 to 72%), yoghurt was two-thirds as effective as metronidazole when compared with the placebo group (relative risk reduction 46%, 95% CI 31 to 58%). [Evidence level 1b]

A systematic review of ten RCTs (n = 4249) found oral or vaginal antibiotics to be highly effective in the eradication of bacterial vaginosis in pregnancy when compared with placebo or no treatment (Peto OR 0.21, 95% CI 0.18 to 0.24)[362] [Evidence level 1a] Antibiotics used in the interventions included oral metronidazole (four RCTs), oral metronidazole plus erythromycin (one RCT), amoxicillin (one RCT), vaginal metronidazole cream (one RCT) and intravaginal clindamycin cream (three RCTs). No significant differences in the rates of preterm birth (birth before 37, 34 or 32 weeks) or perinatal death were observed between the two groups. However, a reduction in risk of preterm premature rupture of membranes was associated with antibiotics (three RCTs, n = 562 women, Peto OR 0.32, 95% CI 0.15 to 0.67). There were no differences in maternal side effects due to treatment found between the treated and non-treated or placebo groups. There was also no evidence of the effect of treatment on the subsequent risk of preterm birth among women with a prior preterm birth (five RCTs, n = 622 women, OR 0.83, 95% CI 0.59 to 1.17). Most women in these trials did not have symptoms of bacterial vaginosis because symptomatic women were treated and therefore excluded.

One trial that was not included in the above systematic review was located.[363] This study identified women between 12 to 22 weeks of gestation with bacterial vaginosis (n = 485) using Nugent's criteria. The study was double blind and women in the intervention group (n = 244) took 300 mg oral clindamycin twice daily for 5 days, while women in the control group (n = 241) took placebos. Women receiving clindamycin had significantly fewer spontaneous preterm deliveries, which were defined as birth occurring between 24 and 37 weeks of gestation, than women in the control group (11 (5%) versus 28 (12%), p = 0.001). [Evidence level 1b] When analysed with the ten trials from the systematic review, the effect of treatment for bacterial vaginosis on preterm birth was not statistically significant (Peto OR 0.93, 95% CI 0.76 to 1.13).

In addition, although oral clindamycin is not known to be harmful in pregnancy, its use as a general antibiotic is limited because of serious adverse effects.[77] In particular, antibiotic-associated colitis may arise and this can be fatal.

Evidence from randomised controlled trials indicates that screening and treating healthy pregnant women (i.e. low risk for preterm birth) for asymptomatic bacterial vaginosis does not lower the risk for preterm birth nor for other adverse reproductive outcomes.

RECOMMENDATION

Pregnant women should not be offered routine screening for bacterial vaginosis because the evidence suggests that the identification and treatment of asymptomatic bacterial vaginosis does not lower the risk for preterm birth and other adverse reproductive outcomes. [A]

10.3   *Chlamydia trachomatis*

Chlamydia trachomatis is a common sexually transmitted infection in European countries.[364] Chlamydia prevalence during pregnancy has been estimated at 6% in one English study.[365] [Evidence level 3] It is more frequent in women who are younger, black, single and those attending genitourinary medicine clinics.[365,366] [Evidence level 3]

Chlamydia infection during pregnancy is associated with higher rates of preterm birth (OR 1.6, 90%CI 1.01 to 2.5) and intrauterine growth restriction (OR 2.5, 90%CI 1.32 to 4.18).[367] [Evidence level 2a] Left untreated, it has also been associated with increased low birthweight and infant mortality.[368] [Evidence level 2b] In a review of randomised control trials, the number of women with positive cultures for chlamydia was reduced by 90% when treated with antibiotics compared with placebo (OR 0.06, 95% CI 0.03 to 0.12).[369] [Evidence level 1a] However this did not alter the incidence of birth before 37 weeks.

In studies of infants born to mothers who have cultured positive to *C. trachomatis*, approximately 25% of the infants have subsequently cultured positive to *C. trachomatis*.[370,371] [Evidence level 3] These infants are also reported to have higher rates of neonatal conjunctivitis, lower respiratory tract infections and pneumonia.[370,371] [Evidence level 3]

Currently, no simple inexpensive laboratory tests for diagnosing *C. trachomatis* exist and different screening tests require samples to be taken from different anatomical sites. Tissue culture is expensive and, although it has good specificity, its sensitivity ranges from 75% to 85% because of inadequate sampling techniques (e.g., not rotating the swab firmly against the tissue for 15 to 30 seconds, removal from os must be without touching vaginal mucosa, use of lubricating jelly decreases chance of detection) and because the bacteria do not always survive transportation to the laboratory.[372] [Evidence level 4] Rapid tests include direct fluorescent antibody staining (50% to 90% sensitive), enzyme-linked immunoassays (sensitivity 75% to 80% and specificity 85% to 100%) and RNA-DNA hybridisation (sensitivity 70% to 85%).[364,372] [Evidence level 4] Direct fluorescent antibody staining, however, is labour intensive and therefore unsuitable for large numbers of samples.[364] [Evidence level 4] Serology is not useful in the diagnosis of acute chlamydial infection.[364,372] [Evidence level 4]

Nucleic acid amplification has sensitivity of 70% to 95% and specificity of 97% to 99%, with the advantage of being able to test invasive as well as noninvasive samples (e.g. urine) and it is suitable for large numbers of samples. However, it is an expensive test and inhibitors may be a problem in urine samples in pregnancy.[364,372] [Evidence level 4]

Due to the high rates of chlamydial infection observed among 16- to 24-year-olds in England, Wales and Northern Ireland, the UK Department of Health (DoH) has initiated a national opportunistic screening programme for all men and women under the age of 25 years. The first phase to roll out this programme has commenced in ten areas in England and the second phase is expected to commence by 2004. One of the healthcare settings for opportunistic screening is antenatal clinics. Therefore, when the roll out is complete, all pregnant women under the age of 25 years attending antenatal clinics will be offered screening for chlamydia.

Further information on screening for chlamydia in pregnant women can be found in the Scottish Intercollegiate Guidelines Network (SIGN) guideline, *Management of genital chlamydia trachomatis infection.*[373]

RECOMMENDATION

Pregnant women should not be offered routine screening for asymptomatic chlamydia because there is insufficient evidence on its effectiveness and cost effectiveness. However, this policy is likely to change with the implementation of the national opportunistic chlamydia screening programme. [C]

Future research

Further investigation into the benefits of screening for chlamydia in pregnancy is needed.

10.4   Cytomegalovirus

Cytomegalovirus (CMV) is a member of the herpesvirus family. It remains latent in the host after primary infection and may become active again, particularly during times of compromised immunity.

In England and Wales in 1992 and 1993 (n = 1.36 million live births) there were 47 reported cases of CMV infections in pregnant women with 22 resulting in intrauterine death or stillbirth.[374] [Evidence level 3] Congenital infection is thought to occur in 3/1000 live births.[375,376] [Evidence level 3] This is likely to be an underestimate, as women who suffer a stillbirth or intrauterine death are more likely to be investigated for CMV infection.

At present, antenatal screening for this condition is thought to be inappropriate, as it is not currently possible accurately to determine which pregnancies are likely to result in the birth of an infected infant,[376] [Evidence level 3] there is no way to determine which infected infants will have serious sequelae, there is no currently available vaccines or prophylactic therapy for the prevention of transmission and no way to determine whether intrauterine transmission has occurred.[377,378] [Evidence level 4]

RECOMMENDATION

The available evidence does not support routine cytomegalovirus screening in pregnant women and it should not be offered. [B]

10.5   Hepatitis B virus

Hepatitis B is a virus that infects the liver and many people with hepatitis B viral infection have no symptoms. The hepatitis B virus has an incubation period of 6 weeks to 6 months, it is excreted in various body fluids including blood, saliva, vaginal fluid and breast milk; these fluids may be highly infectious.

The prevalence of hepatitis B surface antigen (HBsAg) in pregnant women in the UK has been found to range from 0.5% to 1%.[379–381] [Evidence level 3] An older study of the prevalence of hepatitis B virus in pregnant women in the West Midlands from 1974–1977 reported a lower rate of 0.1%.[382] [Evidence level 3] The range in prevalence rates is most likely due to wide variation in prevalence among different ethnic groups, as Asian women in particular appear to have a higher prevalence of HBsAg.[379] [Evidence level III] Consequently, Asian babies also have higher rates of mother-to-child transmission of HBsAg.[382] [Evidence level 3]

As many as 85% of babies born to mothers who are positive for the hepatitis e antigen (eAg) will become HBsAg carriers and subsequently become chronic carriers, compared with 31%

of babies who are born to mothers who are eAg negative (RR 2.8, 95% CI 1.69 to 4.47).[383] [Evidence level 3] It has been estimated that chronic carriers of HBsAg are 22 times more likely to die from hepatocellular carcinoma or cirrhosis than noncarriers (95% CI 11.5 to 43.2).[384] [Evidence level 2b]

Approximately 21% of hepatitis B viral infections reported in England and Wales among children under the age of 15 years is due to mother-to-child transmission.[385] [Evidence level 3] mother-to-child transmission of the hepatitis B virus is approximately 95% preventable through administration of vaccine and immunoglobulin to the baby at birth.[386-392] [Evidence level 1b]

To prevent mother-to-child transmission, all pregnant women who are carriers of hepatitis B virus need to be identified. Screening of blood samples is the accepted standard for antenatal screening for hepatitis B virus. Screening consists of three stages: screening for HBsAg, confirmatory testing with a new sample upon a positive result and, where infection is confirmed, testing for hepatitis B e-markers in order to determine whether the baby will need immunoglobulin in addition to vaccine.[393] Using risk factors to identify 'high-risk' women for HBsAg screening would miss about half of all pregnant women with HBsAg infection.[394] [Evidence level 3] Screening for HBsAg in saliva samples found a sensitivity of 92% (95% CI 84.5% to 99.5%) and a specificity of 86.8% (95% CI 76.0% to 97.6%) when compared with serum samples.[395] [Evidence level 3] Because of the high proportion of cases of mother-to-child transmission that can be prevented through vaccination and immunisation and because risk factor screening fails to identify carriers, the UK National Screening Committee recommends that all pregnant women be screened for hepatitis B virus (Health Services Circular 1998/127).

RECOMMENDATION

Serological screening for hepatitis B virus should be offered to pregnant women so that effective postnatal intervention can be offered to infected women to decrease the risk of mother-to-child transmission. [A]

10.6   Hepatitis C virus

As one of the major causes of liver cirrhosis, hepatocellular carcinoma and liver failure, hepatitis C virus (HCV) is a major public health concern.[396] Acquisition of the virus can occur through infected blood transfusions (pre-1992 blood screening), injection of drugs, tattooing, body piercing and mother-to-child transmission. HCV prevalence observed in studies of antenatal populations in England ranges from 0.14 in the West Midlands (95% CI 0.05 to 0.33) to 0.8 in London (95% CI 0.55 to 1.0).[397] Based on estimates from other European countries, the risk of mother-to-child transmission in the UK is estimated to lie between 3% and 5%.[397] Another study estimated that 70 births each year are infected with HCV as a result of mother-to-child transmission in the UK, which represents an overall antenatal prevalence of 0.16% (95% CI 0.09 to 0.25).[398] [Evidence level 3]

Although there is consistent evidence that the risk of mother-to-child transmission of HCV increases with increasing maternal viral load,[399,400] whether a threshold level for transmission exists remains unknown. [Evidence level 3]

A higher proportion of infected babies has been observed among those delivered vaginally compared with those delivered by caesarean section but only one study has demonstrated a statistically significant difference.[401] [Evidence level 3]

The clinical course of HCV in infants who have acquired the disease through mother-to-child transmission is unclear. Among 104 children studied who were infected through mother-to-child transmission, two developed hepatomegaly with no other clinical symptoms related to HCV infection reported.[402] [Evidence level 3] It has also been suggested that a proportion of infected children subsequently become HCV-RNA negative. In one study of 23 infants, five infants tested HCV-RNA positive 48 hours after birth. All five infants became HCV-RNA negative and lost HCV antibodies by 6 months after birth.[403] [Evidence level 3] Although HCV infection in infants may be benign in the short to medium term, given that HCV infection in adults has a long latency period, it is possible that infected children may develop long-term clinical outcomes.

Screening for HCV in the UK involves detection of anti-HCV antibodies in serum by enzyme immunoassays (EIAs) or enzyme-linked immunosorbent assays (ELISA). Upon a positive result, a second ELISA or a confirmatory recombinant immunoblot assay (RIBA) is performed on the same sample. If the second test is positive, the woman is informed and a second sample is taken to confirm the diagnosis. Using polymerase chain reaction (PCR) as the gold standard, the sensitivity and specificity of third-generation assays are reported to be 100% and 66%, respectively.[404] [Evidence level 3] Other estimates of specificities from studies of blood donors using ELISA and RIBA report ranges between 96% and 99%.[405,406] Upon confirmation of a positive screening test, a woman should be offered post-test counselling and referral to a hepatologist for management and treatment of her infection.

RECOMMENDATION

Pregnant women should not be offered routine screening for hepatitis C virus because there is insufficient evidence on its effectiveness and cost effectiveness. [C]

10.7 HIV

Infection with human immunodeficiency virus (HIV) begins with an asymptomatic stage with gradual compromise of immune function eventually leading to acquired immunodeficiency syndrome (AIDS). The time between HIV infection and development of AIDS ranges from a few months to as long as 17 years in untreated patients.[353]

The prevalence of HIV infection in pregnant women in London in 2001 was about 1/286 (0.35%), a 22% increase from the year 2000 (1/349 or 0.29%). Elsewhere in England, the prevalence of HIV infection is reported to be around one in 2256 (0.044%).[407,408] [Evidence level 3]

In the absence of intervention, mother-to-child transmission was reported to occur in 25.5% of deliveries and was reduced to 8% with antiretroviral treatment with zidovudine.[409] [Evidence level 1b] The combination of interventions (i.e. combination antiretroviral therapy, caesarean section and avoidance of breastfeeding) can further reduce the risk of transmission to 1%.[410] In the UK, mother-to-child transmission rates were 19.6% (95% CI 8.0% to 32%) in 1993 and declined to 2.2% (95% CI 0% to 7.8%) in 1998.[411]

By the end of January 2001, a total of 1036 HIV-infected children had been reported in the UK (excluding Scotland). mother-to-child transmission of HIV accounted for about 70% of the cases.[412] [Evidence level 3] Some 1885 children have been born in the UK (excluding Scotland) to HIV-positive mothers, of which 712 were known to be HIV positive (457 indeterminate, 716 not infected) by the end of January 2001.[412] [Evidence level 3]

In the year 1999, there were 621,872 live births in England and Wales (ONS Birth Statistics, 2000). In the same year, 404 babies were born to HIV infected mothers resulting in 66 HIV-positive babies, 244 not infected and 94 as yet undetermined.[412] [Evidence level 3]

The most common way to diagnose HIV infection is by a test for antibodies against HIV-1 and HIV-2. HIV antibody is detectable in at least 95% of patients within 3 months of infection.[353] Early HIV diagnosis improves outcomes for the mother and can reduce the rate of disease progression.

Currently available HIV tests are more than 99% sensitive and specific for the detection of HIV antibodies.[413] The sensitivities and specificities of various commercial HIV screening assays can be found at the Medicines and Healthcare Products Regulatory Agency website at www.medical-devices.gov.uk. Available tests for HIV diagnosis in pregnant women include the EIA and Western blot protocol, which is at least 99% and 99.99% sensitive and specific,[413] and the 'two-ELISA approach' protocol.[414] [Evidence level 3]

In both protocols, an EIA is initially used and if the results are unreactive, a negative report may be generated.[415] [Evidence level 4]

If the reaction is positive, further testing with different assays (if EIA, then at least one of which is based on a different principle from the first) is warranted. If both confirmatory tests are nonreactive, a negative report may be issued. If the confirmatory tests are reactive, one more test with a new specimen should be obtained in order to ensure no procedural errors have occurred.

mother-to-child transmission of HIV infection can be greatly reduced through diagnosis of the mother before the baby's birth so that appropriate antenatal interventions can be recommended.[416] [Evidence level 1a] [417] [Evidence level 1b] Interventions to reduce mother-to-child transmission of HIV during the antenatal period include antiretroviral therapy, elective caesarean section delivery and advice on avoidance of breastfeeding after delivery (see evidence table).

The risk of infant mortality and maternal death was found to be reduced with zidovudine treatment compared with treatment with placebo (infant mortality: OR 0.57, 95% CI 0.38 to 0.85, maternal death: OR 0.30, 95% CI 0.13 to 0.68). All other outcomes measured (i.e. incidence of stillbirth, preterm delivery, low birthweight, side effects in child, side effects in mother) did not show a significant difference between the treated and untreated groups.[416] [Evidence level 1a] Similarly, nevirapine compared with zidovudine did not show any significant difference in the above mentioned outcomes.[416] [Evidence level 1a] There were also no significant adverse effects reported when caesarean section was compared with vaginal delivery.[418] [Evidence level 1b] Newer antiretrovirals, which are likely to be in use in developed countries, exist. However, these treatments have not yet been evaluated in RCTs.

The use of antiretrovirals to reduce mother-to-child transmission has resulted in resistant mutations. This has raised concerns about the efficacy of antiretroviral treatment decreasing with time.[419,420] [Evidence level 3] In a substudy to the Pediatric AIDS Clinical Trials Group Protocol, 15% of the women (95% CI 8 to 23%) developed nevirapine resistant mutations by 6 weeks' postpartum.[419] [Evidence level 3] In another study, although 17.3% of the women and 8.3% of the HIV infected infants developed zidovudine- or nucleotide reverse-transcriptase inhibitor-resistant mutations, respectively, there was no significant association detected between perinatal transmission and the presence of any resistant mutations.[420] [Evidence level 3]

Since 1999, the NHS has recommended that all pregnant women (i.e., not just in areas of higher prevalence as recommended in 1992) be offered and recommended an HIV test as an integral part of antenatal care, and that the offer be recorded (Health Service Circular 1999/183). The Expert Advisory Group on AIDS (www.doh.gov.uk/eaga/) and the UK National Screening Committee (www.nsc.nhs.uk/) websites can be checked periodically for updates on HIV screening information.

RECOMMENDATIONS

Pregnant women should be offered screening for HIV infection early in antenatal care because appropriate antenatal interventions can reduce mother-to-child transmission of HIV infection. [A]

A system of clear referral paths should be established in each unit or department so that pregnant women who are diagnosed with an HIV infection are managed and treated by the appropriate specialist teams. [D]

10.8 Rubella

The aim of screening for rubella in pregnancy is to identify susceptible women so that postpartum vaccination may protect future pregnancies against rubella infection and its consequences. Hence, rubella screening does not attempt to identify current affected pregnancies.

Rubella infection is characterised by a febrile rash but may be asymptomatic in 20% to 50% of cases.[421] There is no treatment to prevent or reduce mother-to-child transmission of rubella for the current pregnancy.[422] [Evidence level 4] Detection of susceptibility during pregnancy, however, enables postpartum vaccination to occur to protect future pregnancies.

Surveillance in England and Wales by the National Congenital Rubella Surveillance Programme (NCRSP) indicates that susceptibility in the antenatal population varies with parity as well as with ethnicity. Susceptibility is slightly higher in nulliparous women (2%) than in parous women (1.2%).[423] [Evidence level 3] Certain ethnic groups also appear to have higher susceptibility, such as women from the Mediterranean region (4%), Asian and black women (5%) and Oriental women (8%), compared with less than 2% in white women, with an overall susceptibility of about 2.5% reported for pregnant women.[424] [Evidence level 3]

In 1995, the incidence of rubella in susceptible nulliparous women was 2/431 (risk/1000 = 4.6) and 0/547 in parous women, resulting in an overall risk of 2/1000 susceptible women.[423] [Evidence level 3]

From 1976 to 1978, among 966 pregnant women in England and Wales with confirmed rubella infection, 523 (54%) had elective abortions, 36 (4%) had a miscarriage, 9 women had stillbirths (4 of which had severe anomalies) and 5 infants died in the neonatal period.[425] [Evidence level 2b]

Since the introduction of the measles, mumps and rubella vaccine, an average of three births affected by congenital rubella a year and four rubella-associated terminations were registered with the NCRSP (births) and Office for National Statistics (terminations) from 1996 to 2000.[422] [Evidence level 4]

For pregnant women who are offered a rubella susceptibility test, the protective level of antibodies was originally set at 15 international units (iu). However, newer, more sensitive screening tests[426] [Evidence level 2a] have resulted in the detection of women with low but protective levels of antibodies being reported as rubella susceptible and therefore a lower cutoff of 10 iu is the level recommended in the National Screening Committee draft document for the UK in 2002.[422] [Evidence level 4] Results of rubella screening should be reported as rubella antibody detected or not detected as opposed to reports of 'immune' or 'susceptible', to avoid misinterpretation.[422] [Evidence level 4] If rubella antibody is **not** detected, rubella vaccination after pregnancy should be advised.[427]

A Public Health Laboratory service (PHLS) guideline offers an algorithm for the management of pregnant women who present with rash illness.[427]

Detection of rubella does not protect against mother-to-child transmission in the current pregnancy. However, protection of subsequent pregnancies against the rubella virus will prevent future mother-to-child transmission of rubella and reduce the risk of stillbirth and miscarriage due to rubella infection.

In a cohort study of pregnant women with confirmed rubella infection at different stages of pregnancy, a follow-up of nearly 70% of the surviving infants (n = 269) found that 43% (n = 117) of infants were congenitally infected.[425] [Evidence level 2b] Congenital infection in the first 12 weeks of pregnancy among mothers with symptoms was over 80% and reduced to 25% at the end of the second trimester. 100% of infants infected during the first 11 weeks of pregnancy had rubella defects.[425] [Evidence level 2b]

In another study, a decline in the rate of infection was seen from weeks 9 to 16 of gestation (rate of infection 57% to 70%) compared with weeks 17 to 20 (22%) and weeks 21 to 24 (17%) and a minimal risk of deafness only was observed in the children who were born to mothers infected during the 17th to 24th weeks of gestation.[428] [Evidence level 2b]

About 10% of congenital rubella cases reported since 1990 are associated with maternal reinfection[422] [Evidence level 4] and maternal reinfection is usually diagnosed through changes in antibody concentration only.[427] In a study of seven asymptomatic rubella reinfections in early pregnancy, six pregnant women went to term and the infants showed no evidence of intrauterine infection. One pregnancy was terminated and the rubella virus was not identified in the products of conception.[429] [Evidence level 3] Symptomatic maternal reinfection is very rare and risk of fetal damage, which is presumed to be significant, has not been quantified.[427]

Vaccination during pregnancy is contraindicated because of fears that the vaccine could be teratogenic.[422] [Evidence level 4] However, in an evaluation of surveillance data from the USA, UK, Sweden and Germany of 680 live births to susceptible women who were inadvertently vaccinated during or within 3 months of pregnancy (with HPV-77, Cendehill or RA27/3), none of the children was born with congenital rubella syndrome.[430] [Evidence level 3]

Screening for the rubella antibody in pregnancy helps to identify susceptible women so that rubella vaccination can be offered postpartum to protect future pregnancies.

RECOMMENDATION

Rubella susceptibility screening should be offered early in antenatal care to identify women at risk of contracting rubella infection and to enable vaccination in the postnatal period for the protection of future pregnancies. [B]

10.9 Streptococcus group B

Group B streptococcus (GBS), *Streptococcus agalactaie*, is the leading cause of serious neonatal infection in the UK.[431] Although GBS can affect a pregnant woman or her fetus or both, it may exist in the genital and gastrointestinal tract of pregnant women with no symptoms and may also exist without causing harm.

It is estimated that GBS can be recovered from 6.6% to 20% of mothers in the USA.[432,433] [Evidence level 3] In the UK, the prevalence has been estimated at 28%, with no association to maternal age or parity.[434] [Evidence level 3] Maternal intrapartum GBS colonisation is a risk factor for early-onset disease in infants.[435] [Evidence level 3] Early-onset GBS disease (occurring in infants within the first week of life) can result in many conditions, including sepsis, pneumonia and meningitis.[436] The prevalence of early-onset GBS disease in England and Wales is estimated to range from 0.4/1000 to 1.4/1000 live births,[435,437,438] [Evidence level 3] which is equivalent to approximately 340 babies per annum. A 2001 UK surveillance study identified 376 cases of early-onset GBS (prevalence in England 0.5, 95% CI 0.5 to 0.6), among which 39 infants died.[431] [Evidence level 3] In 2000, there were 2519 neonatal deaths from all causes in the UK.

The collection of cultures between 35 and 37 weeks of gestation appears to achieve the best sensitivity and specificity for detection of women who are colonised at the time of delivery.[439] [Evidence level 3] Swabs of both the vagina and rectum provide the highest predictive value for identification of women colonised by GBS.[440] [Evidence level 3] Studies have also indicated that women who obtain their own screening specimen, with appropriate instruction, have comparable sensitivity to specimens collected by a physician. With any positive culture used as the reference standard, self-collected sensitivity ranged from 79% to 97% and physician sensitivity was 82% to 83%.[441,442] [Evidence level 3] When asked about preference, 75% of women either preferred to collect their own specimen or were indifferent as to who collected their swab.[441] [Evidence level 3]

A comparison of screening methods (obtaining cultures from all pregnant women or identifying women for intrapartum treatment through clinical risk factor assessment) in a large interstate study in the USA found that the risk of early-onset disease was more than 50% lower in the universally screened group compared with those screened by assessment of clinical risk factors to identify candidates for intrapartum antibiotics (adjusted relative risk 0.46, 95% CI 0.36 to 0.60).[443] [Evidence level 2b]

However, a systematic review of RCTs of intrapartum antibiotics for the reduction of perinatal GBS infection have not yet demonstrated an effect on neonatal deaths from infection (Peto OR 0.12, 95% CI 0.01 to 2.0), although a reduction in infant colonisation rate (Peto OR 0.10, 95% CI 0.07 to 0.14), as well as a reduction in early-onset neonatal infection with GBS, was observed (Peto OR 0.17, 95% CI 0.07 to 0.39).[444] [Evidence level 1a] A review of trials of antibiotics administered in the antenatal period found that two of four studies reported a reduction in maternal colonisation at delivery and that results from five other trials showed a reduction of 80% in early-onset GBS with intrapartum treatment.[445] [Evidence level 2a] In a trial that compared 5 ml 2% clindamycin cream intravaginally with no treatment in women admitted in labour who had had a positive culture for GBS at 26 to 28 weeks of gestation, no difference was found in the reduction of colonisation.[446] [Evidence level 1b]

With an assumption of 80% effectiveness for the prevention of early-onset GBS disease in infants with intrapartum antibiotics, the number of babies affected each year will decrease from an estimated 340 to 68. This means that for every 1000 women treated with intrapartum antibiotics for GBS, 1.4 cases of early-onset disease may be prevented. However, this estimate assumes that screening will identify all GBS carriers and therefore, in practice, the number of women treated to prevent one case is most likely higher.

No trials comparing antenatal screening with no antenatal screening have been conducted, nor have any trials comparing different screening strategies been identified. Therefore, estimates of efficacy of screening strategies are based only on observational studies. In the USA, an analysis of the incidence of early-onset GBS disease from 1993 to 1998 found a decline from 1.7/1000 live births in 1993 to 0.6/1000 live births in 1998 (65% decrease, p < 0.001),[447] [Evidence level 3] which is the incidence observed in the UK in 2001.[431] [Evidence level 3] This 65% decrease in early-onset GBS disease coincided with efforts in the USA to promote the wider use of intrapartum antibiotics for the prevention of GBS disease in infants less than 7 days old. An Australian study that determined the incidence of GBS in the population before implementing a screening programme found a significant decrease from 4.9/1000 to 0.8/1000 live births after the intervention.[448] [Evidence level 3]

Further information on GBS, such as guidance for when GBS is incidentally detected during pregnancy, can be found in the forthcoming RCOG guideline on the prevention of early onset neonatal Group B streptococcal disease (due for publication late 2003; draft document available for information on the RCOG website at www.rcog.org.uk/resources/Public/Group%20B%20Strep_draft.DOC).

Economic considerations (see Appendix 2)

The review of the economic literature on GBS found 26 articles including the guideline published by the Royal College of Obstetrics and Gynaecology on the prevention of early onset neonatal Group B streptococcal disease. Of these studies, 25 were relevant to the topic and were examined in detail. However, almost all the economic studies were conducted in the USA setting (one was from Australia). The extrapolation and generalisability of the results of the US studies was limited also because the prevalence of the disease used was not comparable with a UK setting. Four of the US studies were of sufficient quality to extrapolate data for the economic model.

An economic model was constructed to estimate the number of early-onset GBS cases in infants averted due to screening and treatment. The model also took into consideration how many cases of early-onset GBS were missed following each screening method and how many cases of early-onset GBS were prevented through the screening and subsequent treatment of the pregnant women. The benefit or harm to the pregnant women and infants over and above the financial costs to the NHS were not included in the model because of the lack of data. The only unit of benefit included in the model was 'case of early-onset GBS averted'. This is a limitation of the model.

The model set out to calculate the following outcomes:

- the number of pregnant women treated per case of early-onset GBS averted
- the number of cases of early-onset GBS averted by screening and subsequent treatment
- an estimate of the total financial cost to the health service provider of the different screening methods
- the average cost per case prevented and the incremental cost effectiveness of the two screening methods.

During the course of developing this model, it became clear that data on a number of crucial parameters in the model were not available in the clinical literature. These were:

- the prevalence of early-onset GBS in infants of women who have been screened positively using the universal (bacteriological) screening strategy
- the number of women screened as falsely negative (who have the disease but are screened as negative) in the universal screening strategy
- the prevalence of GBS among the women with the risk factors (the proportion of 'true positive' women who have risk factors for GBS).

The true prevalence of GBS among women with risk factors would indicate the proportion of women treated unnecessarily for GBS (who have risk factors but do not have the disease). This would probably give an idea of the avoidable cases of severe anaphylaxis due to treatment of women in the risk factor group.

Without good estimates of the prevalence of disease, it was not possible to calculate the overall number of cases of early-onset BGS avoided and costs of implementing each screening strategy.

Early-onset GBS is a severe disease and the treatment has very high costs for the NHS. Therefore, missing even one case could presumably change the cost effectiveness of the two methods. More clinical evidence is required in order to undertake an economic model of different screening methods for GBS.

RECOMMENDATIONS

Pregnant women should not be offered routine antenatal screening for group B streptococcus (GBS) because evidence of its clinical effectiveness and cost effectiveness remains uncertain. [C]

Future research

Further research into the effectiveness and cost effectiveness of antenatal screening for GBS are needed.

10.10   Syphilis

Syphilis is a sexually acquired infection caused by *Treponema pallidum*. The body's immune response to syphilis is the production non-specific and specific treponemal antibodies. The first notable response to infection is the production of specific anti-treponemal immunoglobulin M (IgM), which is detectable towards the end of the second week of infection. By the time symptoms appear, most people infected with syphilis have detectable levels of immunoglobulin G (IgG) and IgM.[449] [Evidence level 4] However, syphilis may also be asymptomatic and latent for many years.[353]

The incidence of infectious syphilis in England and Wales is low, but four outbreaks of infectious syphilis occurred in England from 1997 to 2000.[450] In the USA, an epidemic of syphilis translated into an epidemic of congenital syphilis with rates increasing from 4.3/100,000 live births in 1982 to 94.7/100,000 in 1992.[451]

The prevalence of syphilis in pregnant women as estimated by reports from genitourinary medicine clinics in England and Wales was 0.068/1000 live births (95% CI 0.057 to 0.080) from 1994 to 1997, ranging from zero in East Anglia to 0.3/1000 live births in the North East Thames region.[452] [Evidence level 3] [453] [Evidence level 4] Thirty-four cases of early congenital syphilis (under age 2 years) were reported by genitourinary medicine clinics in England and Wales between 1988 and 1995,[453] [Evidence level 4] and 35 cases were reported from 1995 to 2000,[454] [Evidence level 3] giving an incidence of 0.92/100,000 live births per year (calculated with livebirth rates from ONS Birth Statistics, 2000).

In pregnant women with early untreated syphilis, 70% to 100% of infants will be infected and one-third will be stillborn.[455] [Evidence level 3] [456,457] [Evidence level 4]

mother-to-child transmission of syphilis in pregnancy is associated with neonatal death, congenital syphilis (which may cause long-term disability), stillbirth and preterm birth. However, because penicillin became widely available in the 1950s, no data from recent prospective observational studies in developed countries are available. Data from two observational studies in the USA in the 1950s and, more recently, from developing countries, provide a picture of the effects of untreated syphilis compared with women who did not have syphilis or who had been treated for syphilis. Among pregnancies in women with early untreated syphilis, 25% resulted in stillbirth compared with 3% among women without syphilis; 14% died in the neonatal period compared with 2.2% among women without syphilis and 41% resulted in a congenitally infected infant (compared with 0% among women without syphilis).[455] [Evidence level 3] These findings were reported to be significant, but the level of significance was not specified in the study. In the other US study, 25% of babies were born preterm to mothers with syphilis compared with 11.5% among women without syphilis. The sample size was small and this finding was not reported to be significant.[458] [Evidence level 3] The risk of congenital transmission declines with increasing duration of maternal syphilis prior to pregnancy.

Among 142 pregnant women in South Africa who tested positive for syphilis, 99 were 'adequately' treated with at least two doses of 2.4 mega-units of benzathine penicillin and 43 received 'inadequate' treatment of less than two doses. Among inadequately treated women, perinatal death occurred in 11 (26%) cases compared with 4 (4%) cases among adequately treated women (p < 0.0001).[459] [Evidence level 3]

There are two main classifications of serological tests for syphilis: non-treponemal and treponemal. Non-treponemal tests detect non-specific treponemal antibodies and include the Venereal Diseases Research Laboratory (VDRL) and rapid plasma reagin (RPR) tests. Treponemal tests detect specific treponemal antibodies and include EIAs, *T. pallidum* haemagglutination assay (TPHA) and the fluorescent treponemal antibody-absorbed test (FTA-abs).

EIA tests that detect IgG or IgG and IgM are rapidly replacing the VDRL and TPHA combination for syphilis screening in the UK.[449] [Evidence level 4] Screening with a treponemal IgG EIA is useful for detecting syphilis antibodies in patients who are infected with HIV and is comparable to the VDRL and TPHA combination in terms of sensitivity and specificity.[460,461]

EIAs are over 98% sensitive and over 99% specific. Non-treponemal tests, on the other hand, may result in false negatives, particularly in very early or late syphilis, in patients with reinfection or those who are HIV positive. The positive predictive value of non-treponemal tests is poor when used alone in low prevalence populations. In general, treponemal tests are 98% sensitive at all stages of syphilis (except early primary syphilis) and more specific (98% to 99%) than non-treponemal tests. None of these serological tests will detect syphilis in its incubation stage, which may last for an average of 25 days.[453] [Evidence level 3]

A reactive result on screening requires confirmatory testing with a different treponemal test of equal sensitivity to the one initially used and, preferably, one with greater specificity. A discrepant result on confirmatory testing needs further testing, which is provided by Birmingham Public Health Laboratory (PHL), Bristol PHL, Manchester PHL, Newcastle PHL and Sheffield PHL.[449] [Evidence level 4]

Following confirmation of a reactive specimen, testing of a second specimen to verify the results and ensure correct identification of the person should be done. Whether or not the pregnant woman should then be referred for expert assessment and diagnosis in a genitourinary medicine clinic should be considered. To assess the stage of the infection or to monitor the efficacy of treatment, a quantitative non-treponemal or a specific test for treponemal IgM should be performed.[449] [Evidence level 4]

Not all women who test positive will have syphilis, as these serological tests cannot distinguish between different treponematoses (e.g. syphilis, yaws, pinta and bejel). Therefore, positive results should be interpreted with caution.

In the UK, the Clinical Effectiveness Group of the Association for Genitourinary Medicine and the Medical Society for the Study of Venereal Disease recommend screening for syphilis at the first antenatal appointment.[456] [Evidence level 4]

Parenteral penicillin effectively prevents mother-to-child transmission of syphilis, although available evidence is insufficient to determine whether or not the current treatment regimens in use in the UK are optimal.[462] [Evidence level 1a] In a US study of the effectiveness of treatment with penicillin, a 98.2% success rate for preventing congenital syphilis was observed.[463] [Evidence level 2b] Treatment of syphilis in pregnancy with penicillin has not shown any difference in adverse pregnancy outcomes when compared with untreated seronegative women.[464] [Evidence level 2a] Although erythromycin is useful in the treatment of syphilis for non-pregnant women who are allergic to penicillin, treatment of pregnant women with erythromycin has been shown to be ineffective in some cases.[465] [Evidence level 3] The European and UK guidelines on the management of syphilis in pregnant women with penicillin allergy suggest desensitisation to penicillin followed by treatment with penicillin as an alternative.[456,457] All women testing positive for syphilis should be referred to a specialist for treatment.

Economic considerations (see Appendix 2)

An economic model was constructed to consider three screening options: no screening, universal screening and selective, ethnicity-based screening. Clearly, the prevalence of syphilis in each strategy was assumed to be different, higher for the ethnicity-based strategy than for the universal strategy. The ethnicity-based approach will be associated with varying levels of prevalence depending upon how the strategy is constructed, based on geographical location (and proportion of women of specific ethnic origins in each group) or on screening for ethnicity during antenatal check-ups.

The costs incorporated in the model were only the costs incurred by the health service. A societal perspective would increase the overall costs of providing screening and would be greater for the universal group but data do not exist on whether these costs would differ by screening method. If more couples were subject to the test using a universal approach, there would be potentially more harm incurred by undertaking unnecessary tests.

The benefits and harm of syphilis screening (to the couples undertaking the screening test) has not been explored in the literature. The test is not associated with a choice to end the pregnancy and the treatment for syphilis is not associated with adverse effects that should be incorporated into the analysis. However, the psychological cost and benefit of undergoing the test have not been estimated in the model, since these data were unavailable.

The model also incorporated the costs of the economic consequences of syphilis cases missed due to the different screening methods. The economic consequences of syphilis were considered to be preterm birth, miscarriage and fetal death and the lifetime treatment costs of the cases of congenital syphilis.

RECOMMENDATIONS

Screening for syphilis should be offered to all pregnant women at an early stage in antenatal care because treatment of syphilis is beneficial to the mother and fetus. [B]

Because syphilis is a rare condition in the UK and a positive result does not necessarily mean that a woman has syphilis, clear paths of referral for the management of women testing positive for syphilis should be established. [Good practice point]

10.11 Toxoplasmosis

Caused by the parasite *Toxoplasma gondii*, primary toxoplasmosis infection is usually asymptomatic in healthy women. Once infected, a lifelong antibody response provides immunity from further infection.

A total of 423 cases of toxoplasmosis related to pregnancy were reported to the PHLS, Communicable Disease Surveillance Centre (PHLS CDSC) in England and Wales from 1981 to 1992, during which time there was an average of 667,000 live births per year (ONS, Population Trends). A systematic review from 1996 identified 15 studies that reported toxoplasmosis incidence among susceptible (i.e., antibody negative) women in Europe.[466] [Evidence level 3] Although no data specific to England or Wales were found, incidence rates for other countries ranged from 2.4/1000 women in Finland to 16/1000 women in France. Approximately 75% to 90% of pregnant women in the UK are estimated to be susceptible to toxoplasmosis.[467,468] The prevalence of congenital toxoplasma infection was recently reported to be approximately 0.3/1000 live births in Denmark.[469] [Evidence level 3]

Toxoplasmosis infection is acquired via four routes in humans:

- ingestion of viable tissue cysts in undercooked or uncooked meat (e.g., salami, which is cured) or tachyzoites in the milk of infected intermediate hosts
- ingestion of oocytes excreted by cats and contaminating soil or water (e.g., unwashed fruit or vegetables contaminated by cat faeces)
- transplanted organs or blood products from other humans infected with toxoplasmosis
- mother-to-child transmission when primary infection occurs during pregnancy.

A study in six European centres identified undercooked meat and cured meat products as the principal factor contributing to toxoplasma infection in pregnant women.[470] [Evidence level 3] Contact with soil contributed to a substantial minority of infections.

When primary infection with *T. gondii* occurs during pregnancy, the risk of mother-to-child transmission increases with gestation at acquisition of maternal infection.[471–473] [Evidence level 3] The reported overall risk of congenital toxoplasmosis ranges from 18% to 44%. The risk is low in early pregnancy at 6% to 26% from 7 to 15 weeks of gestation and rising to 32% to 93% at 29 to 34 weeks of gestation.[471–473] [Evidence level 3]

Clinical manifestations of congenital toxoplasmosis include inflammatory lesions in the brain and retina and choroids that may lead to permanent neurological damage or visual impairment. Reported overall rates of clinical manifestations range from 14% to 27% among infants born to infected mothers.[472,473] [Evidence level 3] In contrast to the risk of transmission, the risk of an infected infant developing clinical signs of disease (hydrocephalus, intracranial calcification, retinochoroiditis) is highest when infection occurs early in pregnancy, declining from an estimated 61% (95% CI 34 to 85%) at 13 weeks to 9% (95% CI 4% to 17%) at 36 weeks.[472] [Evidence level 3]

As primary toxoplasma infection is usually asymptomatic, infected women can only reliably be detected by serological testing. Antenatal screening for toxoplasma infection involves initial testing to determine IgG and IgM positivity. Subsequently, in women in whom antibodies are not detected (i.e., susceptible), monthly or three-monthly re-testing to determine seroconversion is necessary. Positive results should then be confirmed by multiple tests.[474] [Evidence level 3] However, available screening tests to determine seroconversion cannot distinguish between infection acquired during pregnancy or up to 12 months beforehand and women who have acquired the infection before conception are not at risk of fetal infection.[475]

For pregnant women with a diagnosis of primary toxoplasma infection, an informed decision as to whether or not to undergo prenatal diagnosis needs to be made. To calculate the risk of clinical signs in a fetus born to an infected woman, it is possible to multiply the risk of congenital infection by the risk of signs among congenitally infected children. For example, at 26 weeks of gestation the risk of maternal–fetal transmission is 40% and the risk of clinical signs in an infected fetus is 25%. The overall risk is therefore 10% (0.4 x 0.25). If this calculation is repeated for all gestational ages, a positively skewed curve results that reaches a maximum of 10% at 24 to 30 weeks of gestation. In the second and third trimesters, the risk never falls below 5% and is 6% just before delivery.

Knowledge of these risks allows women to balance the risks of harm and benefit when deciding about treatment, amniocentesis or ending the pregnancy. The possible reduction in this risk that might be achieved by prenatal treatment must be balanced against the risk of fetal loss of 1% associated with amniocentesis.[307] Most importantly, they need to know the risk of disability due to neurological damage or visual impairment. Unfortunately, information on these latter outcomes is less reliable and the effect of gestation is not known.

Primary prevention of toxoplasmosis with the provision of information about how to avoid toxoplasma infection before or early in pregnancy should be given. Women should be informed about the risks of not cooking meat thoroughly, possible contact with cat faeces, not washing their hands after touching soil, not washing vegetables thoroughly and eating cured meat products.

Of two systematic reviews on the effects of antiparasitic treatment on women who acquire primary toxoplasmosis infection during pregnancy, the first identified no RCTs.[476] The second identified nine cohort studies that compared treatment (spiramycin alone, pyrimethamine-sulphonamides or a combination of the two) with no treatment.[477] [Evidence level 2a] Five of the studies reported a treatment effect and four reported no treatment effect and none of the studies accounted for the rise in the risk of transmission with gestation at maternal infection.

Treatment with spiramycin and pyrimethamine-sulphonamides is reported to be well tolerated and non-teratogenic, although sulpha drugs may carry a risk of kernicterus in infants and also of bone marrow suppression in the mother and infant.[478]

In a comparison of antenatal screening strategies for toxoplasmosis in pregnancy, although universal screening with antenatal treatment reduced the number of cases of congenital toxoplasmosis, an additional 18.5 pregnancies were lost for each case avoided.[479] [Evidence level 3] Other costs include the unnecessary treatment or termination of uninfected or unaffected fetuses and the distress and discomfort of repeated examinations and investigations, both antenatal and postnatal. A further problem is that, even when antenatal diagnostic tests are negative, absence of congenital toxoplasmosis cannot be confirmed until the child is 12 months old. Finally, children with confirmed congenital toxoplasmosis, most of whom are asymptomatic, are labelled as at risk of sudden blindness, or even mental impairment, throughout childhood and adolescence.

An alternative to antenatal screening for toxoplasmosis is neonatal screening. Neonatal screening aims to identify neonates with congenital toxoplasmosis in order to offer treatment and clinical follow up. The vast majority of congenitally infected infants are asymptomatic in early infancy and would be missed by routine paediatric examinations. Neonatal screening is based on the detection of toxoplasma-specific IgM on Guthrie-card blood spots and has been found to detect 85% of infected infants. There are no published studies that have determined the effect of postnatal treatment compared with no treatment, or treatment of short duration compared with 1 year or more on the risk of clinical signs or impairment in children with congenital toxoplasmosis in the long term.

The UK National Screening Committee recently reported that screening for toxoplasmosis should not be offered routinely.[475] There is a lack of evidence that antenatal screening and treatment reduces mother-to-child transmission or the complications associated with toxoplasma infection.

There are also important and common adverse effects associated with antenatal screening, treatment and follow up for mother and child. Antenatal screening based on monthly or 3-monthly re-testing of susceptible women would be labour intensive and would require substantial investment without any proven benefit. Primary prevention of toxoplasmosis through avoidance of undercooked or cured meat may prove a good alternative to antenatal screening, which cannot currently be recommended.

RECOMMENDATION

Routine antenatal serological screening for toxoplasmosis should not be offered because the harms of screening may outweigh the potential benefits. [B]

Pregnant women should be informed of primary prevention measures to avoid toxoplasmosis infection such as:

- washing hands before handling food
- thoroughly washing all fruit and vegetables, including ready-prepared salads, before eating
- thoroughly cooking raw meats and ready-prepared chilled meals
- wearing gloves and thoroughly washing hands after handling soil and gardening
- avoiding cat faeces in cat litter or in soil. [C]

11. Screening for clinical conditions

11.1   Gestational diabetes mellitus

There is no consensus on the definition, management or treatment of gestational diabetes mellitus (GDM).[480] According to WHO, GDM is defined as "carbohydrate intolerance resulting in hyperglycaemia of variable severity with onset or first recognition during the pregnancy".[481] This definition, however, encompasses women diagnosed with diabetes mellitus or impaired glucose tolerance (IGT) during pregnancy, using the same cut-off levels as for non-pregnant women.[482] In pregnancy, glucose levels are usually raised above the level considered 'normal' in non-pregnant women. Therefore, GDM, by the WHO definition, includes all IGT pregnancies and is based on non-pregnant standards that do not take into account the physiological increase in glucose levels during pregnancy. This results in a large range of women who will have gestational 'diabetes' and who may not be at increased risk for adverse pregnancy outcomes.

In a review commissioned by the NHS, it was concluded that there remains considerable debate regarding the definition of gestational diabetes. There is no evidence-based threshold for diagnosis and no standardisation for the use of the terms GDM and IGT in pregnancy.[483]

The incidence of GDM varies according to how it is defined but is reported to range from 3% to 10% in developed countries[484] and to be around 2% in the UK.[483] Women who develop GDM are more likely to develop type-2 diabetes later in life.[485] [Evidence level 2a] However, it is unclear whether the detection of GDM delays or prevents the subsequent development of diabetes mellitus and there are potentially increased adverse outcomes associated with screening, such as increased obstetric intervention.[486] [Evidence level 3] Therefore, without specific advantages for the mother, pregnancy is not an ideal time to conduct population screening for diabetes mellitus.

Observational studies indicate an association between GDM and an increase in mortality rates in babies.[487] [Evidence level 3] Because mortality is rare, measuring more common adverse events as a composite measure of perinatal morbidity has also been used. Morbidity measures include factors such as neonatal encephalopathy, neonatal seizures and birth trauma. GDM has been shown to be associated with fetal macrosomia;[486] [Evidence level 3] fetal macrosomia may be associated with birth trauma as a result of shoulder dystocia. However, while macrosomia may be associated with some poor outcomes (as a marker) there is not a direct causal relationship between macrosomia, shoulder dystocia and birth trauma. Factors such as maternal size and post-maturity are also closely associated with macrosomia.[488] The use of macrosomia as a surrogate outcome is further complicated by the variation in definitions used.[483]

To be effective, a screening programme should identify women at risk and there should be an effective intervention that improves the pregnancy outcome. The rationale for screening for gestational diabetes is to reduce poor perinatal outcome. There is global variation in screening patterns, which reflects the lack of evidence about the value of screening.[489] There are several methods used for GDM screening, which may be used independently or in combination.

Risk-factor screening

The use of risk-factor screening has led to high numbers of diagnostic tests being performed but high proportions of women with GDM being missed. In one US study, 42% of pregnant women had risk factors for GDM, but the same proportion of women with GDM was found among women with risk factors as women without risk factors (3.2% versus 2.4%, p = 0.57).[490]

[Evidence level 2b] There was also no association found between the number of risk factors and risk of GDM.[490] [Evidence level 2b] In an older US study, similar results were reported with 44% of pregnant women without GDM having at least one risk factor.[491] [Evidence level 2a] Risk factor screening on its own is 50% sensitive and 58% specific.[490] [Evidence level 2b]

Universal screening

In Canada, a comparison was made with an area of universal screening and an area that did not implement screening for GDM. From 1990 to 1996, the incidence of GDM increased in the area of universal screening but not in the area of no screening (1.6% to 2.2% versus 1.4% to 1.0%, respectively). Rates of pre-eclampsia, fetal macrosomia, caesarean delivery, polyhydramnios and amniotic infections, however, remained the same in both regions.[492] [Evidence level 3]

Urinalysis

Urine testing has low sensitivity and is a poor screening test for GDM. Reported sensitivities for urine testing for the presence of glucose range from 7% to 46%, but with high specificities ranging from 84% to 99% when compared with the 50-g glucose challenge test (GCT).[493] [Evidence level 2b] [494,495] [Evidence level 3] Glucosuria is also common in pregnant women unaffected by GDM (i.e., a high number of false positives).[493] [Evidence level 2b]

Blood tests

Blood tests include the measurement of glucose in the blood or plasma, with or without prior intake of oral glucose, and the measurement of fructosamine and glycosylated haemoglobin levels (HbA1c). There exists debate regarding cutoff levels for diagnosis, the amount of oral glucose that should be administered and whether glucose testing should be preceded by fasting.

Random plasma glucose (RPG), which measures non-fasting glucose levels, is measured without administration of a glucose load and at no particular fixed time after meals. Analysis can be on plasma or whole blood. Wide variations in the sensitivity of this test have been reported, depending upon the time of day the test is administered and the threshold that is used. One study reported a sensitivity of 46% and specificity of 86% (at a threshold of 6.1 mmol/l) with the RPG in pregnant women who had eaten in the last two hours.[496] [Evidence level 2b] Another study reported a range of sensitivities and specificities, depending upon what time the test was taken. For a threshold of 5.6 mmol/l, sensitivity was 29% to 80% and specificity was 74% to 80%. For a threshold of 6.1 mmol/l, sensitivity ranged from 41% to 58% and specificity ranged from 74% to 96%. The highest sensitivity for both thresholds was found at 3 p.m.[497] [Evidence level 3]

Fasting plasma glucose is meant to be measured after a period of fasting, usually overnight. The following studies that reported sensitivities and specificities did not report the period of fasting used. In Brazil, examining a range of thresholds, maximum sensitivity (88%) and specificity (78%) was found at 4.9 mmol/l.[498] [Evidence level 2a] In Switzerland, maximum sensitivity and specificity (81% and 76%, respectively) was found at a threshold of 4.8 mmol/l.[499] [Evidence level 2a]

The 1-hour, 50-g GCT measures the blood glucose 1 hour after taking 50 g glucose (plus 150 ml fluid) orally; usually performed between 24 and 28 weeks of gestation. The sensitivity and specificity of this test is reported to be 79% and 87%, respectively.[491] [Evidence level 2a] Although glucose testing is usually performed with no regard to fasting status, studies have suggested that time since the last meal affects glucose levels. A test evaluation study compared glucose levels in women with and without GDM after three 50-g GCT tests: one after fasting, 1 hour after a meal and one 2 hours after a meal. In the control group, the fasting GCT was significantly higher than 1 or 2 hours after a meal (p < 0.01), leading to a false positive rate of 58% in the fasting state. Among the women with GDM, glucose levels 2 hours after the GCT were significantly lower than in the fasting state or 1 hour after the test (p < 0.03).[500] [Evidence level 3]

The optimal time for screening in pregnancy has been evaluated in several studies. Screening in the third trimester is reported to be the optimal time for the GCT. However, studies have also shown success with repeat testing during the three trimesters. In studies that only confirmed GDM (with 3-hour, 100-g glucose tolerance test, GTT) in women who screened positive with the 1-hour, 50-g GCT, women were screened three times during pregnancy. In one study, an estimated 11% of the GDM population would have been missed if screening had not continued past 28 weeks.[501] [Evidence level 3] In another study, 33% of the GDM population would have been missed had screening not continued past 31 weeks of gestation.[502] [Evidence level 3]

The GTT is regarded as the gold standard for the diagnosis of GDM after a positive screening result. However, the quantity of glucose load and threshold for diagnosis lack consistency. Commonly used criteria are summarised in Table 11.1.

The first line of intervention for all pregnant women diagnosed with gestational diabetes is diet. However, a systematic review of RCTs found no difference between women treated with diet compared with women who received no dietary advice in frequencies of birthweight greater than 4000 g or 4500 g, caesarean section rates, preterm birth, birth trauma or maternal hypertensive disorders.[504] [Evidence level 1a] Although most pregnant women are treated with diet alone, 15% to 20% are thought to need insulin.[483]

In a trial that randomised women to diet alone or to diet plus insulin, no difference in outcomes was found. However, 14% of the diet-alone group received insulin owing to poor control and this may explain the lack of difference observed between the two groups.[505] [Evidence level 1b] Another study found that, while detection and treatment of GDM normalised birthweights, rates of caesarean delivery were still higher among pregnant women with GDM compared with pregnant women without GDM (34% versus 20%, RR 1.96, 95% CI 1.40 to 2.74).[506] [Evidence level 2a]

In an RCT of exercise as an intervention for GDM, in which only 29 out 144 subjects were successfully recruited and the method of randomisation was not clear, no differences in outcomes were seen.[507] [Evidence level 1b]

Intensive glucose monitoring has been reported to reduce incidence of macrosomia from 24% to 9% ($p < 0.05$) through the detection of women with high glucose levels who were then treated with insulin.[508] [Evidence level 3]

At present, screening for gestational diabetes appears to be hampered by the lack of a clear definition, agreed diagnostic criteria and evidence to show that intervention and treatment for this condition leads to improved outcomes for the mother and fetus. Although fasting plasma glucose and GCT have the highest reported sensitivities and specificities in the literature, there also exists considerable debate about which screening test should be used if there is to be screening. A continuum of risk for GDM should be researched and risk of adverse pregnancy outcomes clarified on such a continuum. This would help to form the basis for diagnosis. The most appropriate strategies for screening, diagnosing and managing asymptomatic GDM remain controversial.

The results of two ongoing studies are expected to resolve some of the issues surrounding the question of whether women should be routinely screened for gestational diabetes. The ACHOIS (Australian Carbohydrate Intolerance in Pregnancy Study) trial is assessing two forms of care for treating women with glucose intolerance of pregnancy detected through screening and includes 1000 women in Australia. The results of this study are expected to be available in 2004. The second trial, the Hyperglycaemia and Adverse Pregnancy Outcomes (HAPO) study, aims to define uniform standards for the detection and diagnosis of diabetes occurring in pregnancy to reduce adverse effects on mother and baby. It is an international study of 25,000 pregnant women and results are also expected to be available in 2004.

Table 11.1 Examples of diagnostic criteria employed for gestational diabetes mellitus

	75-g glucose load (mmol/l)		
	American Diabetic Association[503]	SIGN[480]	WHO[481]
Fasting	5.3	5.5	7.0
1-hour	10.0	–	–
2-hour	8.6	9.0	11.1
Minimum required criteria (n)	2	1	1

RECOMMENDATION

The evidence does not support routine screening for gestational diabetes mellitus and therefore it should not be offered. [B]

11.2 Pre-eclampsia

Pre-eclampsia is a multisystem disorder associated with increased maternal and neonatal morbidity and mortality. The incidence of pre-eclampsia ranges from 2% to 10%, depending upon the population studied and the criteria used to diagnose the disorder. Maternal symptoms of advanced pre-eclampsia may include (www.apec.org.uk/index.html):

- bad headache
- problems with vision, such as blurring or flashing before the eyes
- bad pain just below the ribs
- vomiting
- sudden swelling of face, hands or feet.

Definitions

Pre-eclampsia	Hypertension new to pregnancy manifesting after 20 weeks of gestation that is associated with a new onset of proteinuria, which resolves after delivery.
Pregnancy-induced hypertension	Hypertension new to pregnancy that resolves after delivery but is not associated with proteinuria.
Chronic hypertension	Hypertension that predates a pregnancy or appears prior to 20 weeks of gestation.

This categorisation is helpful as it relates to the prognostic outcome of the pregnancy. Most women with hypertension in pregnancy have no clinical symptoms. Hypertension is frequently the only early sign that predates serious disease. Blood pressure measurement is routinely performed in antenatal care to allow the diagnosis and classification of hypertension in pregnancy.

Pre-eclampsia is thought to be caused by widespread endothelial cell damage secondary to an ischaemic placenta.[509] Hypertension and proteinuria are two easily measured signs associated with pre-eclampsia, although they are surrogate markers indicating end-organ damage.

Eclampsia is rare. It occurs in nearly 1/2000 pregnancies in the UK.[510] It is associated with high maternal morbidity and it accounts for over 50% of the maternal deaths associated with hypertensive disorders in pregnancy. Blood pressure may be of limited importance in identifying women who are going to develop eclampsia as about one-third of first fits occur in women with normal or a mild increase in blood pressure.[510]

Oedema was originally part of the triad of signs describing pre-eclampsia but it occurs in too many pregnant women (up to 80%) to be discriminatory and has been abandoned as a marker in classification schemes.[511a]

Physiological changes to blood pressure during pregnancy

In normal pregnancies, blood pressure usually falls during the first part of pregnancy before rising again towards term to a level similar to the value in the non-pregnant population.[512] Women with chronic hypertension may become normotensive by 10 to 13 weeks of gestation when antenatal care is usually initiated.

Defining hypertension during pregnancy

Blood pressure is a continuous variable and a cutoff point is employed to define 'normal' from 'abnormal' values. In defining an abnormal value, we should aim to identify those women who are at greater risk of an adverse outcome than those who are 'normal'. The conventional definition of hypertension in pregnancy is two readings of 140/90 mmHg taken at least 4 hours apart. Perinatal mortality is increased above this level.[513] However, about 20% of pregnant women in the UK have this reading at least once after 20 weeks of gestation. This will lead to intervention in 10% of all pregnant women but pre-eclampsia will develop only in 2% to 4% of pregnant women.[514] In a case series of 748 women who developed hypertension in pregnancy between 24 and 35 weeks (defined as greater than or equal to 140 mmHg systolic or greater than or equal to 90 mmHg diastolic), 46% later developed proteinuria greater than or equal to 1+ by dipstick on at least two occasions and 9.6% progressed to 'severe pre-eclampsia' (defined as hypertension greater than 160/110 mmHg with proteinuria, greater than 3+ of protein or thrombocytopenia).[515] The rate of progression to proteinuria was greater in those who enrolled in the study before 30 weeks. Pre-eclampsia was associated with a higher stillbirth and perinatal death rate. [Evidence level 3]

A large cohort study (n = 14,833) found that women with mean arterial pressure in the second trimester above 85 mmHg experienced a continuum of increased perinatal death, postnatal morbidity and small-for-gestational-age infants.[516a] In the third trimester, a similar continuum of increasing fetal deaths and morbidity was observed with mean arterial pressure above 95 mmHg.[516b] With or without proteinuria, an increased mean arterial pressure, at or above 90 mmHg, of extended duration in the second trimester, was associated with a higher stillbirth rate, pre-eclampsia and small-for-gestational-age infants. [Evidence level 2a]

The figure of 90 mmHg for the diastolic value corresponds approximately to 3 SD above the mean in early and mid pregnancy, 2 SD above the mean between 34 and 38 weeks of gestation and to 1.5 SD above the mean at term.[517] The finding of such a reading may therefore be more significant at 28 weeks of gestation than at term.

The diagnostic criteria of a 90 mmHg threshold with a 25 mmHg incremental rise is a definition based on evidence,[518–520] rather than the previously recommended diagnostic criteria by the American College of Obstetricians and Gynecologists (ACOG) (a rise in systolic blood pressure of 30 mmHg or of 15 mmHg in the diastolic pressure compared with booking or early pregnancy values),[511b] which included women who were not likely to suffer increased adverse outcomes. Subsequent guidelines from the US National Institutes of Health have advocated the abandonment of the ACOG diagnostic criteria.[511a]

Measuring blood pressure

The diagnosis of hypertension is dependent upon the accurate measurement of blood pressure. This accuracy depends largely on minimising measurement error. Failure to standardise technique will increase error and variability in measurement. A survey of midwives and obstetricians in one UK district general hospital reported in 1991 showed that compliance with recommendations on blood pressure measurement technique in pregnancy was poor.[521] The recommendations below relate to the American Heart Association guidelines produced in 1987,[522] which echoed previous expert opinion,[523] and concur with Shennan and Halligan's recommendations.[524]

- Use accurate equipment (mercury sphygmomanometer or validated alternative method).
- Use sitting or semi-reclining position so that the arm to be used is at the level of the heart. The practice of taking the blood pressure in the upper arm with the woman on her side will give falsely lower readings.
- Use appropriate size of cuff: at least 33 x 15 cm. There is less error introduced by using too large a cuff than by too small a cuff.
- Deflate slowly with a rate of 2 mmHg to 3 mmHg per second, taking at least 30 seconds to complete the whole deflation.
- Measure to nearest 2 mmHg to avoid digit preference.
- Obtain an estimated systolic pressure by palpation, to avoid auscultatory gap.
- Use Korotkoff V (disappearance of heart sounds) for measurement of diastolic pressure, as this is subject to less intra-observer and inter-observer variation than Korotkoff IV (muffling of heart sounds) and seems to correlate best with intra-arterial pressure in pregnancy. In the 15% of pregnant women whose diastolic pressure falls to zero before the last sound is heard, then both phase IV and phase V readings should be recorded (e.g. 148/84/0 mmHg).
- If two readings are necessary, use the average of the readings and not just the lowest reading, in order to minimise threshold avoidance.

As mercury will soon be eliminated from health settings (EU directive, EN 1060-2), a meta-analysis of validation studies of automated devices for blood pressure monitoring in pregnancy was conducted.[525] The findings indicated that, while the automated devices were accurate in pregnancy, they under-read by clinically significant amounts in women with pre-eclampsia. [Evidence level 3] This makes it important for automated devices to be assessed for accuracy before use, by a recognised protocol such as that recommended by the British Hypertension Society, and for readings from automated devices to be interpreted with caution.

A 15-cm cuff size may not be appropriate to use in the case of very thin arms, as blood pressure may be underestimated in those with arm circumferences less than 33 cm. For women with an arm circumference greater than 33 cm but less than 41 cm, a larger cuff should be used. In the case of very obese women, (arm circumference greater than 41 cm) thigh cuffs should be used.[526]

Regarding the use of which sound to use when recording diastolic blood pressure, an RCT of pregnancies managed by Korotkoff phase IV or phase V found that, although more episodes of severe hypertension were recorded with the use of the fourth Korotkoff sound, no differences in requirements for antihypertensive treatment, birthweight, fetal growth restriction or perinatal mortality were reported.[527] [Evidence level 1b] The fifth Korotkoff sound is also closer to the actual intra-arterial pressure and more reliably detected than the fourth Korotkoff sound.[528]

Assessment of risk factors for pre-eclampsia

Risk factors for pre-eclampsia are thought to include older age,[529] nulliparity,[530] long pregnancy interval,[531] a prior history of pre-eclampsia,[530] presence of a multiple pregnancy,[532] genetic susceptibility,[533] high BMI at first contact, and the presence of microvascular medical conditions such as diabetes or hypertension.[534] In the context of frequency of antenatal appointments, the assessment of a pregnant woman's overall level of risk for pre-eclampsia should be assessed at her first antenatal appointment so that a tailored plan of antenatal care can be formulated. Women with any of the following risk factors should be considered for an increased schedule of blood pressure screening [Evidence levels 2b and 3]:[512]

- nulliparity (OR 2.71, 95% CI 1.16 to 6.34)
- age of 40 years and above (nulliparous OR 2.17, 95% CI 1.36 to 3.47; parous OR 2.05, 95% CI 1.47 to 2.87)
- family history of pre-eclampsia (e.g., pre-eclampsia in a mother or a sister, OR 5.27, 95% CI 1.57 to 17.64)
- history of previous pre-eclampsia (in first pregnancy, OR 8.23, 95% CI 6.49 to 10.45)
- BMI at or above 35 at first contact (OR 2.29, 95% CI 1.61 to 3.24)
- presence of multiple pregnancy (OR 2.76, 95% CI 1.99 to 3.82)
- pre-existing vascular disease (e.g., hypertension or diabetes).

Frequency of blood pressure monitoring

No evidence was found on when and how often blood pressure measurements should be taken. However, in a systematic review of RCTs comparing a reduced number of antenatal appointments with the standard number of antenatal appointments, no difference in the rates of pre-eclampsia were reported (pooled OR 0.37, 95% CI: 0.22 to 1.64).[32] [Evidence level 1a]

Urinalysis

The diagnosis of pre-eclampsia depends on the presence of significant proteinuria as well as raised blood pressure. Reagent strips or 'dipsticks' are commonly used to detect proteinuria. The incidence of false positive results in random urine specimens may be up to 25% in trace reactions and 6% with 1+ reactions.[535] Therefore, dipsticks can only be a screening test and will not have much utility when not used in combination with blood pressure measurements.[536] Due to considerable observer errors involved in dipstick urinanalysis, an RCOG Study Group recommended that automated dipstick readers be employed.[537] This can significantly improve false positive and false negative rates. An initial sample of 1+ or greater should be confirmed by a 24-hour urinary protein measurement or protein/creatinine ratio determination.[538] Although a finding of 300 mg/24 hours or more or a protein/creatinine ratio of 30 mg/mmol of creatinine is customarily regarded as significant,[539,540] a proteinuria threshold of 500 mg/24 hours has been suggested to be more predictive in relation to the likelihood of adverse outcome.[537]

RECOMMENDATION

At first contact, a woman's level of risk for pre-eclampsia should be evaluated so that a plan for her subsequent schedule of antenatal appointments can be formulated. The likelihood of developing pre-eclampsia during a pregnancy is increased in women who:

- are nulliparous
- are age 40 years or older
- have a family history of pre-eclampsia (e.g., pre-eclampsia in a mother or sister)
- have a prior history of pre-eclampsia
- have a BMI at or above 35 at first contact
- have a multiple pregnancy or pre-existing vascular disease (for example, hypertension or diabetes). [C]

Whenever blood pressure is measured in pregnancy, a urine sample should be tested at the same time for proteinuria. [C]

Standardised equipment, techniques and conditions for blood-pressure measurement should be used by all personnel whenever blood pressure is measured in the antenatal period, so that valid comparisons can be made. [C]

Pregnant women should be informed of the symptoms of advanced pre-eclampsia because these may be associated with poorer pregnancy outcomes for the mother or baby. Symptoms include headache, problems with vision, such as blurring or flashing before the eyes, bad pain just below the ribs, vomiting, and sudden swelling of face, hands or feet. [D]

Future research

Research is needed to determine the optimal frequency and timing of blood pressure measurement and on the role of screening for proteinuria.

11.3 Preterm birth

Preterm birth, or the birth of a baby before 37 weeks of gestation (less than 259 days) is one of the largest contributors to neonatal morbidity and mortality in industrialised countries. It is estimated to occur in 6% of babies in the UK, although this is difficult to assess since the UK does not collect gestational-age data at a national level.[541] Trials for the antenatal detection of preterm birth through routine cervical assessment or risk factor assessment have proved largely unsuccessful.

Vaginal examination assesses the maturation of the cervix, its dilatation at the internal os, length, consistency and position. Criteria for an abnormal 'test' result vary. A European multicentre RCT of 5440 women compared routine cervical examination at each antenatal appointment with a policy of avoiding cervical examination unless medically indicated.[542] Preterm birth occurred in 5.7% and 6.4% of the women assigned to the two groups (RR 0.88, 95% CI 0.72 to 1.09). The results of this study do not suggest a benefit from routine cervical examination. [Evidence level 1b]

A prospective multicentre study of vaginal ultrasonography assessed the association between cervical length and risk of preterm delivery.[543] A total of 2915 women were assessed at 24 weeks and 2531 of these women were assessed again at 28 weeks. The risk of preterm delivery was found to increase as the length of the cervix decreased. Women with shorter cervices were compared with women whose cervical lengths were above the 75th percentile. The relative risks are shown in Table 11.2. The sensitivity of this method as a screening test, however, was low at 54% and 70% for women with cervical lengths at or below 30 mm for 24 weeks and 28 weeks, respectively. [Evidence level 2a] Although transvaginal ultrasound screening appears to be able to predict increase risk of preterm birth, there is no evidence that this information can be used to improve outcomes.

The same multicentre study also assessed the use of fetal fibronectin to predict preterm birth.[544] Measurements of fetal fibronectin in 10,456 women at 8 to 22 weeks were taken and high values

Table 11.2 Relative risk of preterm delivery at 24 and 28 weeks of gestation by cervical length

Cervical length	24 weeks	28 weeks			
Percentile	(mm)	RR	95% CI	RR	95% CI
≤ 75th	40	1.98	1.2 to 3.27	2.8	1.41 to 5.56
≤ 50th	35	2.35	1.42 to 3.89	3.52	1.79 to 6.92
≤ 25th	30	3.79	2.32 to 6.19	5.39	2.82 to 10.28
≤ 10th	26	6.19	3.84 to 9.97	9.57	5.24 to 17.48
≤ 5th	22	9.49	5.95 to 15.15	13.88	7.68 to 25.10
≤ 1st	13	13.99	7.89 to 24.78	24.94	13.81 to 45.04

after 13 weeks of gestation (with the exception of those from weeks 17 to 18) were found to be associated with a two- to three-fold increased risk of preterm birth (defined as less than 35 weeks of gestation). [Evidence level 2a] A slightly older multicentre cohort study reported that the presence of fetal fibronectin in the cervix and vagina from 22 to 24 weeks of gestation had a sensitivity of 63% for the prediction of preterm birth at less than 28 weeks.[545] [Evidence level 2a]

Using clinical risk assessment at 23 to 24 weeks of gestation, 2929 women were evaluated to assess the ability of this method to predict preterm birth.[546] Demographic factors, socioeconomic status, home and work environment, drug and alcohol use, and clinical history as well as current pregnancy factors were evaluated. Although specific risk factors were highly associated with preterm birth, this risk factor assessment failed to identify most women who subsequently had a preterm delivery. [Evidence level 2a]

RECOMMENDATION

Routine vaginal examination to assess the cervix is not an effective method of predicting preterm birth and should not be offered. [A]

Although cervical shortening identified by transvaginal ultrasound examination and increased levels of fetal fibronectin are associated with an increased risk for preterm birth, the evidence does not indicate that this information improves outcomes; therefore neither routine antenatal cervical assessment by transvaginal ultrasound nor the measurement of fetal fibronectin should be used to predict preterm birth in healthy pregnant women. [B]

11.4   Placenta praevia

Placenta praevia occurs when the placenta covers the internal os and obstructs vaginal delivery of the fetus. A higher rate of pregnancy complications, including abruption placenta, antepartum haemorrhage and intrauterine growth restriction has been reported in women with low-lying placentas identified in the second trimester, despite apparent 'resolution' by the time of delivery.[547] [Evidence level 3]

Evaluation of transvaginal sonography for placental localisation has been shown to be safe in observational studies[599–550] [Evidence level 3] and more accurate than transabdominal sonography in one RCT.[551] [Evidence level 1b] Reported sensitivities range from 88% to 100% and false positives and false negatives are rare.[549,552] [Evidence level 3]

Using ultrasonography, placenta praevia may be detected early in pregnancy. However, many placentas that appear to cover the cervical os in the second trimester will not cover the os at term. In one cohort study (n = 6428 women), 4.5% of women were identified with a placenta extending over the internal os at 12 to 16 weeks of gestation with transvaginal sonographic screening and only 0.16% (10/6428) of these women had placenta praevia at birth. Eight of the ten women with placenta praevia had been identified prior to delivery and, in all eight of these women, the placenta extended 15 mm or more over the internal os at the initial scan.[553] [Evidence level 2b]

In another cohort study, among women scanned transvaginally at 18 to 23 weeks of gestation (n = 3696 women), 1.5% had a placenta extending over the internal os.[554] At delivery, 0.14% of women had placenta praevia and, again, the placenta covered the internal os by 15 mm or more at the time of the first scan for all five of the women. With a cutoff of 15 mm, 0.7% (27/3696) of women would have screened 'positive' and all five cases of praevia at delivery would have been identified (i.e., positive predictive value 19% and sensitivity 100%). [Evidence level 2b]

Similarly, a cross-sectional study which examined 1252 women who underwent ultrasound examination from 9 to 13 weeks of gestation found that although 6.2% (77/1252) of women had a placenta extending over the internal cervical os at initial examination, only 0.32% (4/1252) of the cases persisted to delivery.[555] In all four cases, the edge of the placenta extended over the os by more than 15 mm during the first-trimester ultrasound examination. [Evidence level 3]

With regard to gestational age at the time of detection, later detection appears to be related to likelihood of persisting until delivery. A retrospective study demonstrated that, among women with placenta praevia at 15 to 19 weeks of gestation, 12% persisted until delivery compared with 73% among women in whom placenta praevia was identified at 32 to 35 weeks of gestation.[556] [Evidence level 3]

Symptomatic placenta praevia is associated with the sudden onset of painless bleeding in the second or third trimester. Women with placenta praevia are reported to be 14 times more likely to bleed in the antenatal period compared with women without placenta praevia.[557] Risk factors for symptomatic placenta praevia include prior history of placenta praevia, advancing maternal age, increasing parity, smoking, cocaine use, previous caesarean section and prior spontaneous or induced abortion.[558,559] [Evidence level 2a]

In the case of symptomatic placenta praevia, inpatient management has been recommended[560] [Evidence level 4] and no conclusive evidence contrary to this recommendation was located. A Cochrane review of interventions for the management of placenta praevia compared home with hospitalisation and cervical cerclage with no cerclage.[561] Only three trials with a total of 114 women were identified and although a reduction of length of stay in hospital was observed no other significant differences were found to support inpatient or outpatient management. [Evidence level 1a] Three trials of such small size were considered insufficient evidence to support a change in practice.

RECOMMENDATION

Because most low-lying placentas detected at a 20-week anomaly scan will resolve by the time the baby is born, only a woman whose placenta extends over the internal cervical os should be offered another transabdominal scan at 36 weeks. If the transabdominal scan is unclear, a transvaginal scan should be offered. [C]

12. Fetal growth and wellbeing

12.1 Abdominal palpation for fetal presentation

A study of clinicians using Leopold manoeuvres to assess presentation and engagement of the presenting part found that 53% of all malpresentations were detected and that there was a definite correlation with years of clinical experience and better results.[562] [Evidence level 3] This finding was supported by another study which looked specifically at detection of breech presentation.[563] [Evidence level 3] The sensitivity and specificity of Leopold manoeuvres is reported to be about 28% and 94%, respectively.[564] [Evidence level 3]

One descriptive study reported that women do not enjoy being palpated, finding it uncomfortable and not reassuring or informative.[565] [Evidence level 3]

RECOMMENDATIONS

Fetal presentation should be assessed by abdominal palpation at 36 weeks or later, when presentation is likely to influence the plans for the birth. Routine assessment of presentation by abdominal palpation should not be offered before 36 weeks because it is not always accurate and may be uncomfortable. [C]

Suspected fetal malpresentation should be confirmed by an ultrasound assessment. [Good practice point]

12.2 Measurement of symphysis–fundal distance

Use of measurement of symphysis–fundal height (in centimetres) may assist in recording an objective measure of uterine size. Interpretation of fetal growth from changes in fundal height measurement or palpation should bear in mind the errors intrinsic in the use of this technique in predicting placental insufficiency. Sequential measurements of symphysis–fundal height offer the potential to observe changes in fetal growth rate. The common causes of a size-for-dates discrepancy are:

- small-for-gestational-age
- hydramnios
- multifetal pregnancies
- molar pregnancy
- errors in estimating gestational age.

A systematic review of controlled trials compared symphysis–fundal height measurement with assessment by abdominal palpation alone.[566] Only one trial was included and no differences were detected in any of the outcomes measured, i.e. perinatal mortality, Apgar score less than 4 at 1 minute and 5 minutes, umbilical artery pH less than 7.15, admission to neonatal unit, antenatal hospitalisation for small-for-gestational-age, labour induction for small-for-gestational-age, caesarean section for small-for-gestational-age, birthweight less than tenth centile.

There is not enough evidence to evaluate the use of symphysis–fundal height measurement during antenatal care and it would seem unwise to abandon its use unless a much larger trial shows that it is unhelpful. Symphysis–fundal height measurement is among the least expensive tools in antenatal care, requiring minimal equipment, training and time.

The use of customised fundal height charts as a screening method to detect fetal growth anomalies was assessed in a non-randomised controlled trial.[567] Customised fundal height charts display curves for fetal weight and fundal height while adjusting for maternal height, weight, parity and ethnic group. In this study, fundal height measurements were taken and plotted by community midwives in the intervention area at each antenatal appointment. In the control area, women received usual management, including fundal height assessment by abdominal palpation and standard recording. A significantly higher antenatal detection rate of small- and large-for-gestational-age babies was observed in the group from the study area compared with the women from the control area (OR 2.2, 95% CI 1.1 to 4.5 for small-for-gestational-age; OR 2.6, 95% CI 1.3 to 5.5 for large babies) with no increase in number of scans, but a reduction in the number of referrals for further investigation. No differences in perinatal outcome were reported. [Evidence level 2a] While this study showed that the use of customised growth charts might reduce false positive rates, the benefits of detecting small- or large-for-gestational-age infants without effective interventions remain unclear.

RECOMMENDATION

Pregnant women should be offered estimation of fetal size at each antenatal appointment to detect small- or large-for-gestational-age infants. [A]

Symphysis–fundal height should be measured and plotted at each antenatal appointment. [Good practice point]

Future research

Further research on more effective ways to detect and manage small- and large-for-gestational-age fetuses is needed.

12.3 Routine monitoring of fetal movements

There is often no obvious cause of late fetal death of normally formed singleton births. Many of these deaths are unpredictable and occur in women who are healthy and who have had otherwise uncomplicated pregnancies.

Maternal recognition of decreased fetal movement has long been used during antenatal care in an attempt to identify the jeopardised fetus and intervene to prevent death. Given the low prevalence of fetal compromise and an estimated specificity of 90% to 95%, the positive predictive value of the maternal perception of reduced fetal movements for fetal compromise is low, 2% to 7%.[568]

One RCT was found that assessed the ability of the 'count to ten' method to reduce the prevalence of antenatal fetal death.[569] [Evidence level 1b] The method records on a chart the time interval each day required to feel ten fetal movements. This cluster RCT randomised 68,000 women to either routine formal fetal-movement counting or to standard care. It found that there was no decrease in perinatal mortality in the test group and this policy would have to be used by about 1250 women to prevent one unexplained death.

Following a reduction in fetal movements women should be advised to contact their midwife or hospital for further assessment.

The evidence does not support the routine use of formal fetal movement counting to prevent late fetal death.

RECOMMENDATION

Routine formal fetal-movement counting should not be offered. [A]

12.4 Auscultation of fetal heart

Auscultation of the fetal heart is a component of the abdominal examination and forms an integral part of a standard antenatal examination. Although hearing the fetal heart confirms that the fetus is alive there appears to be no other clinical or predictive value.[570,571] [Evidence level 3] This is because it is unlikely that detailed information on the fetal heart such as decelerations or variability can be heard on auscultation.

There is a perception among doctors and midwives that fetal heart rate auscultation is enjoyable and reassuring for pregnant women and therefore worthwhile. This is not based on published evidence and may not be a correct assumption. Research done on attitudes of women towards auscultation compared with electronic fetal monitoring in labour revealed that many women found the abdominal pressure from auscultation uncomfortable,[572] [Evidence level 3] so perhaps their attitudes to antenatal auscultation cannot be presumed.

RECOMMENDATION

Auscultation of the fetal heart may confirm that the fetus is alive but is unlikely to have any predictive value and routine listening is therefore not recommended. However, when requested by the mother, auscultation of the fetal heart may provide reassurance. [D]

12.5 Cardiotocography

There is no evidence to evaluate the use of antenatal cardiotocography (CTG) for routine fetal assessment in normal pregnancies. RCTs which included women who were healthy and who had uncomplicated pregnancies were not found.

A systematic review of RCTs assessed the effects of antenatal CTG monitoring on perinatal morbidity and mortality and maternal morbidity.[573] [Evidence level 1a] Four trials were included randomising 1588 woman who satisfied the inclusion criteria. In these trials, carried out on high- or intermediate-risk women, antenatal CTG appeared to have no significant effect on perinatal morbidity or mortality. There was no increase in the incidence of interventions such as elective caesarean section or induction of labour.

RECOMMENDATION

The evidence does not support the routine use of antenatal electronic fetal heart rate monitoring (cardiotocography) for fetal assessment in women with an uncomplicated pregnancy and therefore it should not be offered. [A]

12.6 Ultrasound assessment in the third trimester

One systematic review of seven RCTs examined the use of routine ultrasound after 24 weeks in an unselected and designated low-risk population. There was a wide variation in the provision of ultrasound within the studies. The main comparison group of six studies compared routine ultrasound after 24 weeks with no, selective or concealed ultrasound after 24 weeks.[574] [Evidence level 1a]

There were no differences between preterm delivery, birth weight or perinatal mortality. The screened group was less likely to deliver post-term (over 42 weeks), although this may be a result of more accurate dating prior to 24 weeks, as outlined above. Similarly, there were no differences in other outcomes of antenatal, obstetric or neonatal interventions.[574]

RECOMMENDATION

The evidence does not support the routine use of ultrasound scanning after 24 weeks of gestation and therefore it should not be offered. [A]

12.7   Umbilical and uterine artery Doppler ultrasound

One systematic review of five RCTs concluded that routine use of umbilical Doppler ultrasound had no effect on obstetric or neonatal outcomes, including perinatal mortality. The routine use of umbilical Doppler ultrasound increased the likelihood of needing further diagnostic interventions.[575] [Evidence level 1a]

A second systematic review of 27 primary observational studies examined the use of uterine Doppler ultrasound for the prediction of pre-eclampsia, fetal growth restriction and perinatal death in low- and high-risk populations. The predictive value was poor in women who were healthy and who had uncomplicated pregnancies (i.e. low-risk populations).[576] [Evidence level 2a]

RECOMMENDATIONS

The use of umbilical artery Doppler ultrasound for the prediction of fetal growth restriction should not be offered routinely. [A]

The use of uterine artery Doppler ultrasound for the prediction of pre-eclampsia should not be offered routinely. [B]

13. Management of specific clinical conditions

13.1 Pregnancy after 41 weeks

Data from one cohort[577] [Evidence level 2a] revealed that, at 40 weeks of gestation, only 58% of women had delivered. This increased to 74% by 41 weeks and to 82% by 42 weeks. Population studies indicate that in women who are healthy and have otherwise uncomplicated pregnancies perinatal mortality and morbidity is increased in pregnancies of longer duration than 42 weeks. The risk of stillbirth increases from 1/3000 ongoing pregnancies at 37 weeks to 3/3000 ongoing pregnancies at 42 weeks to 6/3000 ongoing pregnancies at 43 weeks.[577] [Evidence level 2a] A similar increase in neonatal mortality is also reported.

Ultrasound assessment of fetal size is associated with a reduction in rates of intervention for post-term pregnancies. One systematic review of nine RCTs found routine ultrasound scanning before 24 weeks to be associated with a reduction in the rate of induced labour for post-term pregnancy when compared with selective use of ultrasound (Peto OR 0.61, 95% CI 0.52 to 0.72). A systematic review evaluated interventions aimed at prevention or improvement of outcomes of delivery beyond term.[578] [Evidence level 1a]

Membrane sweeping

Sweeping the membranes in women at term reduced the delay between randomisation and spontaneous onset of labour, or between randomisation and birth, by a mean of 3 days. Sweeping the membranes increased the likelihood of both spontaneous labour within 48 hours (63.8% versus 83.0%; RR 0.77, 95% CI 0.70 to 0.84; NNT 5) and of birth within 1 week (48.0% versus 66.0%; RR 0.73, 95% CI 0.66 to 0.80; NNT 5). Sweeping the membranes performed as a general policy from 38 to 40 weeks onwards decreased the frequency of prolonged pregnancy: more than 42 weeks: 3.4% versus 12.9%; RR 0.27, 95% CI 0.15 to 0.49; NNT: 11; more than 41 weeks: 18.6% versus 29.87%, RR 0.62; 95% CI 0.49 to 0.79; NNT: 8.[579] [Evidence level 1a]

Membrane sweeping reduced the frequency of using other methods to induce labour ('formal induction of labour'). The overall risk reduction in the available trials was 15%. This risk reduction of a formal induction of labour was 21.3% versus 36.3% (RR 0.59, CI 0.50 to 0.70; NNT 7). The risk of operative delivery is not changed by the intervention. There was no difference in other measures of effectiveness or adverse maternal outcomes. Sweeping the membranes was not associated with an increase in maternal infection or fever rates (4.4% versus 4.5%; RR 0.97, 95% CI 0.60 to 1.57), Similarly, there was no increase in neonatal infection (1.4% versus 1.3%; RR 0.92, 95% CI 0.30 to 2.82). No major maternal side effects were reported in the trials.[579] [Evidence level 1a]

A trial that systematically assessed minor side effects and women's discomfort during the procedure, found women in the "sweeping" group reported more discomfort during vaginal examination. Median pain scores were higher this group. (Pain was assessed by the Short Form of the McGill Pain Questionnaire, that included three scales: a visual analogue scale (0–10 cm), the present pain index (0–5) and a set of 15 descriptors of pain scoring 0–3). In addition, more women allocated to sweeping experienced vaginal bleeding and painful contractions not leading to onset of labour during the 24 hours following the intervention.[580]

There was no difference in any fetal outcome between the membrane sweeping and the non-membrane sweeping groups. These results must be interpreted with caution due to the presence of heterogeneity. The trials included in this review did not report in relevant clinical sub-groups.

Induction of labour after 41 weeks

The benefit of active induction of labour compared with expectant management is derived from trials of routine induction of labour after 41 weeks. With routine induction, perinatal death was reduced (Peto OR 0.23, 95% CI 0.06 to 0.90) and the rate of caesarean section was reduced (Peto OR 0.87, 95% CI 0.77 to 0.99).[578] [Evidence level 1a] There was no effect on instrumental delivery rates, use of epidural analgesia or fetal heart rate abnormalities during labour with a routine policy of induction of labour.[578] [Evidence level 1a] There was a reduction in meconium staining of the amniotic fluid with routine induction (Peto OR 0.74, 95% CI 0.65 to 0.84). However, this finding is probably related to the increase in meconium-stained liquor seen with increasing gestation in the conservative management arm of these trials.[578] [Evidence level 1a] No difference in maternal satisfaction as measured by one trial with either active management or expectant management was found (Peto OR 0.84, 95% CI 0.57 to 1.24).[578] [Evidence level 1a]

Alternative policy of screening pregnancies from 42 weeks

The systematic review included data on one trial comparing complex antenatal fetal monitoring (computerised cardiotocography, amniotic fluid index and assessment of fetal breathing, tone and gross body movements) to simpler monitoring (standard cardiotocography and ultrasound measurement of maximum pool depth) for identification of high-risk pregnancies from 42 weeks. There was no difference between the two policies with respect to perinatal mortality or caesarean section. However, the number of pregnant women included in this trial was small (n = 145) and, hence, the trial was underpowered to detect any significant differences in perinatal mortality.[578] [Evidence level 1a]

Offering routine early pregnancy ultrasound reduces the incidence of induction for perceived prolonged pregnancy. A policy of offering routine induction of labour after 41 weeks reduces perinatal mortality without an increase in caesarean section rates. The type of antenatal monitoring in the identification of high-risk pregnancies beyond 42 weeks is uncertain (but the simpler modalities used have been as effective as the more complex). There has been no detectable difference in effect of simpler modalities compared with more complex modalities.

Comprehensive information on the induction of labour can be found in the RCOG Evidence-based Clinical Guideline Number 9 (June 2001).[612]

RECOMMENDATIONS

Prior to formal induction of labour, women should be offered a vaginal examination for membrane sweeping. [A]

Women with uncomplicated pregnancies should be offered induction of labour beyond 41 weeks. [A]

From 42 weeks, women who decline induction of labour should be offered increased antenatal monitoring consisting of at least twice-weekly cardiotocography and ultrasound estimation of maximum amniotic pool depth. [Good practice point]

See also Section 4.6 Gestational age assessment.

13.2 Breech presentation at term

Evidence from the National Sentinel Caesarean Section Audit indicates that about 4% of singleton pregnancies are breech presentation: 3% of term infants, 9% of those born at 33 to 36 weeks of gestation, 18% of those born at 28 to 32 weeks and 30% of those born at less than 28 weeks.[581]

Breech presentation, but not breech delivery, has been associated with cerebral palsy and handicap, due principally to the association with preterm birth and congenital malformations.[582,583]

Interventions to promote cephalic version of babies in the breech position include external cephalic version (ECV), moxibustion and postural management.

ECV involves applying pressure to the pregnant woman's abdomen to turn the fetus in either a forward or backward somersault to achieve a vertex presentation. Recognised complications of ECV attributable to the procedure (and incidence) include:

- fetal heart rate abnormalities: the most common is transient bradycardia (1.1% to 16%)[584-587]
- placental abruption (0.4% to 1%)[584,586]
- painless vaginal bleeding (1.1%)[586]
- admission for induction of labour (3%).[587]

Success rates for cephalic presentation at delivery following ECV in nulliparous women range from 35% to 57% and from 52% to 84% in parous women.[584-586,588] Caesarean section rates as a complication resulting from the procedure range from 0.4% to 4%.[584,588]

Two systematic reviews identified nine RCTs that examined the effect of ECV for breech at term and before term.[589,590] The trials excluded women with uterine scars or abnormalities, multiple gestations, fetal compromise, ruptured membranes, vaginal bleeding or medical conditions, and those in labour.

ECV before 37 weeks of gestation did not make a significant difference to the incidence of noncephalic births at term (three RCTs, n = 889 women, RR 1.02, 95% CI 0.89 to 1.17) nor to the rate of caesarean section (two RCTs, n = 742, RR 1.10, 95% CI 0.78 to 1.54).[589] [Evidence level 1a] Performing ECV at term (defined as 37 weeks of gestation or more in three RCTs, at least 36 weeks of gestation in two RCTs and between 33 and 40 weeks in one RCT) reduced the number of noncephalic births by 60% when compared with no ECV (six RCTs, n = 612 women, RR 0.42, 95% CI 0.35 to 0.50).[590] [Evidence level 1a] A significant reduction in caesarean section was also observed in the ECV group when compared with no ECV (six RCTs, n = 612, RR 0.52, 95% CI 0.39 to 0.71). Five of the trials used tocolysis routinely or selectively[585,588,591-593] and in one of them,[586] no tocolysis had been used. [Evidence level 1a]

Various interventions have been tried to increase the success rates of ECV. These include the routine or selective use of tocolysis, the use of regional analgesia, the use of vibroacoustic stimulation and amnioinfusion. A systematic review of six randomised and quasi-randomised trials comprising 617 women with a breech presentation at term was identified.[594] Routine tocolysis with betamimetic drugs was associated with a 30% increase in the chances of successful ECV (RR 0.74, 95% CI 0.64 to 0.87). This review also showed that the rate of caesarean section was reduced in the group of women who had tocolysis (RR 0.85, 95% CI 0.72 to 0.99). No differences, however, were reported in rates of noncephalic births at term (RR 0.80, 95% CI 0.60, 1.07). [Evidence level 1a] None of the RCTs used newer tocolytics and the effectiveness of these is uncertain. There is also not enough evidence to evaluate the use of fetal acoustic stimulation in midline fetal spine positions, or epidural or spinal analgesia.

An RCT[595] conducted in the USA evaluated the value of performing pelvimetry in predicting who would deliver vaginally compared with using clinical examination.[235] Women with a breech presentation at term were studied. In the first group, pelvimetry results were revealed to the obstetricians and used as a basis for the decision on mode of delivery. In the second group, pelvimetry results were not disclosed and mode of delivery was decided clinically. Main outcome measures (a priori) were the rates of elective and emergency caesarean section and the early neonatal condition. There was no effect of pelvimetry on the vaginal delivery rate or the overall caesarean section rate but use of pelvimetry lowered the emergency caesarean section rate by half (RR 0.53, 95% CI 0.34 to 0.83). [Evidence level 1b]

It is not certain from this evidence whether magnetic resonance imaging pelvimetry selects cases accurately for vaginal delivery or whether knowledge of pelvic adequacy gives the obstetrician confidence in allowing a trial of vaginal delivery.[596]

ECV at term for women with a singleton breech presentation reduces the number of noncephalic births. When ECV is carried out, tocolysis reduces the chances of failed external cephalic version. ECV is associated with adverse maternal and fetal outcomes, which can be minimised by fetal monitoring during the procedure.

Postural management to promote cephalic version entails relaxation with the pelvis in an elevated position. This is usually achieved either in a knee-to-chest position or in a supine position with the pelvis elevated by a wedge-shaped cushion. Maternal postural techniques have been assessed in a systematic review of RCTs.[597] The size of all the trials was small and no effect on the rate of noncephalic births from postural management was detected between the intervention and control groups (five RCTs, n = 392, RR 0.95, 95% CI 0.81 to 1.11). Nor were any differences detected for caesarean section (four RCTs, n = 292, RR 1.07, 95% CI 0.85 to 1.33). [Evidence level 1a]

Further guidance on ECV and postural management may be found in the RCOG guideline on the management of breech presentation.[631]

Moxibustion refers to the burning of herbs to stimulate the acupuncture points beside the outer corner of the fifth toenail (acupoint BL 67). Two RCTs on moxibustion were located. One trial assessed the efficacy and safety of moxibustion.[598] The other trial assessed efficacy only.[599] In the first trial,[598] primigravidae in the 33rd week of gestation with breech presentation were identified by ultrasound. In the intervention group (n = 130), women were treated with moxibustion for one week and an additional week for those in whom ECV had not yet occurred. Women in the control group (n = 130) received no interventions for breech presentation. All women with persistent breech presentation after 35 weeks of gestation could undergo ECV. At an ultrasound check at the 35th week of gestation, 75% of babies were cephalic in the intervention group compared with 48% in the control group (RR 1.58, 95% CI 1.29 to 1.94). One woman in the intervention group and 24 in the control group underwent ECV after the 35th week of gestation. Version was not obtained in the woman from the intervention group but was obtained in 19 of the women from the control group. Nevertheless, babies in the moxibustion group were still significantly more likely to be cephalic at delivery compared with babies in the control group (RR 1.21, 95% CI 1.02 to 1.43). [Evidence level 1b]

RECOMMENDATIONS

All women who have an uncomplicated singleton breech pregnancy at 36 weeks of gestation should be offered external cephalic version (ECV). Exceptions include women in labour and women with a uterine scar or abnormality, fetal compromise, ruptured membranes, vaginal bleeding and medical conditions. [A]

Where it is not possible to schedule an appointment for ECV at 37 weeks of gestation, it should be scheduled at 36 weeks. [Good practice point]

Future research

Further research is necessary to determine if tocolysis improves the success rate of ECV.

14. Auditable standards

Criterion	Exception	Definition of terms
A pregnant woman has the offer of an HIV test documented in her notes	A woman known to have HIV infection	
A pregnant woman has the offer of a hepatitis B virus test documented in her notes	A woman known to have hepatitis B viral infection	
A pregnant woman has the offer of a syphilis serology test documented in her notes		
A pregnant woman has the offer of a rubella susceptibility test documented in her notes		
A pregnant woman has the offer of a Down's syndrome screening test documented in her notes		An acceptable test is currently one with a detection rate above 60% and a false positive rate of less than 5% (see guideline recommendation in Section 9.2)

Appendix 1

Routine antenatal care for healthy pregnant women. Understanding NICE guidance: information for pregnant women, their families and the public

About this information

This information describes the guidance that the National Institute for Clinical Excellence (called NICE for short) has issued to the NHS on antenatal care. It is based on *Antenatal care: routine antenatal care for healthy pregnant women*, which is a clinical guideline produced by NICE for doctors, midwives and others working in the NHS in England and Wales. Although this information has been written chiefly for women who are pregnant or thinking of becoming pregnant, it may also be useful for family members and anyone with an interest in pregnancy or in healthcare in general.

Clinical guidelines

Clinical guidelines are recommendations for good practice. The recommendations in NICE guidelines are prepared by groups of health professionals, lay representatives with experience or knowledge of the condition being discussed, and scientists. The groups look at the evidence available on the best way of treating or managing a condition and make recommendations based on this evidence.

There is more about NICE and the way that the NICE guidelines are developed on the NICE website (www.nice.org.uk). You can download the booklet *The guideline development process – information for the public and the NHS* from the website, or you can order a copy by phoning 0870 1555 455.

What the recommendations cover

NICE clinical guidelines can look at different areas of diagnosis, treatment, care, self-help or a combination of these. The areas that a guideline covers depend on the topic. They are laid out at the start of the development of the guideline in a document called the scope.

The recommendations in *Antenatal care: routine antenatal care for healthy pregnant women*, which are also described here, cover:

- the care you can expect to receive from your midwife and doctors during your pregnancy, whether you plan to give birth at home or in hospital
- the information you can expect to receive
- what you can expect from antenatal appointments
- aspects of your lifestyle that you may want to consider (such as diet, exercise, alcohol and drug intake, sexual activity and smoking)
- routine screening tests for specific conditions
- occupational risk factors in pregnancy
- what will happen if your pregnancy goes beyond 41 weeks
- what will happen if your baby is bottom first (known as the breech position) for the birth.

They do not cover:

- information on birth or parenthood and on preparing for them

- extra care you may need if you are expecting more than one baby
- extra care you may need if you develop additional problems (such as pre-eclampsia) or if your unborn baby has any abnormalities.

The information that follows tells you about the NICE guideline on antenatal care. It doesn't attempt to explain pregnancy or describe any extra care you may need for specific problems. If you want to find out more about pregnancy and antenatal care, or if you have questions about the specific treatments and options mentioned in this booklet, talk to your local midwife or doctor.

How guidelines are used in the NHS

In general, health professionals working in the NHS are expected to follow NICE's clinical guidelines. But there will be times when the recommendations won't be suitable for someone because of a specific medical condition, general health, their wishes or a combination of these. If you think that the treatment or care you receive does not match the treatment or care described in the pages that follow, you should discuss your concerns with your midwife or doctor.

If you want to read the other versions of this guideline

There are three versions of this guideline:

- this one
- the 'NICE guideline' *Antenatal care: routine antenatal care for healthy pregnant women*, which has been issued to people working in the NHS
- the full guideline, which contains all the details of the guideline recommendations, how they were developed and information about the evidence on which they are based.

All versions of the guideline are available from the NICE website (www.nice.org.uk/). This version and the NICE guideline are also available from the NHS Response Line – phone 0870 1555 455 and give the reference number(s) of the booklet(s) you want (N0310 for this version, N0311 for this version in English and Welsh, and N0309 for the NICE guideline).

Guideline recommendations

The guideline recommendations cover the routine care that all healthy pregnant women can expect to receive during their pregnancy.

You will receive extra care, in addition to what we describe here, if you are pregnant with more than one baby, if you already have certain medical conditions or if you develop a health problem during your pregnancy.

The guideline does not cover the care that women receive during or after a birth.

About antenatal care

Antenatal care is the care that you receive from health professionals during your pregnancy. It includes information on services that are available and support to help you make choices. You should be able to access antenatal care services that are readily and easily available and sensitive to your needs.

During your pregnancy you should be offered a series of antenatal appointments to check on your health and the health of your baby. During these appointments you should be given information about your care.

Your midwife or doctor should give you information in writing or in some other form that you can easily access and understand. If you have a physical, cognitive or sensory disability, for example, or if you do not speak or read English, they should provide you with information in an appropriate format.

A record should be kept of the care you receive. You should be asked to keep your maternity notes at home with you and to bring them along to all your antenatal appointments.

You have a right to take part in making decisions about your care. To be able to do this you will need to feel confident that you:

- understand what is involved
- feel comfortable about asking questions
- can discuss your choices with your antenatal care team.

Your care team should support you in this by making sure you have access to antenatal classes and information that is based on the best research evidence available.

While you are pregnant you should normally see a small number of health practitioners, led by your midwife and/or doctor (GP), on a regular basis. They should be people with whom you feel comfortable.

Antenatal appointments

The exact number of antenatal appointments and how often you have them will depend on your individual situation. If you are expecting your first child, you are likely to have up to ten appointments. If you have had children before, you should have around seven appointments. Some of them may take place at your home if this suits you. Your antenatal appointments should take place in a setting where you feel able to discuss sensitive issues that may affect you (such as domestic violence, sexual abuse, mental illness or drug use).

Early in your pregnancy your midwife or doctor should give you appropriate written or other information about the likely number, timing and purpose of your appointments, according to the options that are available to you. You should have a chance to discuss the schedule with them.

The table on page xx [20] gives a brief guide to what usually happens at each antenatal appointment.

What should happen at the appointments

The aim of antenatal appointments is to check on you and your baby's progress and to provide you with clear information and explanations, in discussions with you, about your care. At each appointment you should have the chance to ask questions and discuss any concerns you have with your midwife or doctor.

Each appointment should have a specific purpose. You will need longer appointments early in your pregnancy to allow plenty of time for your midwife or doctor to assess you and discuss your care. Wherever possible the appointments should include any routine tests you need, to cut down on any inconvenience to you.

Appointments in early pregnancy

Your first appointment should be fairly early in your pregnancy (before 12 weeks). Your midwife or doctor should use it to identify your needs (such as whether you need additional care) and should ask you about your health and any previous physical or mental illness you have had, so that you can be referred for further assessment or care, if necessary.

They should also give you an opportunity to let them know, if you wish, if you are in a vulnerable situation or if you have experienced anything which means you might need extra support, such as domestic violence, sexual abuse or female genital mutilation (such as female circumcision).

Your midwife or doctor should give you information on pregnancy care services and the options available, maternity benefits, diet, other aspects of your life which may affect your health or the health of your baby, and on routine screening tests. They should explain to you that decisions on whether to have these tests rest with you, and they should make sure that you understand what those decisions will mean for you and your baby.

During one of these early appointments your midwife or doctor should check your blood pressure and test your urine for the presence of protein. They should also weigh you and measure your height. If you are significantly overweight or underweight you may need extra care. You should not usually be weighed again.

Appointments in later pregnancy

The rest of your antenatal appointments should be tailored according to your individual health needs. They should include some routine tests (see page 120) which are used to check for certain conditions or infections. Most women are not affected by these conditions, but the tests are offered so that the small number of women who are affected can be identified and offered treatment.

Your midwife or doctor should explain to you in advance the reason for offering you a particular test. When discussing the test with you, they should make it clear that you can choose whether or not to have the test, as you wish.

During your appointments your midwife or doctor should give you the results of any tests you have had. You should be able to discuss your options with them and what you want to do.

Checking on your baby's development

At each antenatal appointment your midwife or doctor should check on your baby's growth. To do this, they should measure the distance from the top of your womb to your pubic bone. The measurement should be recorded in your notes.

The rest of this information tells you more about what you can expect from your midwife and/or doctor during your pregnancy and about the tests that you should be offered. It also tells you what you can expect if your pregnancy continues a week or more beyond your due date or if your baby is in the breech position (that is, bottom first) prior to birth.

Advice on money matters and work

Your midwife or doctor should give you information about your maternity and benefits rights. You can also get information from the Department of Trade and Industry – phone the helpline on 08457 47 47 47, call 08701 502 500 for information leaflets or visit the website at www.dti.gov.uk/er/workingparents.htm. The Government's interactive guidance website (www.tiger.gov.uk) also has information. Up-to-date information on maternity benefits can also be found on the Department for Work and Pensions website (www.dwp.gov.uk).

Your midwife or doctor should ask you about the work that you do, and should tell you about any possible risks to your pregnancy. For most women it is safe to continue working while you are pregnant, but there are hazards in some jobs that could put you at risk. More information about risks at work is available from the Health and Safety Executive; the website address is www.hse.gov.uk/mothers/index.htm or you can phone 08701 545 500 for information.

Lifestyle advice

There are a number of things you can do to help yourself stay healthy while you are pregnant. Your midwife or doctor can tell you more about them.

Exercise

You can continue or start moderate exercise before or during your pregnancy. Some vigorous activities, however, such as contact sports or vigorous racquet games, may carry extra risks, such as falling or putting too much strain on your joints. You should avoid scuba diving while you are pregnant as this can cause problems in the developing baby.

Alcohol

Excess alcohol can harm your unborn baby. If you do drink while you are pregnant, it is better to limit yourself to one standard unit of alcohol a day (roughly the equivalent of 125 ml – a small glass – of wine, half a pint of beer, cider or lager, or a single measure of spirits).

Smoking

Smoking increases the risks of your baby being underweight or being born too early – in both instances, your baby's health may be affected. You will reduce these risks if you can give up smoking, or at least smoke less, while you are pregnant. You and your baby will benefit if you can give up, no matter how late in your pregnancy.

If you need it, your midwife or doctor should offer you help to give up or cut down on smoking or to stay off it if you have recently given up. The NHS pregnancy smoking helpline can also provide advice and support – the phone number is 0800 169 9 169.

Cannabis

If you use cannabis, and especially if you smoke it, it may be harmful to your baby.

Sexual activity

There is no evidence that sexual activity is harmful while you are pregnant.

Travel

When you travel by car you should always wear a three-point seatbelt above and below your bump (not over it).

If you are planning to travel abroad you should talk to your midwife or doctor, who should tell you more about flying, vaccinations and travel insurance.

The risk of deep vein thrombosis from travelling by air may be higher when you are pregnant. Your midwife or doctor can tell you more about how you may be able to reduce the risk by wearing correctly fitted compression stockings.

Prescription and over-the-counter medicines

Only a few prescription and over-the-counter medicines have been shown to be safe for pregnant women by good-quality studies. While you are pregnant, your doctor should only prescribe medicines where the benefits are greater than the risks. You should use as few over-the counter-medicines as possible.

Complementary therapies

Few complementary therapies are known to be safe and effective during pregnancy. You should check with your midwife, doctor or pharmacist before using them.

Diet and food

Folic acid

Your midwife or doctor should give you information about taking folic acid (400 micrograms a day). If you do this when you are trying to get pregnant and for the first 12 weeks of your pregnancy it reduces the risk of having a baby with conditions which are known as neural tube defects, such as spina bifida (a condition where parts of the backbone do not form properly, leaving a gap or split which causes damage to the baby's central nervous system).

Vitamin A

Excess levels of vitamin A can cause abnormalities in unborn babies. You should avoid taking vitamin A supplements (with more than 700 micrograms of vitamin A) while you are pregnant. You should also avoid eating liver (which may contain high levels of vitamin A), or anything made from liver.

Other food supplements

You do not need to take iron supplements as a matter of routine while you are pregnant. They do not improve your health and you may experience unpleasant side effects, such as constipation.

You should not be offered vitamin D supplements as a matter of routine while you are pregnant. There is not enough evidence to tell whether they are of any benefit to pregnant women.

Food hygiene

Your midwife or doctor should give you information on bacterial infections such as listeriosis and salmonella that can be picked up from food and can harm your unborn baby. In order to avoid them while you are pregnant it is best:

- if you drink milk, to keep to pasteurised or UHT milk
- avoid eating mould-ripened soft cheese such as Camembert or Brie and blue-veined cheese (there is no risk with hard cheese such as Cheddar, or with cottage cheese or processed cheese)

- avoid eating paté (even vegetable paté)
- avoid eating uncooked or undercooked ready?prepared meals
- avoid eating raw or partially cooked eggs or food that may contain them (such as mayonnaise)
- avoid raw or partially cooked meat, especially poultry.

Toxoplasmosis is an infection that does not usually cause symptoms in healthy women. Very occasionally it can cause problems for the unborn baby of an infected mother. You can pick it up from undercooked or uncooked meat (such as salami, which is cured) and from the faeces of infected cats or contaminated soil or water. To help avoid this infection while you are pregnant it is best to:

- wash your hands before you handle food
- wash all fruit and vegetables, including ready?prepared salads, before you eat them
- make sure you thoroughly cook raw meats and ready?prepared chilled meats
- wear gloves and wash your hands thoroughly after gardening or handling soil
- avoid contact with cat faeces (in cat litter or in soil).

Screening tests

Early in your pregnancy you should be offered a number of tests. The purpose of these tests is to check whether you have any conditions or infections that could affect you or your baby's health.

Your doctor or midwife should tell you more about the purpose of any test you are offered. You do not have to have a particular test if you do not want it. However, the information they can provide may help your antenatal care team to provide the best care possible during your pregnancy and the birth. The test results may also help you to make choices during pregnancy.

Ultrasound scans

Early in your pregnancy (usually around 10 to 13 weeks) you should be offered an ultrasound scan to estimate when your baby is due and to check whether you are expecting more than one baby. If you see your midwife or doctor for the first time when you are more than 13 weeks pregnant, they should offer you a scan then.

Between 18 and 20 weeks you should be offered another scan to check for physical abnormalities in your baby. You should not have any further routine scans, as they have not been shown to be useful.

Blood tests

Anaemia

You should be offered two tests for anaemia: one at your first antenatal appointment and another between your 28th and 30th week. Anaemia is often caused by a lack of iron. If you develop anaemia while you are pregnant it is usually because you do not have enough iron to meet your baby's need for it in addition to your own; you may be offered further blood tests. You should be offered an iron supplement if appropriate.

Blood group and rhesus D status

Early in your pregnancy you should be offered tests to find out your blood group and your Rhesus D (RhD) status. Your midwife or doctor should tell you more about them and what they are for. If you are RhD negative you should be offered an anti-D injection to prevent future babies developing problems. Your partner may also be offered tests to confirm whether you need an anti-D injection. You can find more information about this in Guidance on the routine use of anti-D prophylaxis for RhD negative women: information for patients, published by NICE in 2002 and available at www.nice.org.uk/pdf/Anti_d_patient_leaflet.pdf.

Early in your pregnancy, and again between your 28th and 36th week, you should be offered tests to check for red cell antibodies. If the levels of these antibodies are significant, you should be offered a referral to a specialist centre for more investigation and advice on managing the rest of your pregnancy.

Screening for infections

Your midwife or doctor should offer you a number of tests, as a matter of routine, to check for certain infections. These infections are not common, but they can cause problems if they are not detected and treated.

Asymptomatic bacteriuria

Asymptomatic bacteriuria is a bladder infection that has no symptoms. Identifying and treating it can reduce the risk of giving birth too early. It can be detected by testing a urine sample.

Hepatitis B virus

Hepatitis B virus is a potentially serious infection that can affect the liver. Many people have no symptoms, however. It can be passed from a mother to her baby (through blood or body fluids), but may be prevented if the baby is vaccinated at birth. The infection can be detected in the mother's blood.

HIV

HIV usually causes no symptoms at first but can lead to AIDS. HIV can be passed from a mother to her baby, but this risk can be greatly reduced if the mother is diagnosed before the birth. The infection can be detected through a blood test. If you are pregnant and are diagnosed with HIV you should receive specialist care.

German measles (rubella)

Screening for German measles (rubella) is offered so that if you are not immune you can choose to be vaccinated after you have given birth. This should usually protect you and future pregnancies. Testing you for rubella in pregnancy does not aim to identify it in the baby you are carrying.

Syphilis

Syphilis is rare in the UK. It is a sexually transmitted infection that can also be passed from a mother to her baby. Mothers and babies can be successfully treated if it is detected and treated early. A person with syphilis may show no symptoms for many years. A positive test result does not always mean you have syphilis, but your healthcare providers should have clear procedures for managing your care if you test positive.

Screening tests for Down's syndrome

Down's syndrome is a condition caused by the presence of an extra chromosome in a baby's cells. It occurs by chance at conception and is irreversible.

In the first part of your pregnancy you should be offered screening tests to check whether your baby is likely to have Down's syndrome. Your midwife or doctor should tell you more about Down's syndrome, the tests you are being offered and what the results may mean for you. You have the right to choose whether to have all, some or none of these tests. You can opt out of the screening process at any time if you wish.

Screening tests will only indicate that a baby may have Down's syndrome. If the test results are positive, you should be offered further tests to confirm whether your baby does, in fact, have Down's syndrome. The time at which you are tested will depend on what kinds of tests are used.

Screening tests for Down's syndrome are not always right. They can sometimes wrongly show as positive, suggesting the baby does have Down's syndrome when in fact it does not. This type of result is known as a 'false positive'. The number of occasions on which this happens with a particular test is called its 'false-positive rate'.

At present you should be offered screening tests with a false-positive rate of less than 5 out of 100 and which detect at least 60 out of 100 cases of Down's syndrome. The tests which meet this standard are:

- from 11 to 14 weeks:
  - nuchal translucency (an ultrasound scan)
  - combined test (an ultrasound scan and blood test)

- from 14 to 20 weeks:
  - triple test (a blood test)
  - quadruple test (a blood test)
- from 11 to 14 weeks and 14 to 20 weeks:
  - integrated test (an ultrasound scan and blood test)
  - serum integrated test (a blood test).

By April 2007 all pregnant women should be offered screening tests for Down's syndrome with a false-positive rate of less than 3 out of 100 and which detect more than 75 out of 100 cases. The tests which meet this standard are:

- from 11 to 14 weeks
  - combined test
- from 14 to 20 weeks
  - quadruple test
- from 11 to 14 weeks and 14 to 20 weeks
  - integrated test
  - serum integrated test.

Pre-eclampsia

Pre-eclampsia is an illness that happens in the second half of pregnancy. Although it is usually mild, it can cause serious problems for you and your baby if it is not detected and treated.

Your midwife or doctor should tell you more about the symptoms of advanced pre-eclampsia, which include:

- headache
- problems with vision, such as blurred vision or lights flashing before the eyes
- bad pain just below the ribs
- vomiting
- sudden swelling of the face, hands or feet.

They should assess your risk of pre-eclampsia at your first antenatal appointment in order to plan for the rest of your appointments.

You are more likely to develop pre-eclampsia when you are pregnant if you:

- have had it before
- have not been pregnant before
- are 40 years old or more
- have a mother or sister who has had pre-eclampsia
- are overweight at the time of your first antenatal appointment
- are expecting more than one baby or you already have high blood pressure or diabetes.

Whenever your blood pressure is measured during your pregnancy, a urine sample should be tested at the same time for protein (as this can be another sign of pre-eclampsia).

Whenever a member of your healthcare team measures your blood pressure they should use the same type of equipment, method and conditions so that the results at different times of your pregnancy can be compared.

Placenta praevia

Placenta praevia is when the placenta is low lying in the womb and covers all or part of the entrance (the cervix). In most women, the placenta usually goes back into a normal position before the birth and does not cause a problem. If it does not, you may need a Caesarean section.

If the 20th week ultrasound scan shows that your placenta extends over the cervix you should be offered another abdominal scan at 36 weeks. If this second abdominal scan is unclear, you should be offered a vaginal scan.

Tests not offered as a matter of routine

There are a number of screening tests which have sometimes been offered to women in the past or have been suggested for routine antenatal care. The following tests should not be offered to you as a matter of routine because they have not been shown to improve outcomes for mothers or babies:

- cardiotocography (a record of the trace of a baby's heartbeat, which is monitored through electronic sensors placed on the mother's abdomen, sometimes called a trace or CTG)
- Doppler ultrasound (an ultrasound scan which measures the blood flow between the baby and the mother)
- vaginal examinations to predict whether a baby may be born too early
- routine breast and pelvic examinations
- screening for gestational diabetes mellitus (a form of diabetes triggered by pregnancy)
- daily counting and recording of the baby's movements
- routine screening for infection with:
  - group B streptococcus (GBS); this is a bacterial infection that can affect the baby (if you have previously had a baby with neonatal GBS, you should be offered treatment around the time of your labour)
  - toxoplasmosis (see page 120)
  - asymptomatic bacterial vaginosis (a vaginal infection which produces no symptoms)
  - cytomegalovirus; infection with this virus can affect the baby
  - chlamydia trachomatis (a vaginal infection) where there are no symptoms (a national screening programme for chlamydia is due to start soon, so arrangements for this will probably change).

There is not enough evidence about the effectiveness or cost effectiveness of routine screening for hepatitis C virus to justify it.

Managing common problems

Pregnancy brings a variety of physical and emotional changes. Many of these changes are normal, and pose no danger to you or your baby, even though some of them may cause you discomfort. If you want to discuss these things, your midwife or doctor is there to give you information and support.

Nausea and sickness

You may feel sick or experience vomiting in the early part of your pregnancy. This does not indicate that anything is wrong. It usually stops around your 16th to 20th week. Your midwife or doctor should give you information about this. You may find that using wrist acupressure or taking ginger tablets or syrup helps to relieve these symptoms. If you have severe problems your doctor may give you further help or prescribe antihistamine tablets for sickness.

Heartburn

Your midwife or doctor should give you information about what to do if you suffer from heartburn during your pregnancy. If it persists they should offer you antacids to relieve the symptoms.

Constipation

If you suffer from constipation while you are pregnant your midwife or doctor should tell you ways in which you can change your diet (such as eating more bran or wheat fibre) to help relieve the problem.

Haemorrhoids

There is no research evidence on how well treatments for haemorrhoids work. If you suffer from haemorrhoids, however, your midwife or doctor should give you information on what you can do to change your diet. If your symptoms continue to be troublesome they may offer you a cream to help relieve the problem.

Backache

Backache is common in pregnant women. You may find that massage therapy, exercising in water or going to group or individual back care classes may help you to relieve the pain.

Varicose veins

Varicose veins are also common. They are not harmful during pregnancy. Compression stockings may relieve the symptoms (such as swelling of your legs), although they will not stop the veins from appearing.

Vaginal discharge

You may get more vaginal discharge than usual while you are pregnant. This is usually nothing to worry about. However, if the discharge becomes itchy or sore, or smells unpleasant, or you have pain on passing urine, tell your midwife or doctor, as you may have an infection.

Thrush

If you have thrush (a yeast infection – also known as *Candida* or vaginal candidiasis) your doctor may prescribe cream and/or pessaries for you to apply to the area for 1 week.

While you are pregnant it is best to avoid taking any medicine for thrush that needs to be swallowed. There is no evidence about how safe or effective these are for pregnant women.

If you are pregnant beyond 41 weeks

If your pregnancy goes beyond 41 weeks there is a greater risk of certain problems for your baby. You should be offered a 'membrane sweep', which involves having a vaginal examination; this stimulates the neck of your womb (known as the cervix) to produce hormones which may trigger spontaneous labour. If you choose not to have a membrane sweep, or it does not cause you to go into labour, you should be offered a date to have your labour induced (started off).

If you decide against having labour induced and your pregnancy continues to 42 weeks or beyond, you should be offered ultrasound scans and may have your baby's heartbeat monitored regularly, depending on your individual care plan.

You can find more information about what induction of labour means from the guideline, which you can find on the NICE website at: www.nice.org.uk/pdf/inductionoflabourinfoforwomen.pdf.

If your baby is positioned bottom first

At around 36 weeks your midwife or doctor will check your baby's position by examining your abdomen. If they think the baby is not in a 'head down' position, which is best for the birth, you should be offered an ultrasound scan to check.

If your baby is bottom first (known as the breech position) your midwife or doctor should offer you a procedure called external cephalic version (ECV). ECV means they will gently push the baby from outside, to move it round to 'head first'. It does not always work.

Your midwife or doctor should give you more information about what ECV involves.

You should not be offered ECV if you:

- are in labour
- have a scar or abnormality in your womb
- have vaginal bleeding
- have a medical condition

or if:

- your waters have broken
- your baby's health seems fragile.

If you choose to have ECV and it cannot be done at 37 weeks, it should be done at 36 weeks.

Where you can find more information

If this is your first pregnancy, your midwife or doctor should give you a copy of *The pregnancy book* (published by Health Departments in England and Wales). It tells you about many aspects of pregnancy including: how the baby develops; deciding where to have a baby; feelings and relationships during pregnancy; antenatal care and classes; information for expectant fathers; problems in pregnancy; when pregnancy goes wrong; and rights and benefits information. It also contains a list of useful organisations.

If you need further information about any aspects of antenatal care or the care that you are receiving, please ask your midwife, doctor or a relevant member of your health team. You can discuss this guideline with them if you wish, especially if you aren't sure about anything in this booklet. They will be able to explain things to you.

For further information about the National Institute for Clinical Excellence (NICE), the Clinical Guidelines Programme or other versions of this guideline (including the sources of evidence used to inform the recommendations for care), you can visit the NICE website at www.nice.org.uk. At the NICE website you can also find information for the public about other maternity-related guidance on:

- pregnancy and childbirth: electronic fetal monitoring (guideline C)
- pregnancy and childbirth: induction of labour (guideline D)
- pregnancy – routine anti-D prophylaxis for rhesus negative women (technology appraisal no. 41).

You can get information on common problems during pregnancy from NHS Direct (telephone 0845 46 47; website www.nhsdirect.nhs.uk).

SUMMARY OF YOUR ROUTINE APPOINTMENTS DURING PREGNANCY

At each appointment, you should be given information with an opportunity to discuss issues and ask questions.
You should usually be asked to keep your own case notes at home with you and bring them to appointments.
Your midwife or doctor should tell you the results of all tests and have a system in place to do this.
As well as face-to-face information you should have access to antenatal classes and written information that is based on the best research evidence available.

Wherever possible you should be cared for by a small group of people with whom you feel comfortable. They should assess your particular needs as an individual and give you continuity of care.

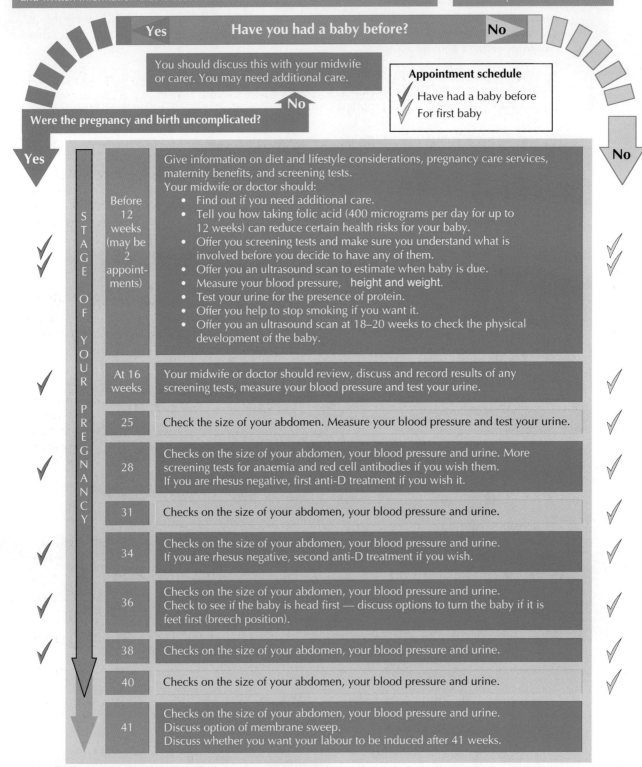

◄ Yes   **Have you had a baby before?**   **No ►**

You should discuss this with your midwife or carer. You may need additional care.

Appointment schedule
✓ Have had a baby before
✓ For first baby

No ▲

Were the pregnancy and birth uncomplicated?

Yes ▼   **No ▼**

	Stage	Details
✓✓	Before 12 weeks (may be 2 appointments)	Give information on diet and lifestyle considerations, pregnancy care services, maternity benefits, and screening tests. Your midwife or doctor should: • Find out if you need additional care. • Tell you how taking folic acid (400 micrograms per day for up to 12 weeks) can reduce certain health risks for your baby. • Offer you screening tests and make sure you understand what is involved before you decide to have any of them. • Offer you an ultrasound scan to estimate when baby is due. • Measure your blood pressure, height and weight. • Test your urine for the presence of protein. • Offer you help to stop smoking if you want it. • Offer you an ultrasound scan at 18–20 weeks to check the physical development of the baby.	✓✓
✓	At 16 weeks	Your midwife or doctor should review, discuss and record results of any screening tests, measure your blood pressure and test your urine.	✓
	25	Check the size of your abdomen. Measure your blood pressure and test your urine.	✓
✓	28	Checks on the size of your abdomen, your blood pressure and urine. More screening tests for anaemia and red cell antibodies if you wish them. If you are rhesus negative, first anti-D treatment if you wish it.	✓
	31	Checks on the size of your abdomen, your blood pressure and urine.	✓
✓	34	Checks on the size of your abdomen, your blood pressure and urine. If you are rhesus negative, second anti-D treatment if you wish.	✓
✓	36	Checks on the size of your abdomen, your blood pressure and urine. Check to see if the baby is head first — discuss options to turn the baby if it is feet first (breech position).	✓
✓	38	Checks on the size of your abdomen, your blood pressure and urine.	✓
	40	Checks on the size of your abdomen, your blood pressure and urine.	✓
	41	Checks on the size of your abdomen, your blood pressure and urine. Discuss option of membrane sweep. Discuss whether you want your labour to be induced after 41 weeks.	

(left column label: STAGE OF YOUR PREGNANCY)

7 : total appointments if you've had a baby before

Total appointments if this is your first baby: **10**

Appendix 2
Economic considerations: economic models

1. Asymptomatic bacteriuria screening programme

The purpose of the model was to compare the cost effectiveness and cost consequences of two different methods for detecting the presence of asymptomatic bacteriuria (ASB). A decision analytic model was created to compare the two strategies:

1. screening with urine culture
2. screening with leucocyte esterase-nitrite dipstick.

These methods have different sensitivities and specificities and associated costs. Untreated ASB can lead to pyelonephritis, which can lead to increased rate of preterm birth. Screening for ASB can lead to the treatment of women for ABS, prevent cases of pyelonephritis and prevent the costs and consequences of preterm birth. The cost consequences of preterm birth by missing one case of ASB have not yet been included in other economic evaluations and may be extremely high. Therefore a model was constructed to include this parameter.

Literature review

Thirteen papers were identified by the search strategy and the abstracts were reviewed. All the papers were retrieved and reviewed using the standard economic evaluation checklist. Of the 13, four papers contained data that were relevant for the economic model. One study[45] considered the cost consequences of preterm birth.

Designing the model

The clinical effectiveness data needed to construct the model were obtained from the guideline. Additional data that had to be collected to construct the model were the prevalence of pyelonephritis and the prevalence of preterm birth. Data on these parameters were derived from a review showing a range of values that were used in the model and subjected to sensitivity analysis.[351] A meta-analysis was also undertaken by the systematic reviewer on the guideline to provide relevant estimates used in the model.

The cost data included in the model were reported for three levels of analysis:

* screening and treatment for asymptomatic bacteriuria
* screening and treatment for asymptomatic bacteriuria and for treatment for pyelonephritis
* screening and treatment for asymptomatic bacteriuria, treatment for pyelonephritis and the cost of preterm birth.

The model reported the cost effectiveness of the two screening options in the following ratios:

* average cost of screening and treating for asymptomatic bacteriuria per person screened
* average cost of screening and treating for asymptomatic bacteriuria and pyelonephritis per person screened
* average cost of screening and treating for asymptomatic bacteriuria, pyelonephritis and the cases of preterm birth per person screened
* total cost per case of pyelonephritis averted
* total cost per case of preterm birth averted
* incremental cost of moving from dipstick test to a culture test screening programme.

Cost data

The cost data used are shown in Table A2.1. All costs apart from the costs of preterm birth were originally reported in US dollars and transformed to UK pounds sterling at the year 2002, using the Purchasing Power Parity Index taken from the website: www.oecd.fr/dsti/sti/it/stats/ppp.htm, and were inflated to year 2002 prices using the Retail Price Index for Health Services.

The baseline model

The sensitivity of the dipstick was assumed to be 0.72 and the sensitivity of the culture method was assumed to be close to 100%. The value used for the prevalence of pyelonephritis in the treatment was 0.04, while the value used for the prevalence of pyelonephritis without treatment was 0.19. The prevalence of preterm birth for the treatment group was 0.088 and for the untreated group 0.155.

The cost of preterm birth was taken from a UK study[601] and was estimated to be around £14,200. This value was subjected to sensitivity analysis. The incremental cost effectiveness analysis shows that, when taking the cost of treating the cases of preterm birth into account, the dipstick screening method would cost an extra £32,357 for each case of preterm birth averted.

Sensitivity analysis

The parameters examined in the model were the sensitivity of the dipstick method, the prevalence of pyelonephritis among women who are treated for ASB, the cost of preterm birth and the prevalence of preterm birth. Increasing the sensitivity of the dipstick by 10% (from 0.72 to 0.82) led to a reduction in the overall difference in costs between the screening tests (savings reduced to £4 to £5 per test). Threshold sensitivity analysis was undertaken to establish the sensitivity of the dipstick test that would have to be reached in order for both the culture and the dipstick test to have equivalent overall costs when taking all costs (screening, treatment and preterm birth) into account. The threshold was 0.91. A greater sensitivity than this for the dipstick test would make it the preferred method of screening. In reality, such sensitivity is considered to be extremely high and reported only in one study (see Section 10.1).

Overall, preterm birth should be included in the analysis, since the relative cost effectiveness of the tests is sensitive to even one additional case of preterm birth at the higher and lower value of the baseline cost. This has not been explored in economic models published in the literature to date and should be explored further in future studies, alongside more robust UK-based estimates of the long-term costs of preterm birth. Increasing and decreasing the cost estimates of preterm birth by as much as 50% did not change the overall results (favouring the culture method).

2. Modelling streptococcus group B screening programme

The purpose of the model was to compare the cost effectiveness and cost consequences of two screening programmes, namely bacteriological screening compared with risk factor screening.

Literature review

Forty-three papers were identified by the search strategy and the abstracts were reviewed. Of these, 19 full papers were retrieved and reviewed using the Drummond checklist. Two unauthored reports were also reviewed.

Table A2.1 Cost data used in the ASB model

Cost item	Range of values used in the model (£)
Cost of screening[600]	1,242 (sensitivity analysis ± 10% of this value)
Cost of pyelonephritis[600]	1,930 sensitivity analysis (± 10% of this value)
Cost of preterm birth[45]	14,000 to 21,000

None of the economic papers was in a UK setting and the majority of them were from a US setting. Sources of effectiveness data and the evidence for the clinical outcomes and all the ranges of their values were based on the clinical effectiveness data of the guideline using the best available data from the literature and expert opinion.

The lack of some definitive effectiveness data, such as the prevalence of early-onset group B streptococcus among positively screened women makes the completeness of the model problematic and therefore no conclusion can be reached from this model as far as the two screening procedures are concerned.

Future cost effectiveness research should include these parameters in order for a model to be estimated.

3. Modelling syphilis screening programme

The purpose of the model was to compare the cost effectiveness and cost consequences of two screening programmes, namely universal screening versus selective screening. The reason for this specific comparison was to consider a change in policy from the current practice of universal screening towards a more limited and potentially more cost effective approach. This is because the prevalence of syphilis is the UK is very low and, in addition, there may be identifiable groups of women who are at higher risk of contracting syphilis. A programme of selective screening could significantly reduce the number of women screened,[602] while at the same time identifying a relatively high proportion of carriers of the disease (100% for universal versus 70% to 78% for selective).

Literature review

In all, 47 papers were identified by the search strategy and the abstracts were reviewed. Of these, 25 full papers were retrieved and reviewed using the Drummond checklist. All the papers had some useful background information and contributed to the general structure of the model.

Data were extracted from one paper only, as it used UK-based cost data, post-1995, and UK effectiveness data, and considered the same screening alternatives.[602] This study identified possible screening strategy for the programme to compare their effectiveness and cost effectiveness to assess whether screening for syphilis is still necessary. Three possible strategic options for antenatal screening were examined:

- to continue the current universal screening programme
- to target the screening programme to pregnant women in high-risk groups
- to stop the screening programme entirely.

The study population comprised pregnant women in the UK, from which three high-risk groups were identified when considering screening strategy options: pregnant women in the Thames region, women from non-white ethnic groups and women born outside the UK.

Although the incremental cost per case detected of universal screening was high and although selectively screening groups by country of birth or by ethnic group could detect at least 70% of cases, this could be politically and practically difficult. Targeting by region would also be effective but difficult to implement.

The published evidence from this study is not ideal because the validity of estimate of measure of effectiveness was not reported. Also, the analysis did not include any cost to pregnant women such as anxiety or time taken to attend clinics and to set up partner notification services. Furthermore, the cost for the treatment of a woman's sexual partner was not calculated.

Designing the model

Because of the lack of data on the parameters discussed above, a model approach similar to the above study was adopted in this guideline. The model set out to estimate the total costs of screening and cost of syphilis treatment in pregnant women positively screened, cost of preterm birth, lifetime cost of congenital syphilis, and cost of spontaneous fetal loss.

Table A2.2 Cost data used in the syphilis model

Cost item	Range of values used in the model (£)
Cost of screening[602]	0.9 to 2.85
Cost of preterm birth[601]	14,000 to 145,000
Lifetime cost of congenital syphilis	Arbitrary value due to lack of literature data (arrived at through consensus with the Guideline Development Group)
Cost of treatment[602]	519 to 1,364

Cost data

The cost data used are shown in Table A2.2.

The evidence for the clinical outcomes and all the ranges of their values were based on the clinical effectiveness data of the guideline using the best available data from the literature and expert opinion.

Baseline results of the model

The model indicated that selective screening could detect from 70% (worse case scenario) to 78% of women affected by syphilis and that it is more cost effective even if preterm birth and lifetime costs of congenital syphilis cases are included. This model did not consider the value forgone of a programme that results in more cases of preventable congenital syphilis. This may be very high and therefore the selective screening programme may not be acceptable because of these losses.

Sensitivity analysis

Parameters examined in the sensitivity analysis were rate of transmission of congenital syphilis from the mother to the fetus (5%, 10%, 15%, 20%, 30%). Keeping all parameters constant, a rate of transmission more than 20% made the universal screening a more cost effective option in comparison with selective screening. The results are found to be insensitive to the sensitivity of the screening test.

Appendix 3

Training and equipment standards for ultrasound screening in pregnancy

Sonography is not recognised as a speciality by the Health Act 1999, so there is no obligation for sonographers to be registered to practise. There is currently no statutory requirement for ultrasound practitioners to receive accredited training.

Many sonographers will have achieved a postgraduate certificate or diploma in clinical ultrasound. Well-established programmes leading to these qualifications are available in a number of universities in the UK and courses are accredited by the Consortium for the Accreditation of Sonographic Education (CASE). Members of the consortium include the British Medical Ultrasound Society, the Royal College of Radiographers (RCR), the Royal College of Midwives and the United Kingdom Association of Sonographers.

To achieve and attain CASE accreditation, an individual course must demonstrate that both its academic and clinical teaching programmes and its assessment methods are sufficiently rigorous to ensure that successful students are safe to practise in the ultrasound areas for which they have studied. Current postgraduate education certificates and diploma training programmes in obstetric ultrasound are designed with the provision of a safe, accurate and efficient screening service for fetal anomaly in mind.

There is a need for practical competence tests at NHS trust level. The RCOG Working Party recommends that local departments monitor standards and keep checks on them.

Trusts should have a process for retraining and updating as required but at present there is little provision for this in trust budgets. Clinical governance provides a facilitating mechanism.

Medical staff who undertake ultrasound scanning for fetal anomalies should ideally hold the Advanced Certificate of Ultrasound Training, which is issued following a 300-hour course held in centres recognised by the RCOG and RCR. Skills should be maintained by performing detailed scans in at least one and preferably two sessions a week.

Medical and midwifery staff should not undertake scans of any sort if they have not been specifically trained.

A scan to perform a fetal structural survey demands the use of modern equipment (not more than 5 years old) of modest sophistication. The scanner must be capable of performing the necessary measurements and should provide good image quality. As always, regards for safety in the use of ultrasound is paramount and minimum output should be used in accordance with the ALARA principle: as low as reasonably attainable.

[Extracted from the recommendations of the Royal College of Obstetricians and Gynaecologists' Working Party on Ultrasound Screening for Fetal Abnormalities.[302]]

Appendix 4
Further information

During the review process of this guideline, various topics were suggested by stakeholders and peer reviewers for inclusion in the guideline. The inclusion or exclusion of any subject not already contained in the guideline was carefully considered by the Guideline Development Group.

Topics that were not originally included in the scope of this guideline and for which guidance already exists are listed in this Appendix, with information on where further information can be obtained. All other topics raised by stakeholders or peer reviewers have been addressed in the main text of the guideline.

Cystic fibrosis   UK National Screening Committee [http://www.doh.gov.uk/nsc/]

Herpes   *Genital Herpes in Pregnancy: Management* (RCOG Guideline No. 30, March 2002). [www.rcog.org.uk/guidelines.asp?PageID=106&GuidelineID=39]

HTLV 1   The UK National Screening Committee position on HTLV1 (human T lymphocyte virus 1) is that screening should not be offered for pregnant women. (www.nelh.nhs.uk/screening/antenatal_pps/htlv1.html)

Thrombophilia   The UK National Screening Committee position on thrombophilia is that there is no evidence to support screening to identify those deemed at increased risk of venous thrombosis in pregnancy. [www.nelh.nhs.uk/screening/antenatal_pps/thrombophilia.html]

Varicella   *Chickenpox in Pregnancy* (RCOG Guideline No. 13, July 2001). [www.rcog.org.uk/guidelines.asp?PageID=106&GuidelineID=7]

Note

RCOG Guidelines (also known as Green-top guidelines) are clinical guidelines produced by the Guidelines and Audit Committee of the Royal College of Obstetricians and Gynaecologists. Guidelines can be accessed online at: www.rcog.org.uk/guidelines.asp?PageID=106.

Evidence tables

Study type codes

CCS	Case–control study
CCH	Controlled cohort study
CH	Cohort study
COM	Comparative study
CR	Case report
CS	Case series
CSS	Cross-sectional study
CSNR	Controlled trial without randomisation
DBP	Double blind parallel trial
DBRP	Double blind randomised placebo controlled trial
EE	Economic evaluation
EV	Evaluation
GL	Guidelines
HTA	Health Technology Assessment
ISNR	Interventional study not randomised
ISS	Interventional study with groups sequentially allocated
LS	Longitudinal study
ME	Model evaluation
NCC	Nested case–control
OB	Observational study
OPC	Open pilot cohort study
PHLS	Report from PHLS AIDS Diagnostic Working Group
QR	Quasi-randomised study
RDBC	Randomised double blind crossover trial
REC	Review by expert committee
RCSS	Review of cross-sectional studies
RCT	Randomised controlled trial
RV	Review
SA	Secondary analysis of RCT data
SR	Systematic review
SSW	Guideline report from PHLS Syphilis Serology Working Group
SV	Surveillance
TES	Test evaluation survey
TESC	Test evaluation survey on crossover
EL	Evidence level

[All other abbreviations will be found in the list of abbreviations on page ix]

Chapter 3 Woman-centred care and informed decision making

Study	Ref.	Population	Intervention	Outcomes	Results	Comments	Study type	EL
Audit Commission, 1997	10	2375 mothers who gave birth during June and July 1995 in England and Wales	Self-completion questionnaires sent to a national sample drawn by ONS	Perceived options in antenatal care Women's assessment of information and communication in antenatal care	Perceived option in where to have antenatal care: 33% yes 63% no 4% don't know Perceived option in which professional provides care: 35% yes 60% no 5% don't know Perceived option in having a scan: 52% yes 31% no 13% partly 4% don't know Perceived option in having a screening test: 60% yes 10% no 8% partly 22% don't know Information on the benefits and risks of various screening tests: 68% reported they had received enough spoken information 60% reported they had received enough written information		CSS	3
Gagnon, 2001	27	6 RCTs, 1443 women	To assess the effects of antenatal education on knowledge acquisition, anxiety, sense of control, pain, support, breastfeeding, infant care abilities, psychological and social adjustment	Satisfaction with maternal role preparation Maternal attachment behaviours Knowledge acquisition	No consistent results were found Maternal role preparation (1 RCT, n = 16): WMD 21.590, 95% CI 11.234 to 31.946 when women who received individual ANC were compared with women who received no organised antenatal education Maternal attachment behaviours (1 RCT, n = 10): WMD 52.600, 95% CI 21.818 to 83.382 when this component was added to antenatal classes compared with antenatal classes without this component Knowledge acquisition (1 RCT, n = 48): WMD 1.620, 95% CI 0.492 to 2.748 in expanded antenatal education classes versus standard antenatal education classes	The largest trial reviewed examined educational intervention to increase vaginal birth after caesarean section (n = 1275) No data from the other 5 trials (n = 168) were reported on labour and birth outcomes, anxiety, breastfeeding success, or general social support	SR	1a

Chapter 3 Woman-centred care and informed decision making (continued)

Study	Ref.	Population	Intervention	Outcomes	Results	Comments	Study type	EL
Thornton et al., 1995	12	1691 pregnant women before 15 weeks gestation in England from 1991 to 1994	Extra information delivered individually (n = 561) vs. extra information delivered in classes (n = 563) vs. information normally given (n = 567) in a routine antenatal clinic on prenatal testing Extra information was delivered at a specifically scheduled class or one-on-one visit for the purpose of covering screening and risks related to: – Down's syndrome – Ultrasound at 18 weeks for fetal abnormalities (esp. neural tube defects) – Haemoglobinopathy (with patients from relevant ethnic groups) – Cystic fibrosis	Uptake rates of prenatal tests Levels of anxiety	Uptake of Down's syndrome screening: 37% vs. 32% vs. 34% Uptake of ultrasonography: 98% vs. 99% vs. 99% Uptake of cystic fibrosis screening: 65% vs. 62% vs. 79% Uptake of amniocentesis: 3% vs. 2% vs. 3% No differences in anxiety at 16 weeks. Anxiety at 20 and 34 weeks was lower among those offered individual information when compared with controls (p < 0.05)	Analysis by intention to treat Randomisation by sealed opaque envelopes	RCT	1b
O'Cathain et al., 2002	13	Women reaching 28 weeks before the intervention (n = 1386) and after (n = 1778) from 13 maternity units in Wales	Maternity units randomised by coin toss. Provision of MIDIRS informed choice leaflets to intervention units vs. no leaflets	Exercising informed choice Changes in women's knowledge Satisfaction with information	Informed choice: OR 1.15, 95% CI 0.65 to 2.06 Antenatal knowledge: mean difference 0.20, 95% CI –0.09, 0.49 Satisfied with amount of information: OR 1.4, 95% CI 1.05 to 1.88		RCT	1b
Hibbard et al., 1979	28	744 primigravid women in Cardiff, Wales	Survey at first attendance (n = 256) Survey at 35 weeks gestation (n = 237) Survey postpartum (n = 251)	Knowledge Anxiety			CSS	3

4.1 Who provides care?

Study	Ref.	Population	Intervention	Outcomes	Results	Comments	Study type	EL
Villar and Khan-Neelofur, 2003	32	3 RCTs, 3041 women	Midwife and GP-managed care vs. obstetrician and gynaecologist-led shared care	Preterm delivery (< 37 weeks)	Preterm birth (2 RCTs, n = 2883): Peto OR 0.79, 95% CI 0.57 to 1.10	All 3 trials conducted in developed countries	SR	1a
				Pre-eclampsia	Pre-eclampsia (2 RCTs, n = 2952): Peto OR 0.37, 95% CI 0.22, 0.64			
				PIH	PIH (3 RCTs, n = 3041): Peto OR 0.56, 95% CI 0.45 to 0.70			
				Caesarean section	Caesarean section (3 RCTs, n = 2972): Peto OR 0.99, 95% CI 0.79 to 1.25			
				Antepartum haemorrhage	Antepartum haemorrhage (2 RCTs, n = 2952): Peto OR 0.79, 95% CI 0.57 to 1.10			
				UTI	UTI (1 RCT, n = 1674): Peto OR 1.23, 95% CI 0.86 to 1.76			
				Anaemia (Hb < 10 g/dl)	Anaemia (2 RCTs, n = 2952): Peto OR 1.00, 95% CI 0.82 to 1.22			
				Perinatal mortality	Perinatal mortality (2 RCTs, n = 2890): Peto OR 0.59, 95% CI 0.28 to 1.26			
				Maternal satisfaction	Satisfaction was similar or higher for those with midwife and GP-led care			

4.2 Continuity of care

Study	Ref.	Population	Intervention	Outcomes	Results	Comments	Study type	EL
Hodnett, 2001	33	2 RCTs, 1815 women	Continuity of care by the same caregiver or small group of caregivers vs. usual care by multiple caregivers throughout pregnancy	Interventions during labour Maternal outcomes Infant outcomes	Clinic waiting times >15 minutes (1 RCT, n=1001): Peto OR 0.14, 95% CI 0.10 to 0.19 Antenatal admission to hospital (2 RCTs, n=1815): Peto OR 0.79, 95% CI 0.64 to 0.97 Failure to attend antenatal classes (1 RCT, n=814): Peto OR 0.58, 95%nCI 0.41 to 0.81 Unable to discuss worries in pregnancy (1 RCT, n=1001): Peto OR 0.72, 95% CI 0.56 to 0.92 Not feel well-prepared for labour (1 RCT, n=1001): Peto OR 0.64, 95% CI 0.48, 0.86 Intrapartum analgesia or anaesthesia (2 RCTs, n=1815): Peto OR 0.53, 95% CI 0.44 to 0.64 Not feel in control during labour (1 RCT, n=1001): Peto OR 0.48, 95% CI 0.34 to 0.68 Failure to enjoy childbirth (1 RCT, n=1001): Peto OR 0.65, 95% CI 0.47 to 0.90 Perceive labour staff as unsupportive (1 RCT, n=1001): Peto OR 0.72, 95% CI 0.56 to 0.92 Episiotomy (2 RCTs, n=1815): Peto OR 0.75, 95% CI 0.60 to 0.94 Unable to discuss postnatal problems (1 RCT, n=1001): Peto OR 0.64, 95% CI 0.49 to 0.85 Feel unprepared for child care (1 RCT, n=1001): Peto OR 0.57, 95% CI 0.41 to 0.80 Neonatal resuscitation (2 RCTs, n=1815): Peto OR 0.66, 95% CI 0.52 to 0.83 Miscarriage (1 RCT, n=814): Peto OR 0.44, 95% CI 0.20 to 0.94 Vaginal or perineal tear (2 RCTs, n=1815): Peto OR 1.28, 95% CI 1.05 to 1.56 First stage labour >6 hours (2 RCTs, n=1815): Peto OR 1.35, 95% CI 1.08 to 1.68 5-minute Apgar score <8 (1 RCT, n=1001): Peto OR 2.63, 95% CI 1.15 to 6.02 No significant difference in the rates of caesarean section, induction of labour, augmentation of labour, amniotomy, stillbirth, neonatal death, preterm birth, intact perineum, admission to NICU, birthweight <2500 g, dissatisfaction with intrapartum pain relief or breastfeeding		SR	1a

4.2 Continuity of care (continued)

Study	Ref.	Population	Intervention	Outcomes	Results	Comments	Study type	EL
Waldenstrom and Turnbull, 1998	34	7 RCTs, 9148 women	Continuity of care by the same caregiver or small group of caregivers vs. usual care by multiple caregivers throughout pregnancy	Interventions during labour Maternal outcomes Infant outcomes	Induction of labour: Peto OR 0.76, 95% CI 0.66 to 0.86 Augmentation of labour: Peto OR 0.78, 95% CI 0.70 to 0.87 Electronic fetal monitoring: Peto OR 0.19, 95% CI 0.17 to 0.21 Epidural: Peto OR 0.76, 95% CI 0.68 to 0.85 Narcotics in labour: Peto OR 0.69, 95% CI 0.63 to 0.77 Instrumental vaginal delivery: Peto OR 0.82, 95% CI 0.70 to 0.95 Episiotomy: Peto OR 0.69, 95% CI 0.61 to 0.77 Perineal tears: Peto OR 1.15, 95% CI 1.05 to 1.26 No significant difference in the rates of caesarean section, intact perineum, admission to NICU, postnatal haemorrhage, manual removal of placenta, antenatal admission to hospital, postnatal complications and readmissions to hospital, or duration of labour No maternal deaths reported Perinatal mortality: Peto OR 1.60, 95% CI 0.99 to 2.59 Satisfaction with care was reported in 6/7 trials but not included in the meta-analysis due to lack of consistency between measures. Women in the intervention group were more satisfied with care during all phases of pregnancy and differences were statistically significant for each study separately. Women in the continuous care group were more pleased with information giving and communication with the caregivers and felt more involved in the decision making and more in control		SR	1a

4.4 Documentation of care

Study	Ref.	Population	Intervention	Outcomes	Results	Comments	Study type	EL
Lovell et al., 1987	44	246 women from antenatal clinic in deprived inner city area in London	Carrying their own case notes vs. cooperation card Questionnaires were administered at 8 to 16 weeks of gestation (before randomisation), 32 to 34 weeks gestation and 2 to 7 days postpartum Clinical and background information was extracted from the case notes and interviews with 20 healthcare professionals involved in maternity care were carried out	Extensive qualitative results on women's perceptions and beliefs Clinical safety of carrying own notes	Women's attitudes towards carrying their own case notes were very positive. Both groups wanted their own notes in future pregnancies. Also would have preferred to have access to notes while in hospital Did not cause anxiety but may reduce it. Experimental group felt their preferences had been taken more into account Women read notes with great interest. No one lost or forgot to bring notes to hospital. More lost notes in control group Women carrying their own notes were more likely to say that they felt in control of their pregnancy: rate ratio 1.45, 95% CI 1.08 to 1.95 and they were more likely to say they found it easier to talk to the doctors and midwives during pregnancy: rate ratio 1.73, 95% CI 1.16 to 2.59 Experimental group less likely to miss antenatal clinic appointments No difference in the availability of notes for clinic appointments but approximately 1 hour of hospital clerical time was saved per week because of not having to retrieve and re-file notes Obstetric outcomes similar in both groups Majority of health professionals and staff in favour of women having their own notes but with reservations. All believed that women liked having them	48 women (19%) dropped out at some stage but all details given in report	RCT	1b

4.4 Documentation of care (continued)

Study	Ref.	Population	Intervention	Outcomes	Results	Comments	Study type	EL
Elbourne et al., 1987	42	290 women attending a rural consultant clinic in Berkshire, England	Carrying full case notes until 10 days after delivery (n = 147) vs. cooperation card while case notes held by hospital (n = 143) Information about women's attitudes and behaviour obtained from 4 questionnaires (booking, 34 weeks, 10 days postnatal, 6 months postnatal) Cotinine assay on polled urine samples from each group at 34 weeks. Clinical information from notes. Observations in medical records department and informal interviews with staff		Two groups of women comparable in terms of sociodemographic characteristics, smoking behaviour and in answers to socio-psychological questions in the recruitment questionnaire Women with own notes nearly 1.5 times more likely to say that they felt in control of their pregnancy (RR1.45 95% CI 1.08 to 1.95) and more than 1.5 times more likely to say that they found it easier to talk to the doctors and midwives antenatally (RR 1.73 95% CI 1.16 to 2.59). No statistically significant differences between groups in terms of women's feelings of being well informed, anxious, confident, depressed, satisfied with their care or about involvement by baby's father, clinical outcomes, women's health-related behaviours. 91% of women in own notes group wanted the same in next pregnancy compared with coop card where 58% wanted a coop card next time. No difference in availability of notes in antenatal clinic. Approx. 1 hour of clerical time saved in peripheral clinic per week	Power calculation shown. 85% response rate at 6 months postnatal. Not as many differences between groups as expected. Possible dilution of difference between groups due to Hawthorn effect and halo effect	RCT	1b
Homer et al., 1999	43	150 English speaking pregnant women from an Australian metropolitan ANC in 1997	holding antenatal record vs. keeping a co-operation card. Questionnaire administered between 34–38 weeks gestation. Audit throughout study period to monitor lost and misplaced records.	Response rate Women's feelings toward carrying their own notes	84% response rate Multiparae who carried notes were significantly more likely to report that the doctors and midwives explained everything in their records to them than multiparae with coop cards or primiparae from either group Open ended questions showed: – 89% of women carrying their own notes felt more in control, felt more informed, liked having access to their results and felt it gave them an opportunity to share information particularly with other family members and partners – 11% of women carrying their own notes thought the record was too bulky, the system inconvenient or were worried they would forget notes – No differences were noted in numbers of lost records in each group – 89% of women in the hand-held notes group wanted to carry their notes in a future pregnancy as well as 52% of the cooperation card group	Power calculation performed. Analysed on intention-to-treat basis	RCT	1b

4.5 Frequency of antenatal appointments

Study	Ref.	Population	Intervention	Outcomes	Results	Comments	Study type	EL
Villar and Khan-Neelofur, 2003	32	7 RCTs	Provision of reduced number of visits compared with standard schedule of visits	Perinatal outcomes Satisfaction outcomes	No significant differences in preterm delivery (< 37 weeks), pre-eclampsia, caesarean section, induction of labour, antenatal haemorrhage, postnatal haemorrhage, low birth weight, SGA, postpartum anaemia, admission to neonatal intensive care unit, perinatal mortality, maternal mortality and UTI found Women from developed countries in the reduced number of visits group were less satisfied with frequency of visits (3 RCTs, n = 3393): Peto OR 0.61, 95% CI 0.52 to 0.72	4 trials in developed countries, 3 in developing countries; same 7 trials as Carroli review[46] exact n not specified and not calculable from 'included trials' tables	SR	1a
Carroli et al., 2001	46	7 RCTs, 57,418 women	Lower number of antenatal visits (n = 30,799) compared with standard antenatal care models (n = 26,620)	Maternal and neonatal clinical outcomes Perceived satisfaction	No differences found in pre-eclampsia, urinary tract infection, postpartum anaemia, maternal mortality, low birthweight or perinatal mortality Women from developed countries in the intervention group were less satisfied with frequency of visits: rate difference –8.5%, p = 0.001	4 trials in developed countries, 3 in developing countries; the same 7 trials as Villar review[32] outcome data available for n = 26,619 in intervention group and n = 25,821 in control group	SR	1a
Petrou et al., 2003	45	17,765 women with a singleton pregnancy from England and Wales from 1994 to 1995	Data from an audit from 9 maternity units were retrospectively analysed	Range of number of visits Odds ratios for adverse perinatal outcomes by unit increase in antenatal visits for nulliparae (n = 7255) and multiparae (n = 10,510)	1 to 25 antenatal care visits Delivery by caesarean section: – primiparae OR 1.04 (95% CI 1.02 to 1.06) – multiparae OR 1.02 (95% CI 1.00 to 1.04, p = 0.036) Low birthweight (< 2500 g): – primiparae OR 1.03 (95% CI 1.00 to 1.07, p = 0.032) – multiparae OR 1.02 (95% CI 0.99 to 1.05) Admission to SCBU: – primiparae OR 1.0 (95% CI 0.97, 1.03) – multiparae OR 0.99 (95% CI 0.97, 1.02) Perinatal mortality: – primiparae OR 1.03 (95% CI 0.94, 1.12) – multiparae OR 1.0 (95% CI 0.91, 1.10)		CSS	3

4.5 Frequency of antenatal appointments (continued)

Study	Ref.	Population	Intervention	Outcomes	Results	Comments	Study type	EL
Hildingsson et al., 2002	48	3061 women attending antenatal care clinics in Sweden from 1999 to 2000	Questionnaire mailed shortly after first antenatal care visit	Preference with number of visits	Multiparous women preferred both more (RR 1.3, 95% CI 1.1 to 1.4) and fewer (RR 2.0, 95% CI 1.5 to 2.7) visits compared with primiparous women Younger women (< 25 years) preferred more visits (RR 1.2, 95% CI 1.1 to 1.4) and older women (> 35 years) fewer visits (RR 1.9, 95% CI 1.3 to 2.6) compared with 25- to 35-year-olds Single women preferred more visits when compared with married or cohabitating women (RR 1.9, 95% CI 1.3 to 2.7) Women with less education preferred fewer visits (RR 1.7, 95% CI 1.1 to 2.6) Women with a prior history of miscarriage, abortion, stillbirth or assisted conception preferred more visits	In an uncomplicated pregnancy in Sweden, a woman sees the midwife 8 to 9 times and a doctor once	CSS	3

4.6 Gestational age assessment

Study	Ref.	Population	Intervention	Outcomes	Results	Comments	Study type	EL
Neilson, 1999	57	9 RCTs	Routine use of ultrasound vs. selective use of ultrasound at < 24 weeks	Induction rates for post-term pregnancy Detection of multiple pregnancy Perinatal mortality Neurobehavioural outcome and school function	Induction rates (6 RCTs, n = 24,195): Peto OR 0.61, 95% CI 0.52 to 0.72 Undiagnosed twins by 26 weeks (6 RCTs, n = 220): Peto OR 0.08, 95% CI 0.04 to 0.16 Perinatal mortality (8 RCTs, n = 34,245): Peto OR 0.86, 95% CI 0.67 to 1.12 Poor oral reading at school (1 RCT, n = 1,993): Peto OR 1.02, 95% CI 0.72 to 1.45 Poor reading comprehension at school (1 RCT, n = 1984): Peto OR 0.82, 95% CI 0.54 to 1.23 Poor spelling at school (1 RCT, n = 1982): Peto OR 0.73, 95% CI 0.53 to 1.0 Poor arithmetic at school (1 RCT, n = 1993): Peto OR 0.90, 95% CI 0.59 to 1.37 Reduced hearing in childhood (2 RCTs, n = 5,418): Peto OR 0.90, 95%CI 0.67, 1.21 Reduced vision in childhood (2 RCTs, n = 5417): Peto OR 0.82, 95% CI 0.66 to 1.01 Use of spectacles (2 RCTs, n = 5331): Peto OR 0.87, 95% CI 0.72 to 1.05		SR	1a
Crowther et al., 1999	52	648 women at a tertiary level hospital in Australia	Women attending for their first antenatal visit at less than 17 weeks of gestation were randomised into ultrasound (n = 321) or no ultrasound (n = 327)	Proportion of women who needed EDD adjusted due to ≥10-day discrepancy at 18 to 20 weeks Feelings about pregnancy Pregnancy outcomes	EDD adjusted: 9% vs. 18%, RR 0.52 (95% CI 0.34 t to 0.79) Concerned about wellbeing of pregnancy: RR 0.98 (95% CI 0.90 to 1.08) Feel worried about pregnancy in any way: RR 0.80 (95% CI 0.65 to 0.99) Do not feel relaxed about pregnancy in any way: RR 0.73 (95% CI 0.56 to 0.96) Do not feel excited about pregnancy in any way: RR 0.73 (95% CI 0.50 to 1.08) Nonviable pregnancy: RR 0.97 (95% CI 0.52 to 1.81)	Menstrual dates were not available for 16 women in the intervention group	RCT	1b

4.6 Gestational age assessment (continued)

Study	Ref.	Population	Intervention	Outcomes	Results	Comments	Study type	EL
Savitz et al., 2002	53	3655 pregnant women in the USA from 1995 to 2001	Women at 24 to 29 weeks of gestation were recruited and gestational age estimates were compared to actual delivery dates by four algorithms Group 1: LMP only Group 2: ultrasound only Group 3: LMP except when a discrepancy ≥ 7 days existed in which case ultrasound dating was used Group 4: same as Group 3 but for ≥ 14 days	Differences in estimates between 4 groups Proportion of preterm births predicted (< 37 weeks) Proportion of post-term births predicted (> 41 weeks) Deviation between predicted and actual delivery dates	Mean duration of gestation estimate: – Group 1: 277.1 days – Group 2: 274.3 days – Group 3: 274.1 days – Group 4: 274.5 days Proportion preterm: no difference between the 4 groups, kappa = 0.72, 95% CI 0.68 to 0.75 Proportion post-term: LMP 12.1%; all other groups 3.4% to 4.5%, kappa = 0.16, 95% CI 0.11 to 0.20 Predicted vs. actual delivery: – Group 1, within 1 week, 48% – Groups 2 to 4, within 1 week, 55% to 58% predicted correctly – A further 15.7% within 2 weeks later for group 1 – A further 15.6% to 16.4% 2 weeks later for groups 2-4 – At more than 2 weeks afterward, 11.5% for group 1 and 2.3% to 3.2% for groups 2 to 4		CH	2a
Tunon et al., 1996	55	14,167 pregnant women in Norway from 1987 to 1992	Ultrasound examination at 18 weeks of gestation compared to LMP for prediction of date of delivery. LMP only used if reliable and menstrual cycle was regular	Prediction of day of delivery for term birth (282 days)	Proportion of women who delivered within 1 week of prediction for term: 61% for ultrasound and 56% for LMP calculation Proportion of women who delivered within 2 weeks of prediction for term: 88% for ultrasound and 84% for LMP calculation Estimated number of post-term births: 4.1% for ultrasound and 9.8% for LMP, p < 0.001		CH	2a

4.6 Gestational age assessment (continued)

Study	Ref.	Population	Intervention	Outcomes	Results	Comments	Study type	EL
Backe and Nakling, 1994	54	1341 pregnant women in Norway from 1988 to 1989	Ultrasound performed before 20 weeks of gestation compared to LMP for prediction of term birth date	Prediction compared to actual day of delivery for term birth (280 days)	Ultrasound prediction was closer to actual day of delivery, p = 0.03 Proportion of women who delivered within 2 weeks of prediction for term: 87.5% for ultrasound and 79.3% for LMP calculation, chi ^{2} = 33, p < 0.001 Delivered more than 2 weeks after predicted date: 3% with ultrasound estimation and 13.9% with LMP, chi^2 = 103, p < 0.001		CH	2a
Blondel et al., 2002	56	44,623 births in Canada from 1978 to 1996	Comparison of 6 algorithms to assess gestational age 1: LMP 2: LMP unless discrepancy greater than 14 days; then, ultrasound 3: LMP unless discrepancy greater than 10 days; then, ultrasound 4: LMP unless discrepancy greater than 7 days; then, ultrasound 5: LMP unless discrepancy greater than 3 days; then, ultrasound 6: ultrasound alone	Rates of preterm and post-term births (< 32, 34, and 37 weeks and ≥ 41 and 42 weeks) Concordance between LMP and ultrasound estimates	At < 37 weeks: 1. 7.6% 2. 7.8% 3. 8.1% 4. 8.5% 5. 9.0% 6. 9.1% At ≥ 41: 1. 20.9% 2. 16.9% 3. 15.1% 4. 13.4% 5. 13.4% 6. 11.2% Concordance within 14 days for 90.7% of births		CH	2a

5.10 Exercise in pregnancy

5.10.1 What exercises are of benefit during pregnancy?

Study	Ref.	Population	Intervention	Outcomes	Results	Comments	Study type	EL
Kramer, 2002	101	10 RCTs, 688 pregnant women	Regular aerobic exercise (at least 2 to 3 times/week) vs. reduction in frequency or intensity of such exercise	Maternal physical fitness Pregnancy outcome Self-perceived body image	5 trials (n = 171) report significant improvement in physical fitness in the exercise group but difference in measures prevents meta-analysis of results; 2 trials (n = 36) reported no significant increase in fitness in the exercise group Gestational age (3 RCTs, n = 416): WMD 0.02, 95% CI −0.4, 0.4 Preterm birth (3 RCTs, n = 421): RR 2.29, 95% CI 1.02, 5.13 Birthweight (5 RCTs, n = 476): WMD 28.64, 95% CI −65.85 to 123.13 Pre-eclampsia (2 RCTs, n = 81): RR 1.17, 95% CI 0.44 to 3.08 Body image (1 RCT, n = 15): Physical stamina, WMD −1.7, 95% CI −3.49 to 0.03 Muscular strength, WMD −2.2, 95% CI −3.62 to −0.72 Energy level, WMD −2.2, 95% CI −3.29 to −1.06 Body build, WMD -1.5, 95% CI −2.51 to −0.39	Trials either did not specify method of allocation or alternated	SR	1a

5.10.2 What exercises are associated with adverse maternal and perinatal outcomes?

Study	Ref.	Population	Intervention	Outcomes	Results	Comments	Study type	EL
Camporesi, 1996	102	Three cross-sectional studies: Study 1, 100 women who dived during pregnancy and n = 69 who did not Study 2, 72 women who dived during pregnancy Study 3, 142 dived pregnancies (i.e., some women dived during more than one pregnancy)	Retrospective questionnaires	Malformations, SGA and other infant outcomes Fetal decompression disease	Overall: fetus is at greater risk of malformations and embolisation after decompression bubbles evolve in circulation, owing to lack of pulmonary filtration and inability to resolve gas bubbles in alveoli Study 1: none among non-diving mothers; 7/100 (7%) mothers had babies with congenital abnormalities 1.4% of babies were SGA in non-diving group; 6% in diving group Raised incidence of miscarriage, stillbirth and neonatal death also reported. Study 2: no evidence of increased risk to unborn fetus in mothers who stopped diving during the first trimester and mothers who dived throughout pregnancy Study 3: n = 109 (75%) live births and n = 33 (23%) stillbirths or spontaneous miscarriages, evenly divided among dived pregnancies and non-dived pregnancies	Response rate of 169/208 (81%) in one study and the 72 from the second study were self-selected and from an initial 610 women Third study fails to mention the outcome of 4 births	RCSS	3

5.11 Sexual intercourse in pregnancy

Study	Ref.	Population	Intervention	Outcomes	Results	Comments	Study type	EL
Berghella et al., 2002	105	966 pregnant women randomised to metronidazole in a BV trial and 320 pregnant women randomised to metronidazole in a *Trichomonas vaginalis* trial in the USA	Women identified at 16 to 23 weeks of gestation with BV or *Trichomonas vaginalis* were treated with metronidazole or placebo. Questions about sexual behaviour were asked at two points in the study: before and after treatment. Treatment was 8 capsules taken at randomisation visit and again 48 hours later, repeated at follow-up visit between 24 and 29 weeks, but at least 14 days after initial visit. Analysis includes women who received metronidazole treatment only	Follow-up cultures taken after initial treatment. Before treatment: effect of number of lifetime partners, number of partners since start of pregnancy and episodes of intercourse in the past 4 weeks on incidence of preterm birth. After treatment: intercourse (yes or no) and frequency of intercourse. Effect of sexual behaviour on efficacy of treatment	For BV trial: 846/966. For *Trichomonas vaginalis* trial: 269/320. Sexual behaviour before treatment had no effect on incidence of preterm birth (p > 0.4 for both trials). Intercourse between the first and second dose had no effect in either trial. Intercourse between the second and third dose: – BV trial RR 0.6 (95%CI 0.4, 0.9) – *Trichomonas vaginalis* trial RR 1.0, (95% CI 0.6 to 1.6). Frequency of intercourse between second and third dose: – BV trial, more frequent intercourse associated with lower incidence of preterm birth (p = 0.03) – *Trichomonas vaginalis* trial, p = 0.64. Sexual behaviour had no effect on treatment efficacy		SA	2a
Read and Klebanoff, 1993	103	13,285 women attending antenatal care from 1984 to 1989 in the USA	Frequency of intercourse at 23 to 26 weeks assessed	Association between preterm birth and Intercourse at 23 to 26 weeks (less than once a week used as reference group)	Intercourse 1 to 2 times/week: OR 0.79, 95% CI 0.70 to 0.90. Intercourse 3 or 4 times/week: OR 0.76, 95% CI 0.64 to 0.90. Intercourse ≥ 5 times/week: 0.89, 95% CI 0.70 to 1.14. Less than once per week vs. once a week or more: OR 0.80, 95% CI 0.71 to 0.89	No data on frequency of intercourse for n = 306 women	CH	2a
Klebanoff et al., 1984	104	39,217 singleton, first pregnancies from 1959 to 1966 in the USA	Coital frequency in the previous month reported until 27 weeks, then frequencies reported for the previous two weeks up to 42 to 43 weeks	Association between coital frequency and preterm birth. Association between coital frequency and perinatal mortality. Association between coital frequency and mean duration of gestation	Inverse relationship between frequency of coitus and preterm delivery reported at 28 to 29 weeks and also at 32 to 33 weeks (p < 0.001). No statistically significant association between coital frequency at 28 to 29 weeks, 32 to 33 weeks, and 36 to 37 weeks and perinatal mortality. Mean duration of gestation increased with increasing coital frequency at 28 to 29 weeks, 32 to 33 weeks, and 36 to 37 weeks (p < 0.001)		CH	2a

5.12 Smoking in pregnancy

5.12.1 What are the maternal and perinatal outcomes associated with smoking in pregnancy?

Study	Ref.	Population	Intervention	Outcomes	Results	Comments	Study type	EL
Shah and Bracken, 2000	117	20 cohort studies	Meta-analysis of any maternal smoking vs. no maternal smoking during pregnancy	Preterm delivery	Pooled OR 1.27, 95% CI 1.21 to 1.33	No information regarding the size of the studies was provided in the review	SR of CH (1966 to 1997)	2a
Castles et al., 1999	116	6 studies on placenta praevia; 8 on placental abruption; 9 on ectopic pregnancy; 6 on PPROM; 5 on pre-eclampsia in the USA and Western Europe	Meta-analysis of any maternal smoking vs. no maternal smoking during pregnancy	Placenta praevia (n = 32,444 cases, n = 18,251 controls) Placental abruption (n = 42,207 cases, n = 15,095 controls) Ectopic pregnancy (n = 2831 cases, n = 7801 controls) PPROM (n = 31,639 cases, 3029 controls) Pre-eclampsia (n = 3485 cases, n = 966 controls)	Placenta praevia: pooled OR 1.58, 95% CI 1.04 to 2.12 Abruption placenta: pooled OR 1.62, 95% CI 1.46 to 1.77 Ectopic pregnancy: pooled OR 1.77, 95% CI 1.31 to 2.22 PPROM: pooled OR 1.7, 95% CI 1.18 to 2.25 Pre-eclampsia: pooled OR 0.51, 95% CI 0.38 to 0.64		SR of CH and CCS (1966 to 1995)	2 & 3
Ananth et al., 1999	115	13 studies, 1,358,083 pregnancies	Meta-analysis of any maternal smoking vs. no maternal smoking during pregnancy	Placental abruption	Pooled OR 1.9, 95% CI 1.8 to 2.0		SR of CH and CCS (1966 to 1997)	2 & 3
Wyszynski et al., 1997	118	11 studies (109,831 infants) on cleft lip, among which 9 also looked at cleft palate	Meta-analysis of any maternal smoking vs. no maternal smoking during first trimester of pregnancy	Cleft palate Cleft lip (with and without cleft palate)	CP: pooled OR 1.32, 95% CI 1.10 to 1.62 Cleft lip: pooled OR 1.29, 95% CI 1.18 to 1.42		SR of CH and CCS (1966 to 1996)	2 & 3
Conde-Agudelo et al., 1999	119	28 cohort studies and 7 case-control studies, 833,714 women	Meta-analysis of any maternal smoking vs. no maternal smoking during pregnancy	Pre-eclampsia	Cohort studies (n = 810,649): pooled RR 0.68, 95% CI 0.67 to 0.69 Case-controls (n = 23,065): pooled OR 0.68, 95% CI 0.57 to 0.81		SR of CH and CCS (1966 to 1998)	2 & 3

5.12.1 What are the maternal and perinatal outcomes associated with smoking in pregnancy? (continued)

Study	Ref.	Population	Intervention	Outcomes	Results	Comments	Study type	EL
DiFranza and Lew, 1995	114	13 studies on miscarriage; 23 on low birthweight; 25 on perinatal mortality; and 12 on sudden infant death syndrome	Meta-analysis of any maternal smoking vs. no maternal smoking during pregnancy	Spontaneous abortion Low birthweight Perinatal mortality Sudden infant death syndrome	Spontaneous abortion: 7 cohort (n = 86,632), pooled RR 1.24, 95% CI 1.19 to 1.30 6 case–control (n = 10,535), pooled OR 1.32, 95% CI 1.18 to 1.48 Low birthweight: 22 cohort (n = 346,899), pooled RR 1.82, 95% CI 1.67 to 1.97 1 case–control (n = 654), OR 1.99, 95% CI 1.74 to 2.28 Perinatal mortality: 23 cohort (n = 657,288), pooled RR 1.26, 95% CI 1.19 to 1.34 2 case–control (n = 22,560), pooled OR 1.23, 95% CI 1.12 to 1.41 SIDS: 12 case–control (n = 2340 cases, n = 607,809 controls), pooled OR 2.98, 95% CI 2.51 to 3.54		SR of CH and CCS	2 & 3
Clausson et al., 1998	120	96,662 singleton, live births in Sweden from 1992 to 1993	Maternal risk factors for SGA; data obtained from the Swedish Medical Birth Register	SGA and smoking vs. no smoking	1 to 9 cigarettes/day: OR 1.7, 95% CI 1.6 to 1.9 10+ cigarettes/day: OR 2.4, 95% CI 2.1 to 2.7	Maternal smoking information was missing from n = 4882 births	CH	2a
Raymond et al., 1994	604	638,242 births to women > 20 years of age in Sweden from 1983 to 1989	Risks for stillbirth; data obtained from the Swedish Medical Birth Register	Stillbirth and smoking vs. no smoking	Stillbirth and smoking vs. no OR 1.4, 95% CI 1.2 to 1.4	Maternal smoking information was missing from n = 42,645 births	CH	2a
Kleinman et al., 1988	122	362,261 singleton deliveries in Missouri, USA from 1979 to 1983	Effects of smoking on fetal and infant mortality; data obtained from birth and death certificates and by interviewing mother on smoking habits	Overall fetal and infant mortality rates	For primiparae (n = 134,429): < 1 pack/day, OR 1.25, 95% CI 1.13 to 1.39; ≥ 1 pack/day, 1.56, 95% CI 1.37 to 1.77 For multiparae (n = 227,832): < 1 pack/day, OR 1.30, 95% CI 1.20 to 1.41; ≥ 1 pack/day, 1.30, 95% CI 1.19 to 1.42		CH	2a

5.12.2 and 5.12.3 Do smoking cessation programmes lead to reduction in smoking rates for pregnant women and what are the characteristics of smoking cessation programmes that are most effective in reducing smoking among pregnant women?

Study	Ref.	Population	Intervention	Outcomes	Results	Comments	Study type	EL
Thorogood et al., 2002	127	2 systematic reviews of RCTs and 3 additional RCTs	Smoking cessation programme vs. no programme during pregnancy RCT 1: nicotine patches vs. placebo RCT 2: 10 to 15 minute session with midwife vs. usual care RCT 3: motivational interviewing vs. usual care	Cessation rates	Review A (44 trials, n = 16,916 women): Peto OR 0.53 95% CI 0.47 to 0.60; among trials where cessation was validated by means other than self-report (8 RCTs, n = 3829), Peto OR 0.53 95% CI 0.44 to 0.63 Review B (10 RCTs, n = 4815 pregnant women): 1.9% to 16.7% in no intervention group; 7.1% to 36.1% in intervention group; absolute risk increase with intervention vs. no intervention 7.6%, 95% CI 4.3 to 10.8 RCT 1: NS RCT 2 (1120 pregnant women): NS RCT 3 (269 women in their 28th week of pregnancy): NS		SR	1a

5.12.4 Do smoking cessation programmes decrease perinatal mortality and morbidity?

Study	Ref.	Population	Intervention	Outcomes	Results	Comments	Study type	EL
Thorogood et al., 2002	127	2 systematic reviews of RCTs and 3 additional RCTs	Smoking cessation programme vs. no programme during pregnancy RCT 1: nicotine patches vs. placebo RCT 2: 10 to 15 minute session with midwife vs. usual care RCT 3: motivational interviewing vs. usual care	Low birthweight Preterm birth Very low birthweight Perinatal mortality Mean birthweight	Review A (subset of 10 trials): low birthweight, Peto OR 0.8, 95% CI 0.67 to 0.95; preterm birth, Peto OR 0.83, 95% CI 0.69 to 0.99; birthweight higher among babies from intervention group, mean difference, 28 g, 95% CI 9 to 49; very low birthweight, NS; perinatal mortality, NS RCT 1: birthweight higher in nicotine patch group, mean difference, 186 g, 95% CI 35 g to 336 g		SR	1a

5.15 Car travel during pregnancy

Study	Ref.	Population	Intervention	Outcomes	Results	Comments	Study type	EL
Johnson and Pring, 2000	144	200 women attending their routine mid-pregnancy anomaly scan; UK	Questionnaire on current knowledge and practice among pregnant women about the use of car restraint systems during pregnancy	Seatbelt and airbag use, sources of information about restraint systems and recommendations regarding car safety	98% (159/159) always wore seatbelts in the front		CSS	3
					68% (109/159) always wore seatbelts in the back			
					48% (77/159) correctly identified where to place the seatbelt			
					37% (50/159) could recall receiving being advised on the correct position of seatbelts; of these 50 women, 66% (33/50) had a correct response rate to the correct position of the three-point seatbelt, this was significantly different (p = 0.003) from the women who could not remember receiving any information, who had a 40% (44/109) correct response			
					87% (138/159) thought that wearing a seatbelt was beneficial to them if they were involved in an accident when pregnant			
					62% (98/159) thought that wearing a seatbelt was beneficial to the fetus if they were involved in an accident			
					74% (118/159) knew that a three-point seatbelt was safer than a lap belt for the fetus			
					71% (113/159) thought that airbags increased the safety of a pregnant women in an accident			
					17% (27/159) thought seatbelts were potentially dangerous to a pregnant woman			
Chang et al., 1987	145	89 women and 82 coaches at childbirth classes; USA	Minimal education (pamphlet)	Observation of shoulder strap of seatbelt	Increase in seatbelt use from 19.4 to 28.6% for minimal intervention group, increase of 9.2% (95% CI –3.1 to 21.5)	Group randomisation only 4 groups (no power calculation)	ISS	2a
			Moderate education (lecture and brief discussion, statistics on auto safety pertaining to pregnant women and pamphlet)		13.5 to 24.2% for moderate intervention women, increase of 10.8% (95% CI 0.3 to 21.1)			
			Control (no education)		16.9% to 17.9% for the women in the control group, change of 1% (95% CI –10.3 to 12.3)			

5.15 Car travel during pregnancy (continued)

Study	Ref.	Population	Intervention	Outcomes	Results	Comments	Study type	EL
Klinich et al., 2000	146	Retrospective study of 43 pregnant women involved in road traffic accidents, USA		Adverse fetal outcome, adverse maternal outcome	Study of 43 pregnant women involved in road traffic accidents showed that a increase in adverse fetal outcome with improper maternal restraint use: Minor crashes: 11% (2/18) adverse fetal outcome in properly restrained women, compared to 33% (2/6) improperly restrained women Moderate crashes: 30% (3/10) adverse fetal outcome in properly restrained women, compared to 100% (1/1) improperly restrained woman Severe crashes: 100% (3/3) adverse fetal outcome in properly restrained women, and 100% (5/5) improperly restrained women There is also a correlation of maternal injury level with adverse fetal outcome		CR	3
Wolf et al., 1993	149	Women of 20 weeks gestation or greater who delivered live births or stillbirths from 1980 to 1988 in Washington State, USA, who were involved as drivers in police investigated motor vehicle crashes	Restrained or not restrained with seatbelt	Birth weight Birth within 48 hours of accident Fetal death	Unrestrained pregnant women drivers were 1.9 times more likely to have a low birth weight baby (95% CI = 1.2, 2.9) and 2.3 times more likely to give birth within 48 hours after a motor vehicle crash (95% CI = 1.1, 4.9) than restrained women drivers after adjusting for age and gestational age at crash. Fetal death was 0.5% (7/1349) in unrestrained, and 0.2% (2/1243) in restrained women		CSS	3
Crosby et al., 1972	148	Pregnant baboons, USA	Horizontal sledge accelerated and decelerated similar to head on collision Lap belt vs. three point belt	Fetal death	Fetal death rate was 8.3 % (1/12) among animals impacted with a three point restraint compared to 50% (5/10) fetal death rate of animals impacted with lap belts only	Animal study that probably would not receive ethical approval if carried out now No details of how baboons were selected to be lap belt or three-point belted	ISNR	2a

6.1 Nausea and vomiting in early pregnancy

6.1.1 What is the prevalence of nausea and vomiting in pregnancy?

Study	Ref.	Population	Intervention	Outcomes	Results	Comments	Study type	EL
Whitehead et al., 1992	166	1000 pregnant women at an obstetric clinic in London, England	Survey of women attending for antenatal care in the first half of their pregnancy (904/1000 (90%) between 11 to 20 weeks of gestation)	Frequency of nausea and vomiting Onset of nausea and vomiting Decline of nausea and vomiting Time of day of nausea and vomiting	Nausea: daily, 584/984 (59%); weekly, 98/984 (10%); less often, 145/984 (15%); none, 157/984 (16%) Vomiting: daily, 202/971 (21%); weekly, 90/971 (9%); less often, 215/971 (22%); none, 464/971 (48%) Onset: within 4 weeks of LMP 275/803 (34%); within 6 weeks, 314/803 (39%); within 8 weeks, 171/803 (21%); within 10 weeks 28/803 (4%); within 12 weeks 15/803 (2%) Decline: from 12 to 16 weeks, 77% reported a reduction in vomiting and 83% a reduction in nausea; at 17 to 20 weeks, 16% reported persistent vomiting, 12% reported persistent nausea; at > 20 weeks, 10% reported persistent vomiting, 13% reported persistent nausea Time of day: 148/827 (18%) reported nausea exclusively in the morning; 477/827 (57%) reported symptoms in the morning as well as other times during the day	Denominators vary owing to missing answers on survey All women who reported vomiting reported feeling nausea as well	CSS	3
Gadsby et al., 1993	167	363 consecutive women from a teaching practice in England from 1986 through 1988	Daily symptoms diary kept by women from time of positive pregnancy test until symptoms ceased	Frequency of nausea and vomiting Onset of nausea and vomiting	71/363 (20%) reported no nausea or vomiting throughout their pregnancy; 28% had nausea only; 52% had nausea and vomiting Onset: 94% by 8 weeks Duration: 91% reported no symptoms by 16 weeks	All women who reported vomiting also reported feeling nausea	CSS	3
Feldman, 1989	168			Incidence of hyperemesis gravidum	3.5/1000 deliveries			

6.1.2 What are the adverse maternal and perinatal outcomes associated with nausea and vomiting in pregnancy? (excluding twins, trophoblastic disease, and severity requiring admission to hospital)

Study	Ref.	Population	Intervention	Outcomes	Results	Comments	Study type	EL
Weigel and Weigel, 1989	165	11 studies	Meta-analysis of previously published data on outcomes in women with nausea and vomiting during pregnancy vs. no nausea and vomiting during pregnancy	Miscarriage Perinatal mortality	Miscarriage, (6 studies, n = 14,564): OR 0.36 (95% CI 0.32 to 0.42) Perinatal mortality: too much heterogeneity between studies to assess, but among 3 studies: n = 466, OR 0.18 (95%CI 0.03 to 0.94) n = 10,441, OR 0.72 (95% CI 0.59 to 0.89) n = 903, OR 0.82 (95% CI 0.22 to 3.03)	Only analyses relevant to miscarriage and perinatal mortality reported here, therefore number of studies does not add up to 11	SR (1966 to 1988)	3
Klebanoff and Mills, 1986	169				No increased risk for fetal death, low birthweight, or congenital malformations			3

6.1.3 & 6.1.4 Are there effective interventions to treat nausea and vomiting in pregnancy and what are the maternal and perinatal outcomes associated with these interventions?

Study	Ref.	Population	Intervention	Outcomes	Results	Comments	Study type	EL
Murphy, 1998	174	10 RCTs of various alternative therapies	Alternative medicine (acupressure, ginger, pyridoxine) vs. placebo, dummy acupressure, or no treatment for nausea, vomiting and hyperemesis	Reduction in severity and frequency of nausea and vomiting	7 trials (686 women) concerning P6 pressure point (4 the same as Cochrane, 3 specifically excluded from Cochrane as crossover studies with no separate data from first treatment period); 6/7 showed positive results for reducing nausea or improving symptoms; 2nd largest trial with 161 patients showed no difference even though 92.5% participants completed protocol 1 trial for ginger (same one as in Cochrane); significant reduction of symptoms of hyperemesis, reducing both degree of nausea and frequency of attacks (p = 0.035) 3 trials for pyridoxine (2 included in Cochrane, 1 extra looking at pyridoxine as part of multivitamin preparation) No trials on hypnosis or homeopathy found	11 trials seem to have been included when looking at the narrative	SR (1996 to 1997)	1a&b
Jewell and Young, 2001	173	23 RCTs	Any treatment for persistent nausea and/or vomiting in pregnancy before 20 weeks (anti-histamines, vitamin B6, debendox/Bendectin (doxylamine, dicycloverine, pyridoxine), P6 acupressure (4 RCTs), ginger root, ACTH, oral prednisolone) vs. placebo or (or dummy acupressure)	Reduction in severity and frequency of nausea and vomiting	23 trials included; variable quality Antiemetics (12 RCTs, n = 1505): Peto OR 0.17 95% CI 0.13 to 0.21 1 trial (n = 161) looked at antiemetic effect on miscarriage, neonatal loss and fetal abnormalities, all NS Association with drowsiness (4 RCTs, n = 343): Peto OR 2.19 (95% CI 1.09 to 4.37) Bendectin, as a subset of result for all medication (3 RCTs, n = 240): effect in reducing nausea Peto OR 0.28 (95% CI 0.16 to 0.51) Vitamin B6 (pyridoxine) (2 RCTs): effect on vomiting (n = 392), Peto OR 0.91 (95% CI 0.60 to 1.38); appears to be effective in reducing the severity of nausea at dosages ranging from 10 mg to 25 mg three times daily (n = 395) P6 acupressure (2 RCTS, n = 404): Peto OR 0.35 (95% CI 0.23 to 0.54) Continuous data from 1 trial was NS Last trial not able to be included in meta-analysis and showed no effect ACTH: no evidence of benefit Ginger (1 g daily) may be of benefit based on weak evidence Very little information on effects on fetal outcome		SR	1a&b

6.1.3 & 6.1.4 Are there effective interventions to treat nausea and vomiting in pregnancy and what are the maternal and perinatal outcomes associated with these interventions? (continued)

Study	Ref.	Population	Intervention	Outcomes	Results	Comments	Study type	EL
Vickers, 1996	176	6 RCTs Systematic review, search date 1995	Stimulation of P6 acupuncture point for the treatment of nausea and/or vomiting associated with pregnancy vs. no treatment, placebo or non-acupuncture intervention	Reduction in nausea and vomiting	6 RCTS for nausea and vomiting in pregnancy; same as trials as selected in Murphy's systematic review. All 6 showing positive effect for acupuncture or acupressure or electrical stimulation at P6 point (p < 0.05)		SR	1a
Vutyavanich et al., 2001	172	70 women with nausea during pregnancy attending antenatal clinic in Thailand before 17 weeks of gestation from 1998 to 1999	Ginger (250 mg capsules 4 times daily) (n = 32) vs. placebo (n = 38), for four days	Visual analogue scale for severity of symptoms (0 = no nausea, 10 = nausea as bad as it could be) Likert scales to measure response to treatment Episodes of vomiting Adverse effects on pregnancy outcomes	Nausea severity average over 4 days: 0.9 ± 2.2 vs. 2.1 ± 1.9, p = 0.014 Response to treatment: 28/32 (87.5%) vs. 10/35 (28.6%) reported improvement in symptoms, p < 0.001 Episodes of vomiting after 4 days: 12/32 (37.5%) vs. 23/35 (65.7%) still vomiting, p = 0.021 Spontaneous abortion: 1/32 (3.1%) vs. 3/35 (8.6%), p = 0.615 Caesarean section: 6/32 (18.8%) vs. 4/35 (11.4%), p = 0.509 No congenital abnormalities and all infants discharged in good condition	Double blinded Table of random numbers used for treatment allocation 3 from placebo group lost to follow-up	RCT	1b
Norheim et al., 2001	177	97 pregnant women at 8 to 12 weeks of gestation invited (by flyer) to participate in Norway from 1995 to 1996	Acupressure vs. dummy wristband	Intensity of nausea and vomiting Duration of nausea and vomiting	Intensity: 71% vs. 63% reported a reduction, p = NS Duration: reduced by 2.74 hours vs. 0.85 hours. p = 0.018	Double blind 'Block-randomisation' by groups of 20 (i.e., 10 at a time randomised to either group)	RCT	1b
Mazzotta and Magee, 2000	182	RCTs and cohort studies Systematic review; search date 1998	Safety of antihistamines and pyridoxine and phenothiazines Effectiveness of phenothiazine vs. placebo (3 RCTs, n = 389)	Teratogenicity Malformations Reduction of nausea and vomiting by phenothiazine (3 RCTs, n = 389)	Antihistamines and teratogenicity (24 RCTs, n > 200,000): OR 0.76 (95% CI 0.60 to 0.94) Pyridoxine and major malformations (cohort study): RR 1.05, 95% CI 0.60 to 1.84 (18/458 cases, 34/911controls) Phenothiazines and teratogenicity (7 observational studies, n = 78,440): RR 1.0, 95% CI 0.84 to 1.18 Phenothiazine vs. placebo (3 RCTs, n = 389): RR 0.31 (95% CI 0.24 to 0.42)		SR	1a, 2a & 3

6.2 Heartburn

6.2.1 What is the prevalence of heartburn?

Study	Ref.	Population	Intervention	Outcomes	Results	Comments	Study type	EL
Marrero et al., 1992	184	607 women attending an antenatal clinic in London	Self-administered questionnaire about heartburn and pharyngeal regurgitation	Symptoms of heartburn and pharyngeal regurgitation. Scores for frequency of symptoms (scale 1 = less than once a week; 2 = two or more times a week) and scores for severity of symptoms (scale = 0, no symptoms to 3, constantly disrupting activities)	Prevalence of heartburn increased with gestational age: 22% in first trimester, 39% in second trimester and 72% in third trimester, p < 0.0001 and similarly for severity, p < 0.0001 There was an increased risk of suffering heartburn with increasing gestation, p < 0.0001, a history of prepregnancy heartburn, p < 0.0001, parity, p < 0.0001 and inversely with maternal age, p < 0.05. Not with BMI, race or weight gain in pregnancy	This survey assessed women at varying stages of pregnancy not at a set week	SY	3
Ho et al., 1998	605	47 consecutive, Singaporean pregnant women (in first trimester) attending an antenatal clinic were enrolled, 35 completed the study	Standardised questionnaire Women were interviewed 4 times at first, second, third trimester and in the postpartum period	Percentage with heartburn symptoms alone Regurgitation alone Heartburn and regurgitation Incidence of heartburn during pregnancy	Heartburn symptoms alone 5.7% Regurgitation alone 17.1% Heartburn and regurgitation 17.1% Heartburn symptoms noticed in first trimester (78.6%) Heartburn symptoms disappeared in second trimester (71.4%)	Prevalence of heartburn appears less in Singapore than in UK. Small population assessed (n = 35)	SY	3
Knudsen et al., 1995	185	180 women attending an antenatal clinic at 30 weeks gestation	Self-administered questionnaire to be completed daily from 31 weeks gestation to delivery	Weekly prevalence of heartburn Prevalence of heartburn related to age	Heartburn: weekly prevalence 60% (n = 112) Heartburn positively related to age p = 0.016		SY	3
Bainbridge et al., 1983	186	2 groups: 200 white European women (101 primiparae, 99 multiparae), interviewed at Birmingham Maternity Hospital 100 Asian women (37 primiparae, 63 multiparae) of mixed extract from the Indian subcontinent, interviewed at Birmingham Maternity Hospital and Dudley Road Hospital	Women were interviewed	Incidence of symptomatic gastro-oesophageal reflux in primiparae and multiparae	Incidence of symptomatic gastro-oesophageal reflux: White European women 81.5% Asian women 80%	Details of interview tool not provided	SY	3

6.2.2 Are there effective interventions to treat heartburn in pregnancy?

Study	Ref.	Population	Intervention	Outcomes	Results	Comments	Study type	EL
Shaw, 1978	187	120 women in third trimester diagnosed with symptoms of heartburn (burning sensation in the epigastrum)	60 received compound A (Syn-Ergel, containing aluminium phosphate, an antacid with a protective mucosal coating agent) 60 received compound B (active placebo)	Pain relief after 1 hour	Pain eased or gone after 1 hour: Treatment group n = 40 (80%) Placebo group n = 13 (31%)	No intention to treat analysis	RCT	1b
Kovacs et al., 1990	606	50 women, > 20 weeks pregnant, suffering severe to moderate heartburn at least once in the preceding 7 days Recruited between May 1985 and June 1987	Mucaine (antacid) without oxethazaine (n = 17) Mucaine (n = 15) Placebo (n = 18)	Heartburn severity Heartburn relief Scored on a scale: 1, mild or no relief to 5, severe total relief	Heartburn severity mean scores: Mucaine w/o oxethazaine 3.0 Mucaine 2.9 Placebo 2.9 p = 0.9 Heartburn relief scores: Mucaine w/o oxethazaine 3.3 Mucaine 3.9 Placebo 2.9 p = 0.05	Mucaine containing oxethazaine meant to have anaesthetic properties. The results suggest that Mucaine with oxethazaine has some benefit over the Mucaine that does not	DBP	1b
Briggs and McKay Hart, 1972	607	Pregnant women Numbers not clear	Randomised double blind crossover trial Alcin tablets (aluminium salicylate) (test product) vs. aluminium hydroxide tablets	Episodes of heartburn Intensity of heartburn Relief of heartburn	Numbers not clear to derive accurate figures	It appears that there is no difference in the effectiveness of these treatments. Concern about the carry over effect of the drugs used in this study design Numbers unclear	RDBC	1b

6.2.2 Are there effective interventions to treat heartburn in pregnancy? (continued)

Study	Ref.	Population	Intervention	Outcomes	Results	Comments	Study type	EL
Lang and Dougall, 1989	188	207 pregnant women < 38 weeks gestation recruited 157 women randomised	Prescribed 2 weeks of:10 ml Algicon® (alginate) suspension (n = 79) vs. 10 ml magnesium trisilicate (n = 78) To be taken after meals and at bedtime	Numbers cured or improved in daytime and night time Numbers complaining of adverse events	Numbers cured or improved in daytime after 1 week: Algicon group n = 38/61 who completed week 1 Magnesium trisilicate n = 38/58 who completed week 2 Numbers cured or improved in daytime after 2 weeks: Algicon group n = 36/50 who completed week 2 Magnesium trisilicate n = 38/47 who completed week 2 Numbers cured or improved at night time after 1 week: Algicon group n = 46/61 who completed week 1 Magnesium trisilicate n = 46/58 who completed week 2 Numbers cured or improved at night time after 2 weeks: Algicon group n = 41/50 who completed week 2 Magnesium trisilicate n = 36/47 who completed week 2 Number of adverse events: Algicon group n = 18 Magnesium trisilicate n = 15	No significant difference in improvement of symptoms between the two groups	RCT	1b
Atlay et al., 1978	190	55 pregnant women complaining of heartburn (41 completed the trial and took the 3 interventions for the required time)	Crossover trial (random) Acid mixture vs. alkali mixture vs. placebo mixture 10 ml before and after meals and before bed, for 7 days with 4 day interval between each intervention	Disappearance of heartburn symptoms	Symptoms disappeared or improved: Acid treatment n = 28 (68%) Alkali treatment n = 21 (51%) Placebo n = 18 (44%) Alkali v acid p = 0.18 Alkali v placebo p = 0.66 Acid v placebo p = 0.045	Acid and alkali mixtures no difference in relief of symptoms but better relief achieved than using a placebo	RCT (cross over)	1b

6.2.2 Are there effective interventions to treat heartburn in pregnancy? (continued)

Study	Ref.	Population	Intervention	Outcomes	Results	Comments	Study type	EL
Rayburn et al., 1999	191	Pregnant women > 20 weeks of gestation	50 patients recruited to receive one week antacid therapy only; 30 patients experiencing > 4 episodes moderate–severe heartburn were randomised to antacids and liquid ranitidine vs. antacids and placebo liquid for a further 2 weeks	Heartburn intensity Global assessment of improvement	Mean heartburn intensity scores: Baseline: 7.7 Week 1: (antacid only) mean score reduced to 6.5 (p < 0.05) Week 2: antacid and placebo and antacid and ranitidine mean score 4.4 (p < 0.01) Heartburn intensity change in scores change from baseline to week 2 for antacid and ranitidine group: 7.7 to 3.7, p < 0.001 Global assessment of improvement: Baseline vs. placebo p < 0.05 Baseline vs. single pm dose ranitidine p < 0.001 Baseline vs. double dose ranitidine am and pm p < 0.001		RCT	1b
Magee et al., 1996	193	178 pregnant women who contacted a Motherrisk programme between 1985-1993 for information on gestational exposure to H₂ receptor antagonists 71% reported exposure to ranitidine (mean dose 258 ± 99 mg/day), cimetidine 16%, (487 ± 389 mg/day), famotidine 8%, (32 ± 10 mg/day) and nizatidine (5%,283± 139 mg/day) 178 controls (selected from Motherrisk database) were matched to cases	Telephone interviews	Major malformations (those having an adverse effect in either the functional or social acceptability of the individual)	Major malformations for exposure in first trimester: Cases 2.1% (3/142) Controls 3.5% (5/143) Mean difference, 1.38%, 95% CI –5.2% to 2.4%) Major malformations for exposure anytime: Cases 3% (5/165) Controls 3.1% (5/161)		CCS	3
Nikfar et al., 2002	194	5 cohort studies	Exposure to proton pump inhibitors (n = 593,593 infants) vs. no exposure (n = 15,330 infants)	Major malformations	For any exposure to proton pump inhibitors (mostly omeprazole): summary relative risk 1.18, 95% CI 0.72 to 1.94 For exposure to omeprazole: 1.05, 95% CI 0.59 to 1.85		MA of 5 CH	2a

6.3 Constipation

6.3.1 What is the prevalence of constipation in pregnant women?

Study	Ref.	Population	Intervention	Outcomes	Results	Comments	Study type	EL
Meyer et al., 1994	195	1860 consecutive series of pregnant women attending antenatal clinic in London between August 1982 and March 1984	Structured questionnaires on symptoms, health problems, at 17, 28 and 36 weeks of gestation	Prevalence of constipation at 14, 28 and 36 weeks pregnancy (several other outcomes reported)	% with constipation: 14 weeks 39% (from sample n = 1513) 28 weeks 30% (from sample n = 1463) 36 weeks 20% (from sample n = 1433)		SY	3

6.3.2 Intervention for the treatment of constipation

Study	Ref.	Population	Intervention	Outcomes	Results	Comments	Study type	EL
Jewell and Young, 2003	196	Pregnant women (in last trimester)	10 g fibre supplements (n = 27) vs. placebo (n = 13)	Increased stool frequency	OR 0.18 (95% CI 0.05 to 0.67)		SR	1a
Jewell and Young, 2003	196	Pregnant women	Stimulant laxatives (n = 70) Bulk-forming laxatives (n = 70)	Constipation not resolved Poor acceptability of treatment Effect on side effects	OR 0.3 (95% CI 0.14 to 0.61) OR 0.89 (95% CI 0.46 to 1.73) OR 2.08 (95% CI 1.27 to 3.41)		SR	1a

6.4 Haemorrhoids

6.4.1 Prevalence of haemorrhoids in pregnancy

Study	Ref.	Population	Intervention	Outcomes	Results	Comments	Study type	EL
Abramowitz et al., 2002	197	165 pregnant women in the last 3 months of pregnancy, who gave consent for proctological examination before and after delivery between December 1996 and April 1997	Proctological examination during last 3 months pregnancy, after delivery and at any time symptoms were suggestive of anal disease (bleeding or pain)	Incidence of anal disease (thrombosed external haemorrhoids and anal fissures)	Women presenting with thrombosed external haemorrhoids (n = 13) (7.8%)		CSS	3

6.4.2 Intervention for the treatment of haemorrhoids

Study	Ref.	Population	Intervention	Outcomes	Results	Comments	Study type	EL
Wijayanegra et al., 1992	198	100 pregnant women (12 to 34 weeks of gestation) recruited from an antenatal clinic with first- to third-degree severity of haemorrhoids	500 mg oral (hydroxyethyl)rutosides, oral tablet, twice daily for 1 month (n = 48) vs. placebo (n = 49)	Symptomatic improvement Side effects Fetal outcome (n = 97)	Symptomatic improvement after 2 weeks: 84% improvement in treatment group and 12% improvement in placebo group. After 4 weeks: 94% improvement in treatment group and 14% improvement in placebo group. Treatment group: abdominal discomfort (n = 1) palpitations after 2 weeks (n = 2). For all 3 patients side effects resolved by 4 weeks. Treatment group (n = 48) 46 normal outcome, 1 preterm delivery, 1 congenital anomaly (mother treated at 34 weeks post-organogenesis). Placebo group (n = 49): 46 normal outcome, 1 fetal death, 1 preterm delivery, 1 SGA	Data evaluated on 97 patients	DBRP	1b

6.4.2 Intervention for the treatment of haemorrhoids (continued)

Study	Ref.	Population	Intervention	Outcomes	Results	Comments	Study type	EL
Buckshee et al., 1997	199	50 pregnant women (amenorrhoea > 28 weeks) with history of acute internal haemorrhoids	Micronised flavonoid therapy Oral tablets (micronised diosmin 450 mg (90% and hesperidin 50 mg (10%) Three phase treatment: First phase: 6 tablets for 4 days and 4 tablets for 3 days, divided dose after lunch and dinner Second and third phase: up to 30 days after delivery, maintenance dose; 2 tablets per day, divided lunch and supper	Self-assessment of acute symptoms (0 absent to 3 severe) Relapses in the antenatal period and the postnatal period Side effects Infant outcomes	Median symptom scores assessed before and after first phase (7 day treatment) for: bleeding reduced by 1 (range 1 to 2), 95% CI, p < 0.001, pain reduced by 1, 95% CI, p < 0.001) rectal exudation reduced by 1, 95% CI p < 0.05 and rectal discomfort reduced by 1, 95% CI p < 0.01 Maintenance treatment: relapses per month before treatment 90% compared with after treatment (maintenance dose) in the antenatal period, 36.3% p < 0.001 Postnatal assessment: pretreatment (history 1 year prior pregnancy), % history with relapse 42% compared with assessment at 30 days post delivery % with relapses 12% Side effects: nausea and diarrhoea (n = 6) Congenital malformation (n = 1) Intrauterine death (n = 1) Birthweight: median 2.9 kg (range 2.7 to 3.1)	Recruitment to study: 50 eligible consecutive patients	CSS	3
Saleeby et al., 1991	200	25 pregnant women (age range 21 to 34 years) 22 were in 3rd trimester, 80% multiparous 88% presented with thrombosed or gangrenous haemorrhoids	Closed haemorrhoidectomy. Removal of symptomatic disease 3 quadrants removed (n = 14), 2 quadrants removed (n = 7), one quadrant removed (n = 4)	Pain relief Long term follow up (range 6 months to 6 yrs) mean 30 months Fetal outcomes	Pain relief in 24 hours (n = 24) Persistent rectal bleeding (n = 1) Additional haemorrhoidal treatment required at follow up (n = 6) No surgical related fetal outcomes		CSS	3

6.5 Varicose veins

Study	Ref.	Population	Intervention	Outcomes	Results	Comments	Study type	EL
Bergstein, 1975 (taken from review Young and Jewell, 2003)	211	69 pregnant women at 28 weeks gestation in the Netherlands	300 mg rutoside, three times/day for 8 weeks vs. a placebo	Reduction in ankle circumference Subjective improvement in symptoms	Not estimable Improvement in symptoms: Peto OR 0.3, 95% CI 0.12 to 0.77	Paper derived from systematic review	RW of 3 RCTs	1a
Jacobs, 1996 (taken from review Young and Jewell, 2003)	211	35 healthy women with normal pregnancies and ankle oedema in the USA	EPIC for 30 minutes resting in the left-lateral position vs. 30 minutes resting in the left-lateral position (no EPIC)	Reduction in lower leg volume	Reduction in lower leg volume (WMD, fixed) −258.800 95% CI 566.914 to 49.314]	Paper derived from systematic review		1a
Katz 1990 (taken from review Young and Jewell, 2003)	211	Pregnant women, 34 to 38 weeks gestation, singleton pregnancies Numbers entered into study are not clear; only 11 completed the study	50 minutes bed rest in the lateral supine position versus the same time immersed to the waist with legs horizontal in water at 32 degrees Celsius versus the same time immersed to the shoulders in water at 32 degrees Celsius. Each crossover was done 2 to 4 days later. Only the shoulder immersion comparison is used in this review	Urine output (diuresis) one hour after treatment Participants (n = 11) Blood pressure at the end of the 50-minute treatment period Participants (n = 11)	Urine output (diuresis) one hour after treatment: WMD (fixed), −137.000 (95% CI −236.283 to −37.717) Mean arterial pressure at the end of 50 minute treatment period: WMD (fixed), −11.000 (95% CI −18.951 to −3.049)			1a

6.7 Backache

Study	Ref.	Population	Intervention	Outcomes	Results	Comments	Study type	EL
Young and Jewell, 2003	211	3 RCTs RCT 1: 92 pregnant women at 36 weeks of gestation RCT 2: 258 women attending hospital in Sweden for an ultrasound scan RCT 3: 60 women in Sweden with pelvic or back pain arising before 32 weeks of gestation	RCT 1: Ozzlo pillow used for 1 week to support the pregnant abdomen when lying in a lateral position vs. a standard hospital pillow (control) RCT 2: 20 1-hour weekly water gymnastic classes involving exercise and relaxation in water vs. no intervention RCT 3: 10 acupuncture sessions vs. 10 physiotherapy group sessions	RCT 1: moderate or better improvement in backache; relief of insomnia RCT 2: number of days of sick leave due to back pain after 32 weeks of gestation RCT 3: numbers of women rating treatment as good or excellent	RCT 1: Effect of Ozzlo pillow on backache: (n = 184) (improvement less than moderate) OR 0.32 (95% CI 0.18 to 0.58) Effect of Ozzlo pillow on sleep: (n = 184) (benefit rated less than moderate) OR 0.35 (95% CI 0.20 to 0.62) RCT 2: Effect of water gymnastics on sick leave days due to back pain (n = 241) OR 0.38 (95% CI 0.16 to 0.88) RCT 3: Effect of acupuncture vs. physiotherapy on back pain (treatment rated as good or excellent) OR 6.58 (95% CI 1.00 to 43.16)		SR	1a
Kristiansson et al., 1996	206	200 consecutive women attending an antenatal clinic. Average age 27.9 years	Survey during pregnancy questionnaires and physical examinations	Frequency of back pain	Onset of back pain before pregnancy: 25.6% Onset of back pain during pregnancy: 61% Prevalence of back pain during weeks of pregnancy: 12 weeks: 19% 24 weeks: 47% 36 weeks: 49%		SY	3
Ostgard et al., 1991	207	950 pregnant women attending an antenatal clinic in Sweden	Women were reviewed at 12th week and every second week until delivery	Incidence of back pain	49% complained of back pain during pregnancy but half of these had back pain before pregnancy Onset of back pain during pregnancy 27% (n = 210)		SY	3
Fast et al., 1987	208	200 women (black, white, Hispanic and oriental origin) interviewed within 24 to 36 hours after giving birth on a maternity ward (of a county hospital in the USA)	Questionnaire relating to personal data and occurrence and manifestation of low back pain	Frequency of back pain during pregnancy Month of onset of back pain	56% complained of back pain during pregnancy 48% no back pain during pregnancy 60.7% of women with back pain onset was between 5th to 7th month of pregnancy		SY	3

6.7 Backache (continued)

Study	Ref.	Population	Intervention	Outcomes	Results	Comments	Study type	EL
Stapleton et al., 2002	209	1530 respondents to a South Australian Omnibus Population Survey, 1120 (73%) had had at least one pregnancy > 20 weeks	Population survey including specific questions on back pain during pregnancy	Incidence of back pain during pregnancy Severity of back pain during pregnancy	397/1120 (35.5%) reported back pain during one or more pregnancies 61.8%(n = 246) had at least moderately severe backache 9% (n = 35) were disabled by the pain	Survey on backache questions was dependent upon retrospective recall. Therefore reliability is unclear	SY	3
Mantle et al., 1977	210	180 women (mean age 26 years) delivering at a London Hospital between May 1973 and August 1973	Questionnaire administered to women within 24 hours of delivery, asking about back pain during pregnancy	Incidence of back pain and severity of backache during pregnancy Month of onset of backache Time of day when backache most troublesome	48% (n = 87) troublesome or severe backache 52% (n = 92) none or not worth troubling about backache Peak month of onset of pregnancy: 54% (n = 47) onset of mild or severe backache during 5th to 7th month Time of day backache most troublesome: 40% evening and 26% night		SY	3
Field et al., 1999	212	26 pregnant working women, between 14 and 30 weeks of gestation, with an interest in relaxation exercises	Randomly assigned: Massage therapy (n = 14) (x 10, 20-minute massages over 5 weeks) vs. progressive muscle relaxation class (n = 12) (a 20-minute relaxation class and encouraged to do these at home twice a week for 5 weeks)	Relief of back pain Pregnancy anxiety Sleep scale disturbance	Back pain relief scores: For massage group: first day (pre- or post-massage) 4.6/2.2 (p = 0.005) Last day (pre- or post-massage) 3.8/2.1 (p = 0.01) For relaxation group: first day (pre- or post-relaxation) 3.4/3.3 not significant Last day (pre- or post-relaxation) 3.2/3.5 (p = 0.01)	Method of randomisation not stated	RCT	1b
Ostgaard et al., 1994	213	407 pregnant women at a maternity care unit in Sweden	Random allocation (quasi) to 3 groups Group A: control group no extra intervention; any development of back or pelvic pain treated according to usual routine Group B: two 45-minute classes of back care in pregnancy Group C: five 30-minute individual lessons on back care in pregnancy	Improvement with back or posterior pelvic pain Sick leave frequency	Improvement with back or posterior pelvic pain following information on muscular training and body posture difference between group A and B (p < 0.05); group A and C (p < 0.05) Improvement with back or posterior pelvic pain following information on vocational technique training between group A and B (NS); group A and C (p < 0.05) Improvement with back or posterior pelvic pain and affect on sick leave: between group A and B (NS); between group A and C (p < 0.05)	Quasi-randomised (allocation by day of birth in month 1 to 10 Group A 11 to 20 Group B 21 to 31 Group C)	RCT	1b

6.7 Backache (continued)

Study	Ref.	Population	Intervention	Outcomes	Results	Comments	Study type	EL
Noren et al., 1997	214	Pregnant women with any type of back pain attending an antenatal clinic in Sweden between April 1991 to February 1993	Intervention group 54 women: individually designed physiotherapy programme of 5 visits (including teaching on anatomy, posture, vocational ergonomics, gymnastics, relaxation) and an exercise programme versus control group of 81 pregnant women with back pain; no specific intervention given	Duration of sick leave	Average number of sick leave days: Intervention group: 30.4 days/woman vs. control group 53.6 days; difference in sick leave (p < 0.001)		CCH	2a
Tesio et al., 1994	215	16 pregnant women between 12 and 30 weeks gestation with back and/or sciatica pain onset during pregnancy and unremitting for 4 weeks	Autotraction, a mechanical treatment for back pain. Consists of a 3- to 6-second maximal pulling effort followed by 1-to 2-minute rest period for 25 minutes Three treatments every, 3 days	Pain relief recovery	Recovery: Fully recovered (n = 5) Improved (n = 8) No change (n = 3) Change in pain scores from before to after treatment: Median pain intensity as a group at start 50/100 and at end 15/100 (p < 0.001)	No control group	OPC	3
Guadagnino III, 1999	216	12 pregnant women (age range 14 to 34 years) with back pain attributed to pregnancy	Spinal manipulative therapy (1 to 3 techniques applied) and received treatment 2 to 3 times/week until delivery Postal questionnaire sent to mothers at end of pregnancy	Pain intensity (scale 1 to 10)	Average pain score when treatment sought: 7.58 Average pain score when maintained under care: 4.25	Method of recruitment is unclear The questionnaire included several questions that required retrospective memory of the symptoms they experienced while receiving treatment Significant bias affect in this study. Authors conclude that an RCT is required	CH	3

6.7 Backache (continued)

Study	Ref.	Population	Intervention	Outcomes	Results	Comments	Study type	EL
McIntyre and Broadhurst, 1996	217	20 pregnant women reporting low back pain in the second or third trimester	Rotational mobilisation exercise carried out at 3 antenatal visits	Resolution of pain	15 patients had complete resolution of pain 3 patients had 50-80% resolution 2 patients unaccounted for	Methods of study unclear	CH	3
Requejo et al., 2002	218	A 28-year-old primigravida, 20 weeks gestation with low back pain beginning at 18 weeks gestation Presented with pain limiting her to sit for 20 minutes and restricted ability to bend forward	Treatment 4 episodes during 2 weeks of manual joint mobilisation applied to symptomatic vertebral segment	Resolution of pain improved mobility	Improved mobility (able to bend forward without pain and sit longer than 1 hour without discomfort) Oswestry score reduced from 38/100 to 10/100		CR	3

8.1 Anaemia

8.1.1 Is anaemia in pregnancy associated with adverse maternal and perinatal outcomes?

Study	Ref.	Population	Intervention	Outcomes	Results	Comments	Study type	EL
Zhou et al., 1998	272	829 pregnant women in China from 1991 to 1992	Women divided into 6 groups based on their 1st-trimester Hb) concentrations (<9.0, 9.0 to 9.9, 10.0 to 10.9, 11.0 to 11.9, 12.0 to 12.9, ≥13.0 g/dl) Vitamin C, iron sulphate and folic acid treatment was offered to all women with Hb levels <110 g/dl (defined as anaemia)	Prevalence of anaemia Based on initial Hb concentrations: Risk of low birthweight Risk of preterm birth Risk of SGA	49% at enrolment; 66% in 2nd trimester; 67% in 3rd trimester Low birthweight: > 11.9 g/dl, NS; 10.0 to 10.9, RR 2.7 (95% CI 1.01 to 7.39); 9.0 to 9.9, RR 3.3 (95% CI 1.09 to 9.77); < 9.0, RR 3.0 (95% CI 0.60 to 14.76) Preterm birth: >11.9 g/dl, NS; 10.0 to 10.9, NS; 9.0 to 9.9, RR 2.6 (95% CI 1.17 to 5.90); < 9.0, RR 3.7 (95% CI 1.36 to 10.23) SGA: NS for all groups		CH	2a
Steer et al., 1995	271	153,602 pregnancies in North West Thames region, England	Retrospective analysis of information on database to determine association of lowest Hb level in pregnancy and birthweight and rates of low birthweight and preterm delivery in different ethnic groups	Birth weight, rates of low birthweight, preterm labour	Maximum mean birth weight (3483 g ± 565) achieved with lowest Hb 8.6 g/dl to 9.5 g/dl Lowest incidence of low birth weight and preterm labour occurred with lowest Hb 9.5 g/dl to 10.5 g/dl Similar for all ethnic groups		CSS	3

8.1.2 Does routine iron supplementation during pregnancy improve maternal and perinatal outcomes?

Study	Ref.	Population	Intervention	Outcomes	Results	Comments	Study type	EL
Mahomed, 2001	74	20 RCTs	Iron vs. no iron or placebo (except one trial: selective vs. routine iron) in pregnant women	Haemoglobin Measures of iron status Pregnancy outcome Side effects of treatment	Low (< 10 g or 10.5 g) predelivery Hb (12 RCTs, n = 1802): Peto OR 0.15 (95% CI 0.11 to 0.20) Low predelivery serum iron (4 RCTs, n = 726): Peto OR 0.19 (95% CI 0.12 to 0.29) Low (< 10 mg/dl) predelivery serum ferritin (4 RCTs, n = 481): Peto OR 0.12 (95% CI 0.08 to 0.17) Caesarean section (1 RCT, n = 2694): Peto OR 1.36 (95% CI 1.04 to 1.78) Blood transfusion (1 RCT, n = 2694): Peto OR 1.68 (95% CI 1.05 to 2.67) Preterm delivery (1 RCT, n = 2694): Peto OR 1.41 (95% CI 0.94 to 2.12) Low birthweight (1 RCT, n = 2694): Peto OR 1.12 (95% CI 0.72 to 1.75) SGA (1 RCT, n = 2690): Peto OR 1.10 (95% CI 0.79 to 1.52) Admission to neonatal unit (1 RCT, n = 2694): Peto OR 1.06 (95% CI 0.80 to 1.40) Congenital malformations (1 RCT, n = 2694): Peto OR 1.01 (95% CI 0.77 to 1.33) Stillbirths and deaths in first week of life (1 RCT, n = 2694): Peto OR 0.33 (95% CI 0.11, 0.99) Side effects in mothers (3 RCTs, n = 7098): Peto OR 0.41 (95% CI 0.34 to 0.50)	All pregnancy outcome results were from the trial that compared selective vs. routine iron in pregnancy	SR	1a

8.1.2 Does routine iron supplementation during pregnancy improve maternal and perinatal outcomes? (continued)

Study	Ref.	Population	Intervention	Outcomes	Results	Comments	Study type	EL
Mahomed, 2001	76	8 RCTs (5449 pregnant women with haemoglobin level > 10 g/dl	Iron and folate supplementation vs. no iron and folate or placebo	Haemoglobin Measures of iron and folic acid status	Low (<10 g or 10.5 g) predelivery Hb (6 RCTs, n = 1099): Peto OR 0.19 (95% CI 0.13 to 0.27) Low predelivery serum iron (3 RCTs, n = 277): Peto OR 0.14 (95% CI 0.08 to 0.24) Low (<10 mg/dl) predelivery serum ferritin (1 RCT, n = 48): Peto OR 0.04 (95% CI 0.01 to 0.14) Low (<2.5 microgrammes/ml) predelivery serum folate (3 RCTs, n = 501): Peto OR 0.11 (95% CI 0.06 to 0.21) Low predelivery serum red cell folate (1 RCT, n = 46): Peto OR 0.12 (95% CI 0.02 to 0.89) Caesarean section (2 RCTs, n = 104): Peto OR 0.16 (95% CI 0.03 to 0.82) Preterm delivery (1 RCT, n = 48): Peto OR 8.08 (95% CI 0.80 to 81.60) Low birthweight (1 RCT, n = 48): Peto OR 7.72 (95% CI 0.47 to 127.14) Admission to neonatal unit (1 RCT, n = 48): Peto OR 7.39 (95% CI 0.15 to 372.41) Stillbirth and neonatal death (1 RCT, n = 48): Peto OR 7.72 (95% CI 0.47 to 127.14)		SR	1a

8.1.3 What are the side effects of iron supplementation in pregnancy and how can they be minimised?

Study	Ref.	Population	Intervention	Outcomes	Results	Comments	Study type	EL
Cuervo and Mahomed, 2001	274	5 RCTs, 1234 pregnant women with anaemia (Hb <11 g/dl) in pregnancy	14 variations of interventions for anaemia, including all types of iron preparations (oral, slow release, intramuscular and intravenous iron, blood transfusions, and recombinant erythropoietin)	Women with anaemia Maternal morbidity and mortality Neonatal morbidity and mortality	Oral iron vs. placebo: anaemia (1 RCT, n = 125) Peto OR 0.12 (95% CI 0.06 to 0.24); no published data on clinically relevant outcomes	All trials were assessed to be of poor quality	SR	1a

8.2 Haemoglobinopathies

8.2.1 What is the prevalence of haemoglobinopathies in pregnant women in the UK?

Study	Ref.	Population	Intervention	Outcomes	Results	Comments	Study type	EL
Davies et al., 2000	275	20,333 pregnancies in Brent, England from 1986 to 1995	Universal antenatal screening for haemoglobinopathies	Prevalence	n = 1688/20,333 pregnancies tested positive for haemoglobinopathy trait or disease (8.3%): 751/20,333 with sickle trait or disease (3.7%) 265/20,333 with beta-thalassaemia trait or disease (1.3%) 272 other haemoglobinopathy 400 alpha-thalassaemia		CSS	3

8.2.2 What are the adverse maternal and perinatal outcomes associated with haemoglobinopathies?

Study	Ref.	Population	Intervention	Outcomes	Results	Comments	Study type	EL
Davies et al., 2000	275	751 pregnant women with sickle trait or disease and 265 pregnant women with beta-thalassaemia trait or disease from 1986 to 1995	Women attended counselling (n = 623/751 (83%) in sickle cases; n = 246/265 (93%) in beta-thalassaemia cases), partners tested (n = 481/623 (77%) in sickle cases; n = 234/246 (88%) in beta-thalassaemia cases), postnatal diagnosis offered	Pregnancies at risk Outcomes of pregnancies at risk Estimates of prevalence among all live births in England	Sickle cell pregnancies at risk: 113/481 (23%) Beta-thalassaemia pregnancies at risk: 22/234 (9.4%) Outcomes of at risk pregnancies: Sickle cell: 16 of 108 women who returned for follow-up accepted prenatal diagnosis (15%) 3 terminations from 4 affected pregnancies 22 affected births from 92 of 108 women who did not accept prenatal diagnosis 5 affected births among 142/623 partners not tested Beta-thalassaemia: 19 of 22 women who returned for follow-up accepted prenatal diagnosis (86%) 4 terminations from 4 affected pregnancies 0 affected births from 3 of 22 women who did not accept prenatal diagnosis 0 affected births among 12/246 partners not tested 1 beta-thalassaemia birth among 15 unaffected pregnancies Prevalence estimates: 17 infants born each year with beta-thalassaemia (0.03/1000 live births) 160 infants born each year with sickle cell disorder (0.25/1000 live births)	The prevalence estimates allow for terminations	HTA RW CSS	3

8.2.3 Does recording of racial background in the notes of pregnant women help in selective screening for haemoglobinopathies?

Study	Ref.	Population	Intervention	Outcomes	Results	Comments	Study type	EL
Aspinall et al., 2003	281	N/A	Assessing effectiveness of questions about ethnic origin	Quality of data collected	Risk group misclassification as high as 20% June quarter 2000 data from Hospital Episode Statistics indicate ethnic group data missing from 43% of records in London and 37% in England		RW	3
Modell et al., 2000	276	400 pregnancies in 138 women in the UK from 1990 to 1994	Audit to evaluate the quality of antenatal screening for haemoglobinopathy and genetic counselling	Haemoglobinopathy affected Screening offered Risk recognition	138/400 (35%) pregnancies with haemoglobinopathy 68/138 (49%) of affected pregnancies had been offered screening at first pregnancy Risk recognised in 27/63 (43%) pregnancies before 1990 and in 41/74 (55%) pregnancies after 1990	This study assumes that antenatal screening for Hb disorders is standard practice in the UK	CSS	3

8.2.4 What tests are available for detecting maternal haemoglobinopathies?

Study	Ref.	Population	Intervention	Outcomes	Results	Comments	Study type	EL
Zeuner et al., 1999	279	N/A		Screening and diagnosis algorithm	1. Estimation of red blood cell indices. MCH <27 pg indicates thalassaemia trait 2. Subsequent quantification of HbA and HbF for thalassaemia trait (via HPLC) and identification of Hb structural variants for sickle cell traits (via isoelectric focusing) 3. If HbA and HbF > 3.5% is indicative of thalassaemia trait 4. Partner testing initiated 5. DNA analysis used when assessment of at-risk pregnancy cannot be adequately obtained by phenotyping	p. 5, 8–10	HTA	RW 4

8.2.5 Do effective interventions exist to improve outcomes for these women?

Study	Ref.	Population	Intervention	Outcomes	Results	Comments	Study type	EL
Modell et al., 1997	277	2068 cases of prenatal diagnosis in England from 1974 to 1994	Comparison of prenatal diagnosis for Hb disorders with annual number of pregnancies at risk for these disorders (ethnic group data from 1991 census)	Utilisation of prenatal diagnosis Termination of pregnancy Proportion of referrals in the first trimester	Utilisation for thalassaemias: 55% (range 10% among Bangladeshis to 89% among Cypriots) Use for sickle cell disorders: 13% by black Africans and black Caribbeans 296/305 (97%) pregnancies with fetuses diagnosed as homozygous were terminated		CSS	3
Modell et al., 2000	276	400 pregnancies in 138 women in the UK from 1990 to 1994	Audit to evaluate the quality of antenatal screening for haemoglobinopathy and genetic counselling	Uptake of prenatal diagnosis	80% uptake when offered among British Pakistanis, 35/48 (73%) agreed to prenatal diagnosis in first trimester, with 11/12 affected pregnancies terminated, compared with 11/28 (39%) accepting prenatal diagnosis in the second trimester, with 4/7 affected pregnancies terminated	This study assumes that antenatal screening for Hb disorders is standard practice in the UK	CSS	3
Ahmed et al., 2000	284	300 couples requesting prenatal diagnosis of beta-thalassaemia during 3.5 years in Pakistan	Counselling and prenatal diagnosis of beta-thalassaemia between 10 and 16 weeks (n = 15 diagnosed after 16th week)	Termination of affected pregnancies	47/53 (89%) of affected pregnancies were terminated 6/53 terminations declined for religious reasons		CSS	3

9.1 Screening for structural abnormalities

Study	Ref.	Population	Intervention	Outcomes	Results	Comments	Study type	EL
Williamson et al., 1997	298	148 births involving neural tube defects in England and Wales from 1990 to 1991	Pregnancies of neural tube defect affected births reported to the Office of Population Census Survey were retrospectively reviewed through obstetric records	Sensitivity of ultrasound screening for anencephaly between 14 to 22 weeks (90/148 pregnancies were screened by ultrasound)	100%		CSS	3
Bricker et al., 2000	297	96,633 babies from 11 studies (1 RCT, 11 cohort) from 1986 to 1996 in Europe, USA and Korea	Literature review to assess the clinical effectiveness of routine ultrasound in pregnancy	Prevalence of fetal anomalies Sensitivity and specificity of detection with ultrasound Proportion of structural abnormalities detected with scan at less than 24 weeks	Overall: 2.09%, range 0.76 to 3.07% Detection at less than 24 weeks: 41.3% (range 15% to 71.5%) and 99.9% (range 99.4% to 100%) Detection at greater than 24 weeks: 18.6% (sensitivity only), range 18.2% to 21.7% Overall detection rate: 44.7% (sensitivity only), range 15.0% to 85.3% Structural abnormalities: Central nervous system 76.4% Pulmonary 50% Cardiac 17.4% Gastrointestinal 41.9% Urinary tract 67.3% Skeletal 23.8%	HTA report	SR	1b & 2a
Saari-Kemppainen et al., 1994	299	9310 women pregnant women from two hospitals in Finland from 1986 to 1987	Routine early ultrasound between 16 to 20 weeks gestation (n = 4691) vs. selective ultrasound (n = 4619)	Termination of pregnancy after detection of anatomical malformations in the fetus Perinatal mortality (per 1000) Screening sensitivity for major malformations	Terminations: 11 vs. 0 (no p value reported) Perinatal mortality among singleton births: 4.2 vs. 8.0, p < 0.05 Sensitivity: 40% vs. 27.7% Sensitivity per hospital: 75% (9/12 cases detected) and 35% (9/26 cases detected)		RCT	1b
Whitlow et al., 1999	300	6634 women carrying 6443 live fetuses in London, England	Ultrasound scan at 12 to 13 weeks of gestation	Detection rate for major structural abnormalities	Overall detection rate: 59% (37/63), 95% CI 46.5 to 72.4: CNS 84% (16/19) Face 0% (0/2) Neck 100% (13/13) Cardiac 40% (4/10) Pulmonary 33% (1/3) Gastrointestinal 100% (7/7) Urinary tract 60% (3/5) Skeletal 0% (0/7)		CSS	3

9.2 Screening for chromosomal anomalies

Study	Ref.	Population	Intervention	Outcomes	Results	Comments	Study type	EL
ONS, 2000	303	All children in England and Wales	Notification of Down's syndrome	Incidence of Down's syndrome per 10,000 live and still births	1986: 6.7 1988: 6.1 1990: 5.9 1992: 5.7 1994: 4.7 1996: 5.5 1998: 6.2	Report of child health statistics	SV	3
Morris et al., 2002	311	All antenatal or postnatally diagnosed and confirmed cases (via a karyotype) of Down's syndrome in England and Wales from 1989 to 1998	Collection of reports from all regional cytogenetic laboratories of cases found to have a Down's syndrome karyotype	Observed odds of maternal age specific risk of Down's syndrome	Odds at age 20 years: 1:1441 Odds at age 25 years: 1:1383 Odds at age 30 years: 1:959 Odds at age 35 years: 1:338 Odds at age 40 years: 1:84 Odds at age 45 years: 1:32	An estimated 6% of births with Down's syndrome are missed by the National Down Syndrome Cytogenetic Register; therefore, the number of births was increased by 6% to allow for those not included	SV	3

9.2 Screening for chromosomal anomalies (continued)

Study	Ref.	Population	Intervention	Outcomes	Results	Comments	Study type	EL
Smith-Bindman et al., 2001	315	56 studies, 130,365 unaffected fetuses and 1930 cases of Down's syndrome Systematic review; from 1980 to 1999 on Medline only	Articles that assessed second trimester (15 to 24 weeks) ultrasound markers (choroid plexus cyst, nuchal fold thickening, echogenic intracardiac focus, echogenic bowel, renal pyelectasis, shortened humerus, shortened femur, and fetal structural malformations) to detect Down's syndrome fetuses	Sensitivity and specificity of each ultrasonographic marker and associated fetal loss per case diagnosed	Nuchal fold (95% CI): Sensitivity 0.04 (0.02 to 0.10) Specificity 0.99 (0.99 to 0.99) Fetal loss 0.6 Choroid plexus cyst (95% CI): Sensitivity 0.01 (0.0 to 0.03) Specificity 0.99 (0.97 to 1.0) Fetal loss 4.3 Femur length (95% CI): Sensitivity 0.16 (0.05 to 0.40) Specificity 0.96 (0.94 to 0.98) Fetal loss 1.2 Humerus length (95% CI): Sensitivity 0.09 (0.0 to 0.60) Specificity 0.97 (0.91 to 0.99) Fetal loss 1.9 Echogenic bowel (95% CI): Sensitivity 0.04 (0.01 to 0.24) Specificity 0.99 (0.97 to 1.0) Fetal loss 1.0 Echogenic intracardiac focus (95% CI): Sensitivity 0.11 (0.06 to 0.18) Specificity 0.96 (0.94 to 0.97) Fetal loss 2.0 Renal pyelectasis (95% CI): Sensitivity 0.02 (0.01 to 0.06) Specificity 0.99 (0.98, 1.0) Fetal loss 2.6		SR	2a & 3
Dick, 1994	608	4 cohort studies	Comparison of proportion of Down's syndrome pregnancies identified through triple testing with the total number of Down's syndrome pregnancies	Detection rates	Range 48% to 91% with false positive rate of 3.2 to 6%, respectively (cutoff rates from 1/190 to 1/274 used) When varying cutoff rates were accounted for, triple marker screening in the 2nd trimester with AFP, hCG, and uE3 combined with maternal age offered 50% detection rate in women < 35 years with 5% false positive rate		SR of CH	2a

9.2 Screening for chromosomal anomalies (continued)

Study	Ref.	Population	Intervention	Outcomes	Results	Comments	Study type	EL
Conde-Agudelo and Kafury-Geola, 1998	320	20 cohort studies, 194,326 pregnant women	Meta-analysis of effectiveness of triple marker screening for Down's syndrome	Sensitivities and false positive rates	Sensitivities for maternal age ≥ 35 years: For cutoff rates 1/190 to 1/200, 89% (range 78% to 100%), false positive rate 25% (range 20% to 29%) For cutoff rates 1/250 to 1/295, 80% (range 75% to 100%), false positive rate 21% (range 20% to 21%) Sensitivities for maternal age < 35 years: For cutoff rates 1/250 to 1/295, 57% (range 53% to 58%), false positive rate 4% (range 3% to 6%)		SR of CH	2a
Bindra et al., 2002	609	15,030 pregnant women in London from 1999 to 2001	Screening for Down's syndrome by nuchal translucency, free beta-hCG and PAPP-A and maternal age at 11 to 14 weeks	Detection rates at cutoff rate of 1/300 False positive rate for 75% and 85% detection rate Detection rate with false positive rate fixed at 5% Uptake of prenatal diagnosis	82 cases of Down's syndrome identified False positive rate at 75% detection rate: Maternal age alone, 27.7% Maternal age, free beta-hCG, and PAPP-A, 10.1% Maternal age and NT, 2.6% Maternal age, NT, free beta-hCG and PAPP-A, 0.9% False positive rate at 85% detection rate: Maternal age alone, 46.4% Maternal age, free beta-hCG, and PAPP-A, 15.2% Maternal age and NT, 9.1% Maternal age, NT, free beta-hCG and PAPP-A, 3.0% Detection rate for fixed false positive rate of 5%: By maternal age alone, 30.5% maternal age, free beta-hCG and PAPP-A, 60% Maternal age and NT, 79% Maternal age, NT, free beta-hCG and PAPP-A, 90% 89% (73/82) of women in the screen positive group chose invasive testing for prenatal diagnosis		CH	2a

9.2 Screening for chromosomal anomalies (continued)

Study	Ref.	Population	Intervention	Outcomes	Results	Comments	Study type	EL
Wald et al., 2003	316	101 cases from 45,712 singleton pregnancies and 490 matched controls from 28,434 singleton pregnancies at 24 maternity centres in the UK and one in Austria from 1995 to 2000	Women matched on centre, maternal age and crown–rump length or biparietal diameter Comparison of efficacy of various methods and combination of methods for Down's syndrome screening Nuchal translucency obtained at 12 to 13 weeks gestation Serum and urine samples taken at 9 to 13 weeks and also included if taken at 14 to 22 weeks Serum tested for AFP, total hCG, uE$_3$, PAPP-A) free beta-hCG and dimeric inhibin A Urine tested for ITA, beta-core fragment, total hCG and free beta-hCG	False positive rate for 75% and 85% detection rate Detection rate with false positive rate fixed at 5% Estimates of fetal loss (stillbirth or miscarriage) due to amniocentesis or chorionic villus sampling at 85% detection rate, 80% uptake rate and 0.9% fetal loss rate attributable to procedure Outcomes of Down's syndrome pregnancies	False positive rate at 75% detection rate: Integrated test 0.3% Serum integrated test 0.8% Combined test 2.3% Quadruple test 2.5% Triple test 4.2% Double test 6.6% NT 8.6% False positive rate at 85% detection rate (95% CI): Integrated test 1.2% (1.1 to 1.3) Serum integrated test 2.7% (2.4 to 3.0) Combined test 6.1% (5.7 to 6.5) Quadruple test 6.2% (5.8 to 6.6) Triple test 9.3% (8.8 to 9.8) Double test 13.1% (12.6 to 13.6) NT 20% (18.6 to 21.4) Detection rate for fixed FPR of 5%: Integrated test 92% Serum integrated test 92% Quadruple test 92% Triple test 90% Double test 86% Fetal losses/100,000 women screened (i.e. 173 cases diagnosed) (n): Integrated test 9 Serum integrated test 19 Combined test 44 Quadruple test 45 Triple test 67 Double test 94 NT 144 71 Down's syndrome pregnancies were terminated, 4 miscarried after amniocentesis and 26 resulted in a live birth	Integrated test defined as NT and PAPP-A at 10 weeks and quadruple test markers at 14 to 22 weeks Serum integrated test is the same as above minus the NT Combined test is based on NT, free beta-hCG, PAPP-A and maternal age assessed in the first trimester Quadruple test based on AFP, uE$_3$, free beta-(or total) hCG, and inhibin A measurements with maternal age in the 2nd trimester Triple test based on AFP, uE$_3$, free beta-(or total) hCG, and maternal age in the 2nd trimester Double test based on AFP, free beta-(or total) hCG, and maternal age in the 2nd trimester	CCS	3
Alfirevic et al., 1998	323	3 RCTs, 9067 women	1st trimester CVS vs. 2nd trimester amniocentesis	Sampling failure Total pregnancy loss	Failure (1 RCT, n=3201): Peto OR 2.86, 95% CI 1.93 to 4.24 Pregnancy loss (3 RCTs, n=9067): Peto OR 1.33, 95% CI 1.17 to 1.52		SR	1a

9.2 Screening for chromosomal anomalies (continued)

Study	Ref.	Population	Intervention	Outcomes	Results	Comments	Study type	EL
Alfirevic, 2000	324	3 RCTs, 1832 women	Amniocentesis vs. transabdominal CVS at 9 to 14 weeks gestation	Sampling failure Total pregnancy loss	Failure (3 RCTs, n = 1832): 0.4% vs. 2%, RR 0.23, 95% CI 0.08 to 0.65 Pregnancy loss (3 RCTs, n = 1832): 6.2% vs. 5%, RR 1.24, 95% CI 0.85 to 1.81		SR	1a
RCOG Guideline No. 8, 2000	307	N/A	Amniocentesis vs. no amniocentesis at 16 to 18 weeks (n = 4606 women) Early amniocentesis (before 14 weeks, n = 2183) vs. amniocentesis at 15 weeks or later (n = 2185)	Excess loss rate for amniocentesis vs. no amniocentesis For early amniocentesis vs. late amniocentesis: Rates of fetal loss and fetal talipes following amniocentesis Procedure analysis	Excess miscarriage rate in amniocentesis group: 1% Early vs. late amniocentesis: Total fetal loss, 7.6% vs. 5.9%, p = 0.012 Fetal talipes, 1.3% vs. 0.1%, p = 0.0001 Procedure reported difficult, 10.1% vs. 4.0%, p < 0.0001 Amniotic fluid leakage at <22 weeks, 3.5% vs. 1.7%, p = 0.0007 Multiple needle insertion, 5.4% vs. 2.1%, p < 0.0001 First attempt success, 96.9% vs. 99.6%, p < 0.0001		SR	1b

10.1 Asymptomatic bacteriuria

10.1.1 What is the incidence of asymptomatic bacteriuria in pregnancy?

Study	Ref.	Population	Intervention	Outcomes	Results	Comments	Study type	EL
Foley et al., 1987	331	6883 women attending antenatal clinics; hospital in Ireland	Treatment vs. non-treatment of women with confirmed bacteriuria	Incidence of asymptomatic bacteriuria	220/6883 (3.2%)	Randomisation by coin-tossing	RCT	1b
Little, 1966	329	Women attending two antenatal clinics in two London hospitals	Antibiotic treatment vs. treatment of 'cases' only when symptomatic	Incidence of asymptomatic bacteriuria	265/5000 (5.3%)	No method of randomisation described	RCT	1b
Etherington and James, 1993	342	898 women attending antenatal clinic in a Bristol (UK) hospital	Test evaluation study	Incidence of asymptomatic bacteriuria	27/898 (3%)		TES	2a

10.1.2 What are the maternal and perinatal outcomes associated with asymptomatic bacteriuria?

Study	Ref.	Population	Intervention	Outcomes	Results	Comments	Study type	EL
Little, 1966	329	Women attending two antenatal clinics in two London hospitals 4735 women without bacteriuria 265 women with bacteriuria diagnosed by culture of midstream urine on at least two occasions Screened at first antenatal visit	Antibiotic treatment vs. treatment of 'cases' only when symptomatic Antibiotic used was sulphamethoxypyridazine for 30 days	Maternal: pyelonephritis, toxaemia Fetal: perinatal mortality, preterm birth, fetal abnormalities	Pyelonephritis: more common in women with bacteriuria when untreated (24.8% vs. 0.4% women without bacteriuria) Toxaemia: no difference between groups Perinatal mortality: no difference between groups Preterm birth: higher in the women with bacteriuria (8.7% vs. 7.6%) Fetal abnormalities: no difference between groups	Method of randomisation was not indicated	RCT	1b
Leblanc and McGanity, 1964	332	1325 women attending antenatal clinics in a US hospital; enrolled at first clinic visit Urine samples collected by catheter and initial bacteriuria defined as colony counts of greater than 10^5 of a single organism/ml	Randomisation of women found to be bacteriuric to no drug and three different drug regimens Antibiotics used were: 1. Sulfamethizole and mandelamine combination 2. Nitrofuradantoin 3. Mandelamine alone	Pyelonephritis in pregnancy Prematurity	Group [incidence of pyelonephritis]: Initially negative culture (no Rx) [21/1028 (1.9%)] Initially negative culture and long-term Rx [1/115 (0.9%)] Initial positive cultures and drug Rx [3/69 (4.3%)] Initial positive culture and no long-term Rx [8/41 (19.5%)] Group [incidence of prematurity]: Initially negative culture (no Rx) [117/1003 (11.6%)] Initially negative culture and long-term Rx [16/138 (11.6%)] Initial positive cultures and drug Rx [7/101 (6.9%)] Initial positive culture and no long-term Rx [6/27 (22.1%)]	Method of randomisation was not indicated Follow-up rate of > 90%	RCT	1b

10.1.2 What are the maternal and perinatal outcomes associated with asymptomatic bacteriuria? (continued)

Study	Ref.	Population	Intervention	Outcomes	Results	Comments	Study type	EL
Foley et al., 1987	331	220 women with asymptomatic bacteriuria Hospital in Ireland Bacteriuria defined as more than 10^5 organisms per ml in a single midstream specimen of urine	Treatment vs. non-treatment of women with confirmed bacteriuria; 100 treated, 120 not treated Antibiotics used were either sulphamethizole or nitrofurantoin	Percentage of participants with sterile urine Incidence of symptomatic urinary tract infections Incidence of pyelonephritis	Percentage with sterile urine: Treatment group: 73% Non-treatment group: 48% Incidence of symptomatic UTI: ASB group: 2.3% Sterile urine group: 0.5% Incidence of pyelonephritis: Treatment group: 3/100 (3%) Non-treatment group: 3/120 (2.5%) Peto odds ratio (95% CI): 1.21 (0.24 to 6.13)	Randomisation was by coin-tossing Allocation concealment method not indicated Follow-up rate 81% Method of analysis not indicated	RCT	1b
Kincaid-Smith et al., 1965	333	240 women with bacteriuria 500 women without bacteriuria Bacteriuria defined as 10^5 organisms/ml Confirmed on two counts Australian hospital Women attending before 26 weeks of gestation	Antibiotic treatment vs. no treatment Treatment continued till delivery Antibiotic used was sulphamethoxydiazine, changed to sulphadimidine at week 30 of pregnancy Ampicillin or nitrofurantoin was used if resistance was demonstrated to any of the above	Pyelonephritis Prematurity (excluding twin pregnancies and pregnancies complicated by pre-eclampsia) Pre-eclampsia Fetal loss	Incidence of pyelonephritis: Treated group: 4/133 (3.0%) Placebo group: 41/128 (32.0%) Incidence of prematurity: Treated group: 18/133 (13.5%) Placebo group: 25/129 (19.4%) p value: NS No bacteriuria at first antenatal visit: 13/500 (2.6%); bacteriuria at first antenatal visit: 19/140 (7.9%); p value 0.001 Incidence of pre-eclampsia: No bacteriuria at first antenatal visit: 30/500 (6%) Bacteriuria at first antenatal visit: 26/240 (10.8%) p value: < 0.05 Incidence of fetal loss: No bacteriuria at first antenatal visit: 16/500 (3.2%) Bacteriuria at first antenatal visit: 22/240 (9.2%) p value: < 0.001	Method of randomisation not clear	RCT	1b

10.1.2 What are the maternal and perinatal outcomes associated with asymptomatic bacteriuria? (continued)

Study	Ref.	Population	Intervention	Outcomes	Results	Comments	Study type	EL
Mulla, 1960	337	100 patients with bacteriuria US hospital Urine sample obtained by catheter Culture collected at 30th week of pregnancy	50 patients treated with antibiotic 50 patients not given medication until symptoms appeared Antibiotic used was sulphadimethoxine	Pyelonephritis	Incidence of pyelonephritis: Treatment group: 3/50 (6%) Placebo group: 23/50 (46%)	Method of randomisation not indicated No losses to follow up reported Method of analysis not indicated	RCT	1b
Elder et al., 1971	335	289 patients with bacteriuria diagnosed by a colony count of 10^5 organisms or more in 2 of 3 specimens of urine US hospital Samples taken at first antenatal visit Matched controls	Bacteriuric patients: Antibiotic 133 Placebo 148. Non-bacteriuric patients Antibiotic 147 Placebo 132 Antibiotic: 6 weeks of tetracycline	Pyelonephritis	Incidence of pyelonephritis: Bacteriuric (placebo): 27/148 (18%) Bacteriuric (antibiotic): 4/33 (12%) Non-bacteriuric (antibiotic): 3/146 (2.0%) Non-bacteriuric (placebo): 3/132 (2.3%)	Randomisation was by alternating with placebo and would therefore be predictable and with no allocation concealment	CSNR	2a
Gold et al., 1966	336	65 patients with bacteriuria US hospital Bacteriuria was defined as having 10^5 organisms of the same species/ml of urine on 2 consecutive laboratory reports	35 treated with sulfadimethoxine till delivery 30 treated with placebo	Prevalence of ASB Prematurity Pyelonephritis	Prevalence 65/1281 (5.1%) Incidence of prematurity: Bacteriuric (treated) group: 2/65 (3.1%) Bacteriuric (placebo) group: 0/30 Non-bacteriuric group: 168/1216 (13.9%) Incidence of pyelonephritis: Treatment group: 0/35 Placebo group: 4/30 (13.3%)	Patients were randomised according to 'odd' or 'even' number of allocation	QR	2a

Paper looking specifically at asymptomatic group B streptococcal bacteriuria

Study	Ref.	Population	Intervention	Outcomes	Results	Comments	Study type	EL
Thomsen et al., 1987	334	69 women with GBS in the urine 1 midstream sample between weeks 27 and 31	37 patients treated with penicillin in the antenatal period	Preterm delivery (defined as delivery before the end of week 37 of gestation) Primary rupture of the membranes	Incidence of preterm delivery: Treated group: 2/37 (5.4%) Non-treated group: 12/32 (38%) p value: < 0.002	Prevalence of GBS bacteriuria was 69/4122(1.7%)	RCT	1b

10.1.3 What diagnostic tests are available for the detection of asymptomatic bacteriuria?

Study	Ref.	Population	Intervention	Outcomes	Results	Comments	Study type	EL
Comparing urine culture with reagent strips								
Shelton et al., 2001	343	200 women with attending antenatal clinic 20 identified as having ASB by urine culture US hospital	Urine dipstick–nitrite or LE vs. urine culture Commercially available reagent strips used	Sensitivity Specificity PPV NPV	LE: Sensitivity: 40 (95% CI 19 to 64) Specificity: 63 (95% CI 56 to 70) PPV: 11 (95% CI 5 to 20) NPV: 90 (95% CI 84 to 95) Nitrite: Sensitivity: 15 (95% CI 3 to 38) Specificity: 99 (95% CI 96 to 100) PPV: 60 (95% CI 15 to 95) NPV: 91 (95% CI 86 to 95) LE or Nitrite: Sensitivity: 45 (95% CI 23 to 68) Specificity: 62 (95% CI 55 to 69) PPV: 12 (95% CI 5 to 21) NPV: 91 (95% CI 85 to 95)	Using the dipstick will potentially fail to detect 55% of cases of ASB	TES	2a
McNair et al., 2000	345	528 women at first antenatal visit or admission with possible preterm labour US hospital February 1998 to March 1999	Urine culture compared with reagent strip testing Reagent strip positive if either nitrite or leucocyte esterase positive Commercially available reagent strips used	Sensitivity Specificity PPV NPV	Sensitivity: 47.2% (95% CI 30.8 to 64.3) Specificity: 80.3% (95% CI 76.4 to 83.7) PPV: 14.9% (95% CI 9.2 to 23.1) NPV: 95.9% (95% CI 92.8 to 97.1)		TES	2a
Tincello and Richmond, 1998	348	960 women attending antenatal clinics between June and September 1996	Commercial reagent strip tests for the presence of blood, protein, nitrite and leucocyte esterase vs. microscopy and culture of midstream urine Commercially available reagent strips used	Sensitivity Specificity PPV NPV of reagent strips in diagnosing asymptomatic bacteriuria (defined as 10^5 colony-forming units/ml urine)	Sensitivity: 33.3% (95% CI 26.5 to 40.1) Specificity: 91.1% (95% CI 89.1 to 93.1) PPV: 17.6% (95% CI 9.8 to 25.4) NPV: 96.0 (95% CI 94.6 to 97.4)	Blinding of investigators to the different test results is not indicated	TES	2a

10.1.3 What diagnostic tests are available for the detection of asymptomatic bacteriuria? (continued)

Study	Ref.	Population	Intervention	Outcomes	Results	Comments	Study type	EL
Etherington and James, 1993	342	898 women attending antenatal clinic UK hospital	Urine culture compared with Reagent strip testing (testing for individual reagent strips then in combination) Leuc Leucocyte Nit-Nitrite Pr-Protein Commercially available reagent strips used	Sensitivity Specificity PPV NPV Accuracy	(see table below)		TES	2a

	RT	S	SP	PPV	NPV
Leuc	60.0%	86.1%	16.1%	98.0%	82.3%
Nit	67.5%	99.7%	90.0%	98.5%	98.2%
Pr	57.4%	93.2%	29.7%	97.8%	90.6%
Blood	57.4%	93.2%	29.7%	97.8%	92.0%
All 4	81.8%	79.0%	10.5%	99.3%	73.6%
Leuc	60.0%	86.1%	16.1%	98.0%	82.3%
Nit	67.5%	99.7%	90.0%	98.5%	98.2%
Either+	73.0%	85.9%	15.9%	98.9%	83.0%

Study	Ref.	Population	Intervention	Outcomes	Results	Comments	Study type	EL
Bachman et al., 1993	347	1047 patients attending antenatal clinic US hospital	Urine culture compared with reagent strip testing (testing for nitrites) Commercially available reagent strips used	Sensitivity Specificity PPV	(see table below)	Reagent strip testing using nitrites only will potentially fail to detect 50% of cases of ASB	TES	2a

Test	S	SP	PPV
Nitrite	45.8%	99.7%	78.6%
LE	16.7%	97.2%	12.1%
Both +	12.5%	100%	100.0%
Either+	50.0%	96.9%	27.3%

Study	Ref.	Population	Intervention	Outcomes	Results	Comments	Study type	EL
Robertson et al., 1988	346	750 patients attending an Army Medical Centre in the USA	Urine dipstick-leucocyte esterase and nitrite compared with urine culture ASB defined as two clean-catch midstream urine cultures showing at least 10⁵ cfu/ml of a single uropathogen	Sensitivity Specificity PPV NPV	(see table below)	Sensitivity of either test positive higher in this series than Shelton[343] or Bachman[347]	TES	2a

Test	S	SP	PPV	NPV
Nitrite	43.4%	98.9%	79.4%	95.1%
LE	77.4%	96.1%	64.0%	97.9%
Both +	32.2%	94.2%	100.0%	99.2%
Either+	92.0%	95.0%	62.6%	99.2%

Comparing urine culture with microscopic urinalysis

Study	Ref.	Population	Intervention	Outcomes	Results	Comments	Study type	EL
McNair et al., 2000	345	528 women at first antenatal visit or admission with possible preterm labour US hospital February 1998 to March 1999	Urine culture compared with microscopic urinalysis Urinalysis positive if there was a count of 10 leucocytes/high-power field	Sensitivity Specificity PPV NPV	Sensitivity: 80.6% (95% CI 63.4 to 91.2) Specificity: 71.5% (95% CI 67.3 to 75.4) PPV: 17.2% (95% CI 12.0 to 23.9) NPV 98.1% (95% CI 95.8 to 99.1)		TES	2a

10.1.3 What diagnostic tests are available for the detection of asymptomatic bacteriuria? (continued)

Study	Ref.	Population	Intervention	Outcomes	Results	Comments	Study type	EL
Bachman et al., 1993	347	1047 patients attending antenatal clinic / US hospital	Urine culture compared with microscopic urinalysis / Significant pyuria was inferred by the presence of more than 10 leucocytes/high-power field	Sensitivity / Specificity	Sensitivity 25% / Specificity 99%	Urinalysis will potentially fail to detect 75% of cases of ASB	TES	2a
Abyad, 1991	349	Population taken from 3000 registered patients over 7 years	Urine culture compared with microscopic urinalysis / Bacteriuria > 1000 organisms/ml	Sensitivity / Specificity / PPV / NPV	WBC/HPF — S(%) — SP(%) — PPV(%) — NPV(%); >8: 72.2, 98.6, 76.5, 98.2; ≥5: 94.4, 95.3, 56.7, 99.6; ≥1: 100.0, 66.6, 16.2, 100.0		TES	2a

Comparing urine culture with centrifugation with Gram stain

Study	Ref.	Population	Intervention	Outcomes	Results	Comments	Study type	EL
McNair et al., 2000	345	528 women at first antenatal visit or admission with possible preterm labour / US hospital / February 1998 to March 1999	Urine culture compared with centrifugation with Gram stain	Sensitivity / Specificity / PPV / NPV	Sensitivity: 100% (95% CI 88 to 100) / Specificity: 7.7% (95% CI 5.6 to 10.5) / PPV: 7.3% (95% CI 5.3 to 10.1) / NPV: 100% (95% CI 88.5 to 100)	Centrifugation with Gram staining will potentially detect all cases of ASB but with a poor specificity will incorrectly label over 90% of women as having ASB	TES	2a
Bachman et al., 1993	347	1047 patients attending antenatal clinic / US hospital	Urine culture compared with Gram staining	Sensitivity / Specificity	Sensitivity 91.7% / Specificity 89.2%	Less than 10 % of cases of ASB will potentially be missed and a little over 10% of cases incorrectly labelled as having ASB	TES	2a

Other tests

Study	Ref.	Population	Intervention	Outcomes	Results	Comments	Study type	EL
Shelton et al., 2001	343	200 women with attending antenatal clinic / 20 identified as having ASB by urine culture / US hospital	Urinary interleukin-8 vs. urine culture	Sensitivity / Specificity / PPV / NPV	Sensitivity: 70% (95% CI 46 to 88) / Specificity: 67 %(95%CI 59 to 74) / PPV: 19% (95% CI 11 to 30) / NPV: 95% (95% CI 90 to 98)	Urinary interleukin-8 will potentially fail to detect 30% of women with asymptomatic bacteriuria	TES	2a

10.1.3 What diagnostic tests are available for the detection of asymptomatic bacteriuria? (continued)

Study	Ref.	Population	Intervention	Outcomes	Results	Comments	Study type	EL
Millar et al., 2000	344	383 women attending antenatal clinic US hospital Bacteriuria defined as 10⁴ colony-forming units of a single pathogen	Rapid enzymatic screening test (detection of catalase activity) vs. urine culture	Sensitivity Specificity PPV NPV	Sensitivity: 70% (95% CI 56.5 to 83.5) Specificity: 45% (95% CI 39.5 to 50.5) PPV: 14% (95% CI 9.0 to 19) NPV: 92% (95% CI 88 to 96)	The rapid enzymatic screening test will potentially fail to detect 30% of women with asymptomatic bacteriuria	TES	2a
Graninger et al., 1992	350	1000 women attending antenatal clinic in a German hospital	Bioluminescence assay	Sensitivity Specificity Predictive accuracy	Sensitivity: 93% Specificity: 78% Predictive accuracy: 99%		TES	2a

10.1.4 Does universal screening for asymptomatic bacteriuria during pregnancy (and treatment of those found to be positive) result in improved outcomes compared with no screening?

Study	Ref.	Population	Intervention	Outcomes	Results	Comments	Study type	EL
Smaill, 2002	351	Cochrane review, updated 2000 14 RCTs Women with asymptomatic bacteriuria found on antenatal screening Various countries	Antibiotic treatment vs. placebo or no treatment	Effect of antibiotic treatment on persistent bacteriuria during pregnancy Risk of preterm delivery or low birth weight babies Development of pyelonephritis	Effect of antibiotic treatment on persistent bacteriuria during pregnancy: Treatment group: 38/293 (13%) Control group: 225/300 (75%) Peto odds ratio: 0.07 (95% CI 0.05 to 0.10) Risk of preterm delivery or low birth weight babies: Treatment group: 101/1044 (9.7%) Control group: 127/879 (14.5%) Peto odds ratio: 0.60 (95% CI 0.45 to 0.80) Development of pyelonephritis: Treatment group: 59/1125 (5.2%) Control group: 203/1064 (19.1%) Peto odds ratio: 0.24 (95% CI 0.19 to 0.32) NNT: 7	Study quality was assessed and found to be generally poor Inadequate allocation concealment except in one study No blinding of observer to treatment allocation Results were however consistent from study to study None of the studies collected adverse outcomes of antibiotic treatment	SR	1a

10.1.5 What antibiotic regimens are cost effective in treating asymptomatic bacteriuria in pregnant women?

Study	Ref.	Population	Intervention	Outcomes	Results	Comments	Study type	EL
Villar et al., 2001	352	Cochrane systematic review, updated 2000 8 RCTs comparing different antibiotic regimens	Single dose compared with 4 to 7 day course 2 RCTs	Preterm delivery Pyelonephritis	Preterm delivery: Treatment group: 5/55 (9.1%) Control group: 5/46 (10.9%) Peto odds ratio: 0.81(95% CI 0.26 to 2.57) Pyelonephritis: Treatment group: 5/54 (9.3%) Control group: 5/46 (2.1%) Peto odds ratio: 3.09 (95% CI 0.54 to 17.55)	Only two RCTs reported preterm birth rates and pyelonephritis	SR	1a

10.1.6 What are the outcomes associated with these antibiotic regimens?

Study	Ref.	Population	Intervention	Outcomes	Results	Comments	Study type	EL
Villar et al., 2001	352	Cochrane systematic review, updated 2000 8 RCTs comparing different antibiotic regimens 2 RCTs	Single dose compared with 4 to 7 day course	Gastrointestinal side effects	Treatment group: 16/231 (6.9%) Control group: 29/209 (14%) Peto odds ratio: 0.53 (95% CI 0.31 to 0.91)	Results largely influenced by a trial that was stopped mainly due to side effects of sulphadimidine	SR	1a

10.2 Asymptomatic bacterial vaginosis (BV)

10.2.1 What is the prevalence of asymptomatic BV infection in pregnancy?

Study	Ref.	Population	Intervention	Outcomes	Results	Comments	Study type	EL
Goldenberg et al., 1996	355	13,747 pregnant women from 7 medical centres in the USA from 1984 to 1989	Women at 23 to 26 weeks gestation were grouped according to ethnic origin (white, black, Hispanic, Asian-Pacific islander). BV was diagnosed by Gram stain score ≥ 7 in conjunction with vaginal pH > 4.5	Frequency of BV	White women (n = 4049): 8.8% Black women (n = 5285): 22.7% (p < 0.05 compared with white women) Hispanic women (n = 4240): 15.9% (p < 0.05 compared with white women) Asian-Pacific islander (n = 173): 6.1%		CSS	3
Hay et al., 1994	356	718 women attending an antenatal clinic in North West London	Swabs taken at first visit (< 28 weeks) Gram stained	BV diagnosis	At first visit: 87/718 (12%) diagnosed with BV		CSS	3

10.2.2 What are the diagnostic tests for detecting BV infection and how do they compare in terms of sensitivity and specificity?

Study	Ref.	Population	Intervention	Outcomes	Results	Comments	Study type	EL
Amsel et al., 1983	359			Criteria for BV diagnosis	Presence of 3 of the following required: – Thin white-grey homogeneous discharge – Vaginal fluid pH > 4.5 – Fishy odour on adding of alkali – Clue cells present on direct microscopy			
Nugent et al., 1991	360			Criteria for BV diagnosis	Gram-stained vaginal smear to estimate proportions of bacterial morphotypes to give 0 to 10 score: < 4 normal, 4 to 6 intermediate, > 6 BV			
Mastrobattista et al., 2000	610	69 asymptomatic pregnant women from 1996 to 1997 in the USA	Amsel criteria compared (2 of 3 criteria required) with Gram stain by Nugent criteria as the standard for BV diagnosis in women at 16 weeks gestation (mean)	Sensitivity Specificity	Sensitivity: 56% (95% CI 32 to 78) Specificity: 96% (95% CI 90 to 100)	Character of vaginal discharge not used as criteria because it is less easily characterised in pregnant women than in nonpregnant women	TES	3
Krohn et al., 1990	611	593 pregnant women from 1984 to 1986 in the USA	Clinical diagnosis of BV by Amsel's criteria (standard) compared with Gram stain (Nugent's criteria) and gas-liquid chromatography (Spiegel's criteria)	Sensitivity Specificity	Gram-stained: sensitivity 62%; specificity 95% Gas-liquid chromatography: sensitivity 78%; specificity 81%		TES	3

10.2.3 Is BV infection associated with adverse maternal and perinatal outcomes?

Study	Ref.	Population	Intervention	Outcomes	Results	Comments	Study type	EL
Flynn et al., 1999	357	8 case–control studies and 11 cohort studies	Meta-analysis to determine magnitude of risk associated with BV (vs. no BV) and preterm birth	Preterm birth (defined as < 35 weeks in two studies, < 36 weeks in one study, < 37 weeks in all others)	OR (fixed) 1.85, 95% CI 1.62 to 2.11 OR (random) 2.05, 95% CI 1.67 to 2.50 RR (fixed, 10 cohort studies): 1.56, 95% CI 1.37 to 1.78 RR (random, 10 cohort studies): 1.75, 95% CI 1.34 to 2.29		SR	2 & 3
Gratacos et al., 1998	358	635 women screened for BV in Spain at < 35 weeks	Diagnosis based on Gram-stained smears based on Nugent's criteria Positive women retested within 4 to 8 weeks	BV diagnosis at initial visit Preterm birth	125/635 (19.6%) with BV Repeat sample taken in 92/125 (73.6%) of women 47/92 (51.1%) found still positive for BV Preterm birth: BV+ at initial visit 20/125 (16%) vs. BV– at initial visit 26/510 (5%); RR 3.1, 95% CI 1.8 to 5.4 Preterm birth in BV+ persistent women 8/47 (16%) vs. BV disappearance at second visit 7/45 (15.5%)		CSS	3

10.2.4 & 10.2.5 What are the antibiotic regimens of BV infection in pregnancy and how do they compare in terms of effectiveness and does screening for and treating pregnant women found to have BV infection lead to improved maternal and perinatal outcomes?

Study	Ref.	Population	Intervention	Outcomes	Results	Comments	Study type	EL
McDonald et al., 2003	362	10 RCTs, 4249 pregnant women screened (or treated) for BV at 10 to 26 weeks of gestation	Antibiotic regimen vs. placebo or no treatment	'Test-of-cure' Preterm delivery PPROM	Failure of test-of-cure (8 RCTs, n = 2835): Peto OR 0.21, 95% CI 0.18 to 0.24 Preterm delivery, <37 weeks (8 RCTs, n = 4062): Peto OR 0.95, 95% CI 0.82 to 1.10 Preterm delivery, <34 weeks (5 RCTs, n = 851): Peto OR 1.20, 95% CI 0.69 to 2.07 Preterm delivery, <32 weeks (3 RCTs, n = 3080): Peto OR 1.08, 95% CI 0.70 to 1.68 PPROM (3 RCTs, n = 3080): Peto OR 0.32, 95% CI 0.59 to 1.17		SR	1a

10.3 *Chlamydia trachomatis*

10.3.1 What is the prevalence of chlamydial infection in pregnant women in the UK?

Study	Ref.	Population	Intervention	Outcomes	Results	Comments	Study type	EL
Preece et al., 1989	365	3309 women screened for chlamydial antigen over a one year period District general hospital in Birmingham, England	Cervical swab, ELISA technique	Prevalence of chlamydia in pregnant women	Overall prevalence = 6% (198 women) Prevalence: women under 20 years, 14.5%; single women, 14.2%; black women, 16.8%		CSS	3
Goh et al., 1982	366	53 pregnant women attending GUM clinic at a hospital in London from June to December 1981	cervical swabs	Prevalence of chlamydia	Chlamydia prevalence was isolated in 20/53 (37.7%)		CSS	3

10.3.2 What re the maternal and perinatal outcomes associated with chlamydial infection in pregnancy?

Study	Ref.	Population	Intervention	Outcomes	Results	Comments	Study type	EL
Preece et al., 1989	370	3309 women screened for chlamydia in a district hospital in England, from September 1985 through August 1986	Screening for chlamydia in pregnant mothers on presentation in labour with ELISA. Infants of mothers with chlamydia seen at 3, 6, 12, and 26 weeks	Neonatal *C. trachomatis* infection. Neonatal conjunctivitis. Respiratory infection	198 mothers positive for chlamydial antigen identified. 174 of the 198 infants followed-up. Culture positive 25% (n = 43/174). 11% (n = 20/174) infants had neonatal conjunctivitis. 3% (n = 6/174) infants developed lower respiratory tract infections	Only babies born to women with chlamydia followed up	CSS	3
Schachter et al., 1986	371	131 neonates of 262 pregnant women who tested positive for chlamydia in obstetric clinic in San Francisco hospital, from 1977 to 1983	Screening of all pregnant women who presented for their first antenatal care visit and prospective follow-up of their infants plus 46 control infants whose mothers had negative chlamydia cultures before delivery	Neonatal deaths. Culture positive for chlamydia in newborn. Conjunctivitis in the newborn. Pneumonia in the neonate	Neonatal death 4% (n = 5/131). 36% (n = 47/131) cultured positive for chlamydia. 17.6% (n = 23/131) neonatal conjunctivitis. 16% (n = 21/131) had pneumonia. None of the controls developed any clinical disease due to *C. trachomatis* nor were any cultures positive by 9 months of age	Only 50% of infants born to infected mothers were followed up. All women who were delivered by caesarean section or who refused or had moved were excluded	COM	3

10.3.3 Does screening women for chlamydial infection in pregnancy lead to improved maternal and perinatal outcomes?

Study	Ref.	Population	Intervention	Outcomes	Results	Comments	Study type	EL
Brocklehurst and Rooney, 2002	369	11 RCTs included	Antibiotic therapy or alternative antibiotic therapy vs. placebo or no treatment for chlamydia in pregnant women	Eradication of maternal infection Preterm delivery Side effects, endometritis and neonatal death: no significant difference	Number of women with positive cultures reduced by 90% when treated with antibiotics compared with placebo; OR 0.06 (95% CI 0.03 to 0.12) Preterm delivery OR 0.89 (0.51 to 1.56) Side effects, endometritis and neonatal death: no significant difference	Being updated	SR	1a
Ryan et al., 1990	368	11,544 women cultured at their first prenatal care visit Tennessee, USA, from September 1982 through August 1985	Cervical culture at first antenatal care visit and prospective follow up Women who presented from September 1982 through December 1983 were not treated (n = 1110) Women who presented from Jan 1984 through Aug 1985 were treated with erythromycin (n = 1323)	Prevalence Low birthweight Infant death	21.1% (n = 2433/11544) were positive for chlamydia Increase in low birthweight in untreated group vs. treated group (19.6% vs. 11.0%, p < 0.0001, RR 1.78, 95% CI 1.48 to 2.18) No difference between treated and culture negative group (RR 0.94, 95% CI 0.79 to 1.10) Decrease in survival in untreated group vs. treated group (97.6% vs. 99.4%, p < 0.001, RR 0.98, 95% CI 0.97 to 0.99) Treated also more likely to survive than culture-negative group (99.4% vs. 98.5%, p < 0.01, RR 1.01, 95% CI 1.0 to 1.01)	Historical cohort different calendar periods could explain observed differences Infant death defined as those who did not leave the hospital alive	CH	2b

10.3.4 What methods should be used for screening for *Chlamydia trachomatis* in pregnancy?

Study	Ref.	Population	Intervention	Outcomes	Results	Comments	Study type	EL
Fitzgerald et al., 1998	372	Adults	Culture Enzyme immunoassay Serology	Sensitivities and specificities of various tests	Chlamydia culture Sensitivity 75% to 85% at best, and may be low as 55%, only appropriate for invasive samples, and labour intensive Enzyme immunoassay Sensitivity 75% to 80% compared with culture Suitable for large number of samples, requires invasive samples and high specificity only if positive results are confirmed Serology of no value in diagnosis of acute chlamydial infection	Work carried out in collaboration with Royal College of Physicians Research Unit and Members of Central Audit Group in Genitourinary Medicine	GL	4
Stary, 2001	364	Adults	Culture Direct fluorescent antibody assays Enzyme immunoassays RNA-DNA hybridisation Nucleic acid amplification	Sensitivities and specificities of various tests	Cell culture sensitivity range 40% to 85%, only appropriate for invasive samples Direct fluorescent antibody assays sensitivity range 50% to 90%, suitable for invasive and noninvasive samples, but time-consuming and therefore unsuitable for large numbers Enzyme immunoassays sensitivity range 20% to 85%, suitable for large number of samples, requires invasive samples and high specificity only if positive results are confirmed RNA-DNA hybridisation sensitivity range 70% to 85%, rapid and reliable, suitable for large numbers and requires invasive samples Nucleic acid amplification sensitivity range 70% to 95%, also has high specificity (97% to 99%), suitable for large numbers of samples, invasive and noninvasive samples may be used, but expensive and inhibitors may be a problem in urine samples	Single author, no guideline methodology given	GL	4

10.4 Cytomegalovirus

10.4.1 What is the prevalence of cytomegalovirus (CMV) infection in pregnancy?

Study	Ref.	Population	Intervention	Outcomes	Results	Comments	Study type	EL
Ryan et al., 1995	374	Pregnant women in England and Wales in 1992 and 1993 (1,363,123 live births)	Reports of CMV to laboratories in England and Wales	Number of cases in pregnant women Outcomes of pregnancy	47 reports of CMV infection in pregnancy Intrauterine death or stillbirth in 22 cases	Reports in pregnancy could not be linked to outcomes in live born infants Most infections with CMV in pregnancy are not recognised	SV	3

10.4.2 What is the prevalence of congenital cytomegalovirus (CMV) infection?

Study	Ref.	Population	Intervention	Outcomes	Results	Comments	Study type	EL
Preece et al., 1986	375	23,247 pregnant women 3 London hospitals Dates not given	Infants diagnosed if CMV isolated from throat swab in first week of life	Estimated prevalence of congenital CMV	69/23,247 Prevalence 2.6/1000	Estimated denominator as not all women screened	CSS	3
Peckham et al., 1983	376	14,200 babies born at three London hospitals from Sep 1979 through Aug 1982	Infants diagnosed if CMV isolated in first week of life from throat swab	Congenital infection with CMV	42 live births, rate of 3/1000 None of the 42 mothers had any signs or symptoms of acute CMV infection 26 had been positive at their first antenatal visit	Discrepancy between 14,789 mothers and 14,200 infants, i.e. approx 589 infants unaccounted for	CS	3

10.4.3 Does screening pregnant women for cytomegalovirus (CMV) infection lead to improved maternal and perinatal outcomes?

Study	Ref.	Population	Intervention	Outcomes	Results	Comments	Study type	EL
Bolyard et al., 1998	377				Repeated testing is necessary to identify CMV because it can be shed Seropositivity does not offer complete protection against maternal reinfection and subsequent fetal infection No currently available vaccines or prophylactic therapy		GL	4
Stagno and Whitley, 1985	378				Maternal immunity does not prevent virus reactivation nor transmission to fetus No effective drug therapy for CMV or its transmission exists No ways to determine whether intrauterine transmission has occurred No way to determine whether infected infant will have serious sequelae		RV	4

10.5 Hepatitis B virus

10.5.1 What is the prevalence of hepatitis B viral infection in pregnant women in the UK?

Study	Ref.	Population	Intervention	Outcomes	Results	Comments	Study type	EL
Boxall et al., 1994	379	3522 anonymous serum samples collected from women attending an antenatal clinic in the West Midlands from February 1990 to January 1991	Sera tested for HBsAg using RIA or ELISA and positives confirmed using reverse passive haemagglutination	HBsAg prevalence among women of various ethnic origins	Overall prevalence 0.56% (20/3522) Breakdown: 13/20 Asian 4/20 African-Caribbean 3/20 SE Asian Prevalence in women from immigrant groups 1.04%		CSS	3
Brook et al., 1989	380	6226 women attending antenatal clinic at the Royal Free Hospital, London, from 1983/84 to 1988/89	Screening using HBsAg	Number of mothers HBsAg positive at first antenatal care visit	33/6226 (0.5%) HBsAg positive at first visit		CS	3
Chrystie et al., 1992	381	Stored serum from antenatal clinics 1990 (n = 3760) and 1988 (n = 3975) Sera of women originally collected for rubella in West Lambeth Health authority in London	Serology	Prevalence among women screened	In 1988: 38/3760 (1%) women HBsAg positive In 1990: 35/3975 (0.9%) women HBsAg positive		CSS	3
Derso et al., 1978	382	Approximately 240,000 pregnant women from antenatal clinics in West Midlands, England, from May 1974 to May 1977	Serum screening using HBsAg	Prevalence of HBsAg carriage in pregnant mothers	297 pregnant women were HBsAg positive Overall prevalence of approx 1/850 (0.1%)		CSS	3

10.5.2 What is the prevalence of congenital hepatitis B virus in the UK?

Study	Ref.	Population	Intervention	Outcomes	Results	Comments	Study type	EL
Ramsay et al., 1998	385	England and Wales from 1985 to 1996	Surveillance of laboratory reported cases to PHLS communicable disease surveillance centres	Infection in children (under 15 years) Number of cases due to mother-to-child transmission Estimated annual number of perinatal transmissions which lead to chronic carriage	Total of 173 cases reported 37/173 (21%) due to mother-to-child transmission 93/116 cases of perinatal transmission leading to carriage per year	Assumption that 80% of perinatal infections lead to chronic carriage	CSS	3
Derso et al., 1978	382	Approximately 240,000 pregnant women from antenatal clinics in West Midlands, England, from May 1974 to May 1977	Serum screening using HBsAg	Infants HBsAg positive beyond 3 months of age	Antigen detected in cord blood of 101/219 (46%) of 269 babies delivered 17/122 (14%) babies followed up beyond 3 months of age had persistently high titres of HBsAg; 64% were Chinese, 30% African-Caribbean and 8% Asian (0 European)	The paper states that 297 carrier mothers were discovered but in the table of ethnic distribution of mothers, only 100 mothers are accounted for	COM	3

10.5.3 What are the consequences for the baby of congenital hepatitis B virus?

Study	Ref.	Population	Intervention	Outcomes	Results	Comments	Study type	EL
Beasley and Hwang, 1984	384	22,707 men presenting for routine examination from 1976 to 1978 in Taiwan	Prospective follow-up through 1983	HBsAg carrier state Hepatocellular carcinoma Mortality	3,454 HBsAg positive 113/3,454 HCC cases among HBsAg carriers 3/19,253 cases among non-carriers 103/202 deaths due to cirrhosis or hepatocellular carcinoma in HBsAg carrier group 9/394 deaths due to cirrhosis or hepatocellular carcinoma in non-carrier group RR 22.3 (95% CI 11.5 to 43.2)		CH	2b

10.5.4 What are the diagnostic tests available for detection of hepatitis B viral infection and how do they compare in terms of specificity, sensitivity, and cost effectiveness?

Study	Ref.	Population	Intervention	Outcomes	Results	Comments	Study type	EL
Summers et al., 1987	394	All women attending the antenatal clinic at a US hospital in New Orleans from November 1983 through October 1985	Serum collected at initial prenatal visit Patients interviewed for hepatitis B virus risk factors	Number of women identified with risk factors	136/15399 women found to be HBsAg positive (prevalence 0.88%) No patient symptomatic 54/108 (50%) pregnant women demonstrated risk factors		CSS	3
Chaita et al., 1995	395	88 Thai women attending an antenatal clinic with known HBsAg status (44 HBsAg positive)	Saliva and serum samples were collected and then analysed in Liverpool, England, using ELISA to detect HBsAg	Sensitivity and specificity of screening for HBsAg in saliva compared with serum	Sensitivity 92% (95% CI 84.5 to 99.5) Specificity 86.8% (95% CI 76.0 to 97.6)		CSS	3

10.5.5 What are the interventions to reduce mother-to-child transmission of hepatitis B virus?

Study	Ref.	Population	Intervention	Outcomes	Results	Comments	Study type	EL
Sehgal et al., 1992	386	109 HBsAg positive mothers in India from 1987 through 1989	Group 1: HBV vaccine within 24 hours of birth and 2nd and 3rd dose at 4 and 8 weeks, respectively (n = 24) Group 2: HBV vaccine and HBIG within 24 hours of birth. Further HBV vaccine doses at 4 and 8 weeks respectively (n=27)	HBsAg carrier state in infants at 6 months	HBV carrier rate: Group 1: 1/21* (4.8%) Group 2: 3/24* (12.5%) *3 cases excluded from each group RR 2.6 (95%CI 0.29, 23.4)	58 mothers refused vaccination for their babies	RCT	1b
Xu et al., 1985	392	208 pregnant mothers with HBsAg from antenatal clinics in Shanghai from 1982 to 1984	Group 1: BIVS vaccine for hepatitis B virus within 24 hours of birth and at 1 and 6 months of age (n=60) Group 2: NIAID vaccine for hepatitis B virus within 24 hours of birth and at 1 and 6 months of age (n=60) Group 3: BIVS vaccine for hepatitis B virus plus HBIG within 24 hours of birth and further vaccine only at 1 and 6 months of age (n=60) Group 4: placebo within 24 hours of birth and at 1 and 6 months of age (n=28)	HBsAg carrier state in infants at 6 months (n=5, 5, 4, and 1 lost to follow-up, for each group respectively)	HBV carrier rate: Group 1: 12/56 (21.4%) Group 2: 3/55 (5.4%) Group 3: 2/27 (7.4%) Group 4: 24/55 (43.6%) Group 4 vs. group 1: RR 0.49 (95% CI 0.27 to 0.88) Group 4 vs. group 2: RR 0.13 (95% CI 0.40 to 0.39) Group 4 vs. group 3: RR 0.17 (95% CI 0.04 to 0.67)	BIVS = Beijing Institute of Vaccine and Serum vaccine NIAID = National nstitute of Allergy and Infectious disease vaccine	RCT	1b
Nair et al., 1984	391	20 pregnant women attending antenatal clinic found positive for HBsAg and anti-HBe in USA from 1978 through 1982	HBIG (n=12) or placebo (n=8) within 24 hours after birth and at five week intervals for a total of 6 injections for infants	HBsAg carrier state in infants	1/20 infants became HBsAg and HBeAg positive from the HBIG group		RCT	1b

10.5.5 What are the interventions to reduce mother-to-child-transmission of hepatitis B virus? (continued)

Study	Ref.	Population	Intervention	Outcomes	Results	Comments	Study type	EL
Wong et al., 1984	387	315 pregnant women found positive for HBeAg attending antenatal clinic in Hong Kong from June 1981 to September 1983 from which 262 gave consent	Group 1: HBV vaccine at birth and at 1, 2 and 6 months after birth, plus 7 monthly HBIg injections (n = 36) Group 2: same as above, but only one HBIG injection at birth (n = 35) Group 3: vaccine only at 0, 1, 2, and 6 months (n = 35) Group 4: placebos for both vaccine and HBIg (n = 34)	HBsAg carrier state in infants	HBV carrier rate: Group 1: 2.9% Group 2: 6.8% Group 3: 21.0% Group 4: 73.2% (Rates as calculated by life-table attack-rate analysis)	By September 1983, 216 babies had been born to 262 mothers Infants excluded because of low birthweight, low Apgar score, congenital abnormality, withdrawn from study, stillbirth, or other criteria These results are for 140 babies who were at least 6 months of age by September 1983	RCT	1b
Zhu et al., 1997	388	204 HBsAg positive pregnant women from two hospital obstetric departments in Shanghai, China from February 1991 to February 1994 207 babies were born to the 204 mothers	HBIG given 3, 2 and 1 month before delivery (n = 105) vs. no treatment (n = 102)	Seroconversion to HBeAg in mothers at 3 months before delivery Prevention of intrauterine transmission of HBV	Treatment group: 37/103 (36%) Control group: 32/101 (32%) 6/105 HBsAg positive babies in treatment group (5.7%) vs. 15/102 HBsAg positive babies born in control group (14.7%) p < 0.05 (RR 0.39, 95% CI 0.16 to 0.95)	Method of randomisation not indicated No losses to follow up	RCT	1b
Lo et al., 1985	389	361 HBeAg positive mothers in 3rd trimester at obstetric clinic in Taipei, Taiwan from September 1982 to October 1983	Group 1: HBV vaccine alone (38 infants) Group 2: HBV vaccine and HBIG at birth (36 infants) Group 3: HBV vaccine and HBIG at birth and 1 month of age (38 infants)	Hepatitis B virus in infants at 6 months	HBV carrier rate: Group 1: 9/38 (23.7%) Group 2: 4/36 (11.1%) Group 3: 2/38 (5.3%) Group 1 vs. group 2 RR: 0.47 (95% CI 0.16 to 1.39) Group 1 vs. group 3 RR: 0.22 (95% CI 0.05 to 0.96)	Method of randomisation not specified 112 infants received vaccine and were followed-up for 6 months or longer	RCT	1b

10.5.5 What are the interventions to reduce mother-to-child-transmission of hepatitis B virus? (continued)

Study	Ref.	Population	Intervention	Outcomes	Results	Comments	Study type	EL
Beasley et al., 1983	390	1026 HbeAg positive women from 2 large hospitals in Taipei, Taiwan, attending antenatal clinics from November 1981 through December 1982	Group 1: HBIG at birth and at 3 months at which time vaccination also initiated (n = 51) Group 2: HBIG at birth and vaccine initiated at 4 to 7 days old (n = 50) Group 3: HBIG at births and vaccination initiated at 1 month (n = 58) All initial vaccination followed by booster 1 month and 6 months later 159 infants and 84 controls for analysis at least 9 months of age	Hepatitis B virus in infants at 9 months	HBV carrier rate: Group 1: 1/51 (2.0%) Group 2: 3/50 (6.0%) Group 3: 5/58 (8.6%) Group 3 vs. group 2 RR: 0.70 (95% CI 0.18 to 2.77) Group 3 vs. group 1 RR: 0.23 (95% CI 0.03 to 1.88)	Method of randomisation not indicated 159 infants whose parents gave consent, were not withdrawn from the study, who received the full treatment of the group to which they were assigned and were at least 9 months of age at time of analysis	RCT	1b
Beasley et al., 1977	383	62 asymptomatic HBsAg positive women at an antenatal clinic in Taiwan No date given	Mothers' sera tested either during pregnancy or 1 to 20 months postpartum 20 women eAg positive	Transmission rate	17/20 (85%) of babies from eAg positive mothers became HBsAg positive 13/42 (31%) of infants from eAg negative mothers became HBsAg positive RR 2.8 (95% CI 1.69 to 4.47)		CSS	3

10.7 HIV

10.7.1 What is the prevalence of HIV infection in pregnant women in the UK?

Study	Ref.	Population	Intervention	Outcomes	Results	Comments	Study type	EL
Unlinked Anonymous Surveys Steering Group, 2002	407	426,474 pregnant women in England, plus 52,707 in Scotland, tested in 2001	Survey used leftover blood from samples taken for routine clinical tests	Number HIV-1 infected HIV prevalence	London: 363/103,840 Elsewhere in UK: 143/322,634 London prevalence: 0.35% (0.05 to 0.84) Elsewhere in UK prevalence: 0.04 (0.0 to 0.43)	Results represent 72% of all live births in UK for 2001	CSS	3
Unlinked Anonymous Surveys Steering Group, 1999	613	506,462 pregnant women in Scotland and England, tested in 1998	Survey used leftover blood from samples taken for routine clinical tests	Number HIV-1 infected Prevalence Mother-to-child transmission	HIV-1 infected: London: 224/101,602 Scotland: 13/57,298 Elsewhere in UK: 53/347,562 Prevalence: London: 0.22% (0.0 to 0.62) Scotland: 0.023% (0.0 to 0.079) Elsewhere in the UK: 0.015% (0.0 to 0.12) Infected babies and births in HIV infected women: London: 37/232, 15.9% (95% CI 12.1% to 21.6%) Scotland: 2/13, 15.4% (95% CI 7.7% to 23.1%) Rest of UK: 19/86, 22.1% (95% CI 17.4% to 26.7%)		CSS	3
Unlinked Anonymous Surveys Steering Group, 2001	408	Pregnant women in Scotland and England, 484,563 women tested in 2000	Survey used leftover blood from samples taken for routine clinical tests	Number HIV-1 infected Prevalence (range)	HIV-1 infected: London: 298/103,852 Scotland: 25/53,347 Elsewhere in UK: 89/327,364 London prevalence 0.29% (0.0 to 0.73) Elsewhere in the UK prevalence 0.027% (0.0 to 0.3)		CSS	3

10.7.2 What is the prevalence of congenitally acquired infection in the UK?

Study	Ref.	Population	Intervention	Outcomes	Results	Comments	Study type	EL
Unlinked Anonymous Surveys Steering Group, 2002	407	426,474 pregnant women in England, plus 52,707 in Scotland, tested in 2001	Survey used leftover blood from samples taken for routine clinical tests	Mother-to-child transmission of HIV-1	Infected babies and births in HIV infected women in the UK: 49/561	Estimates are based on the observed proportion of maternal infections diagnosed before delivery and assume that 2% of infants will acquire HIV even if maternal infection is diagnosed before delivery	CSS	3
Unlinked Anonymous Surveys Steering Group, 2001	408	484,563 pregnant women in Scotland and England, tested in 2000	Survey used leftover blood from samples taken for routine clinical tests	Mother-to-child transmission of HIV-1	Infected babies and births in HIV infected women: 45/452	Estimates are based on observed proportions of maternal infections diagnosed before delivery and assumed that about 2% of infants will acquire HIV even if maternal infection is diagnosed prior to delivery	CSS	3
CDR Weekly, 26 April 2001	412	Paediatric surveillance data	None	Confirmed cases of HIV infection in children by the end of January 2001 in the UK (excluding Scotland)	1036 infected children, 68% probably acquired through mother-to-child transmission

1885 children born to HIV infected mothers reported by end of January 2001, 712 known to be infected, 716 known to be uninfected, 457 unresolved or unreported

By the end of 1999, 697 known to be infected, 259 indeterminate, and 659 not infected out of a total of 1615 children born to HIV infected mothers

In 2000, 270 babies were born to HIV infected mothers resulting in 15 HIV-positive babies, 57 not infected and 198 as yet undetermined | | LS | 3 |
| Conner et al., 1994 | 409 | RCT with 477 HIV infected pregnant women enrolled from April 1991 to December 1993 (409 births leading to 415 live-born infants) | Zidovudine vs. placebo | Efficacy of zidovudine in reducing risk of vertical transmission measured by HIV infection status of child | 67.5% (95%CI 40.7 to 82.1) relative reduction in risk of HIV transmission (z = 4.03, p = 0.00006)

Proportion infected at 18 months in zidovudine group 8.3% (95% CI 3.9 to 12.8)

Proportion infected at 18 months in placebo group 25.5% (95% CI 18.4 to 32.5) | | RCT | 1b |

10.7.3 What are the diagnostic tests available for detection of HIV infection and how do they compare in terms of specificity, sensitivity and cost-effectiveness?

Study	Ref.	Population	Intervention	Outcomes	Results	Comments	Study type	EL
Balano, 1998	614		Rapid HIV screening during labour	Performance of rapid HIV 1 antibody testing	Sensitivity 99.9% Specificity 99.6% Positive predictive value exceeds 50% only when prevalence of HIV 1 exceeds 0.5%	Letter This paper only reported the performance of this test, i.e. did not investigate the test's performance itself		
PHLS AIDS Diagnosis Working Group, 1992	415		HIV testing algorithm	Initial assay (EIA or rapid tests). If reaction is positive, further testing with different assays (two). If both confirmatory tests are nonreactive, issue negative report. If confirmatory tests are reactive, one more test with a new specimen should be obtained to ensure no procedural errors have occurred	Available EIAs or rapid tests have similar and adequate sensitivity to be used singly to generate a negative report (unless HIV-2 assay is also needed) HIV culture and tests for p24 antigen are not of much value in diagnostic testing, as they may be insensitive, non-specific and expensive tests	In a low prevalence population such as the UK, high specificity and reasonable sensitivity are important	Report from PHLS AIDS Diagnosis Working Group	IV
Postma et al., 1999	615		Performance of ELISA as initial test for HIV as specified for use in cost effectiveness model		Sensitivity 100% Specificity 99.9%	Unclear, but these values seem to be as reported from the manufacturer		
Van Doornum, 1998	414	Serum specimens from 31,232 pregnant women in Amsterdam between 1988 and 1995	Two ELISA approach (with membrane spot assay to discriminate between infection with HIV-1 or HIV-2) vs. Western blot analysis	Evaluation of confirmatory strategy of two-ELISA approach and resolution of indeterminate results with NASBA and SIA	42 sera that were available for analysis which gave positive or borderline results by ELISA and indeterminate or negative results by Western blot All initially reactive samples (tested by EIA) were retested by a second ELISA (based on a different principle) and the initial screening assay Confirmation of reactivity with a second EIA, enhanced with a membrane spot assay to discriminate between HIV-1 and HIV-2, was necessary and useful for endorsing a negative result and confirming possible cases of HIV 2 infection The importance of requesting a new specimen upon reactive confirmation results to ensure against procedural errors was also demonstrated.		EV	3

10.7.3 What are the diagnostic tests available for detection of HIV infection and how do they compare in terms of specificity, sensitivity and cost-effectiveness? (continued)

Study	Ref.	Population	Intervention	Outcomes	Results	Comments	Study type	EL
Samson and King, 1998	413		Literature review to compile evidence-based guidelines on HIV screening in pregnancy	Recommendations on HIV testing in pregnant women	Third generation EIA kits have sensitivity 99.4%–100% and specificity 99–100% Combined EIA and Western blot protocol has sensitivity 99% and specificity 99.99%	These are guidelines for Canada		

10.7.4 What are the interventions to decrease congenitally acquired HIV?

Study	Ref.	Population	Intervention	Outcomes	Results	Comments	Study type	EL
Brocklehurst and Volmink, 2002	416	8 RCTs, various countries, HIV infected, pregnant women Cochrane review Most recent update 2002	Zidovudine monotherapy vs. placebo Zidovudine vs. zidovudine Short–short vs. long–long Long–short vs. long–long Short–long vs. long–long Nevirapine vs. zidovudine Nevirapine in mothers already taking antiretroviral therapy vs. standard ART Combination therapy (zidovudine and lamivudine) vs. placebo Antenatal and intrapartum Intrapartum and postpartum	HIV infection status of child	Zidovudine vs. placebo, 4RCTs (n = 1379): OR 0.44 (95% CI 0.33 to 0.59) Short–short vs. long–long, 1 RCT (n = 453): OR 2.46 (95% CI 1.15 to 5.27) Long–short vs. long–long, 1RCT (n = 746): OR 0.66 (95% CI 0.35, 1.24) Short–long vs. long–long, 1 RCT (n = 743): OR 1.40 (95% CI 0.82 to 2.38) Nevirapine vs. zidovudine, 1 RCT (n = 496): OR 0.50 (95% CI 0.32 to 0.79) Nevirapine + ART vs. placebo + ART, 1 RCT (n = 1174): OR 1.10 (95% CI 0.42 to 2.87) Zidovudine + lamivudine vs. placebo, 1 RCT (n = 1792): Antenatal and intrapartum: RR 0.52 (95% CI 0.35 to 0.76) Intrapartum and postpartum: RR 0.66 (95% CI 0.46 to 0.94)	In two studies, there was uncertainty about whether randomisation was adequately concealed. Another study was not blind once the randomly allocated packs were opened. The remaining 5 studies were double blind and randomised	SR	1a
Shey Wiysonge et al., 2002	616	1 RCT; 898 HIV-infected pregnant women, conducted in Kenya Cochrane review Most recent update 2002	Vaginal disinfection with disinfectant (chlorhexidine) during labour vs. no disinfection	HIV infection status of child	OR 0.93 (95% CI 0.63 to 1.38)	Generation of allocation sequence and concealment of allocation inadequate	SR	1a

10.7.4 What are the interventions to decrease congenitally acquired HIV? (continued)

Study	Ref.	Population	Intervention	Outcomes	Results	Comments	Study type	EL
European Mode of Delivery Collaboration, 1999	417	436 women between 34 and 38 weeks pregnancy with confirmed HIV-1 diagnosis without indication (or contraindication) for caesarean section delivery in various European countries, including UK	Caesarean section delivery vs. vaginal delivery	HIV infection status of child by 18 months (n = 370)	By intention to treat: adjusted OR 0.2 (95% CI 0.1 to 0.6) By actual mode of delivery: adjusted OR 0.4 (95% CI 0.2 to 0.9)	No woman breastfed. Randomisation through computer-generated lists and analysis by intention to treat and by actual mode of delivery	RCT	1b
Mandelbrot et al., 1998	410	2,834 singleton children born to mothers with HIV infection in 85 perinatal centres in France from 1985 to 1996	Vaginal delivery vs. caesarean section plus zidovudine compared with vaginal delivery vs. caesarean section without zidovudine	HIV infection status of child	Univariate analysis: No zidovudine: RR 1.0 (95% CI 0.6 to 1.6) With zidovudine: RR 0.1 (95% CI 0.0 to 0.8) Multivariate analysis: No zidovudine: OR 1.2 (95% CI 0.6 to 2.3) With zidovudine: OR 0.2 (95% CI 0.0 to 0.9)		Cohort	2b
Kind et al., 1998	617	414 children of mothers in Switzerland known to be HIV infected from 1986 to 1 July 1996	Elective caesarean section plus zidovudine vs. caesarean section and no zidovudine AND Other modes of delivery plus zidovudine vs. other modes of delivery and no zidovudine	HIV infection status of children	Caesarean section + zidovudine: 0/31 infected (0%, 95% CI 0 to 11.0) Caesarean section + no zidovudine: 7/86 infected (8%, 95% CI 3 to 16) Other delivery mode + zidovudine: 4/24 infected (17%, 95% CI 5 to 37) Other delivery mode + no zidovudine: 55/271 infected (20%, 95% CI 16 to 24) Risk difference for zidovudine: −8 (95% CI −14 to −2) for caesarean section −3 (95% CI −19 to 12) for other delivery modes Risk difference for caesarean section: −17 (95% CI −32 to −2) for zidovudine −12 (95% CI −20 to −5) for no zidovudine		NCC	3

10.7.4 What are the interventions to decrease congenitally acquired HIV? (continued)

Study	Ref.	Population	Intervention	Outcomes	Results	Comments	Study type	EL
Shey Wiysonge, et al., 2002	618	2 RCTs, 1813 known HIV infected women who are pregnant Cochrane review Most recent update 2002	Vitamin A supplementation during pregnancy vs. placebo or micronutrient supplementation	HIV infection status of child	OR 1.09 (95% CI 0.81 to 1.45)	Both studies are described as randomised and double blind, although one study did not report the method of allocation concealment. In one study, 7.8% of women were excluded from the analysis and 5% were lost to follow-up in the other	SR	1a
Duong et al., 1999	411	Pregnant women with HIV infection reported through obstetric surveillance in the British Isles	Surveillance of mother-to-child transmission of HIV infection	Mother-to-child transmission rate by infection status of child among women who did not breastfeed Reduction of risk of mother-to-child transmission with no antiretroviral treatment and vaginal or emergency caesarean section vs. elective caesarean section and antiretroviral therapy	Mother-to-child transmission rate by infection status of child among women who did not breastfeed: 19.6% (8.0% to 32%) in 1993; 2.2% (0% to 7.8%) in 1998 Reduction of risk of mother-to-child transmission with no antiretroviral treatment and vaginal or emergency caesarean section vs. elective caesarean section and antiretroviral therapy: 31.6% (13.6% to 52.2%) to 4.2% (0.8% to 8.5%)			

Short–short (treatment with zidovudine) = 35 weeks in pregnancy for mother and until 3 days old for baby

Long–long (treatment with zidovudine) = from 28 weeks in pregnancy for mother and for the baby until 6 weeks old

Long–short (treatment with zidovudine) = from 28 weeks pregnancy for the mother and for the baby until it is 3 days old

Short–long (treatment with zidovudine) = from 35 weeks in pregnancy for the mother and for the baby until 6 weeks old

10.7.5 Does screening for HIV in pregnancy and instituting appropriate interventions lead to improved maternal and perinatal outcomes?

Study	Ref.	Population	Intervention	Outcomes	Results	Comments	Study type	EL
Brocklehurst and Volmink, 2002	416	8 RCTs total, various countries, HIV infected, pregnant women Cochrane review Most recent update 2002	Zidovudine vs. placebo	Infant death within 1 year of birth (n = 1487, 4 RCTs)*	OR 0.57 (95% CI 0.38 to 0.85)	* Significant heterogeneity between RCTs ** Number of maternal deaths small and wide CIs *** This study was double-blind with central randomisation and a non-breastfeeding population. 2% lost to follow-up	SR	1a
			Zidovudine vs. zidovudine Short–short vs. long–long Long–short vs. long–long Short–long vs. long–long	Infant death within 28 days of birth (n = 1210, 3 RCTs)	OR 1.87 (95% CI 0.68 to 5.10)			
			Nevirapine vs. zidovudine	Infant death after 1 year of birth (n = 395, 1 RCT)	OR 1.02 (95% CI 0.14 to 7.28)			
				Incidence of stillbirth (n = 1504, 4 RCTs)	OR 0.83 (95% CI 0.36 to 1.92)			
				Incidence of preterm delivery (n = 757, 2 RCTs)	OR 0.86 (95% CI 0.57 to 1.29)			
				Incidence of low birthweight (n = 1192, 3 RCTs)	OR 0.74 (95% CI 0.53 to 1.04)			
				Any side effects in child (n = 1480, 4 RCTs)	OR 1.27 (95% CI 0.87 to 1.87)			
				Sufficient side effects in child to stop or change treatment (n = 415, 1 RCT)	OR 1.02 (95% CI 0.43 to 2.40)			
				Maternal death (n = 1391, 4 RCTs)**	OR 0.30 (95% CI 0.13 to 0.68)			
				Any side effect in mother (n = 1085, 3 RCTs)	OR 1.01 (95% CI 0.66 to 1.53)			
				Sufficient side effects in mother to change or stop treatment (n = 1506, 4 RCTs)	OR 1.42 (95% CI 0.64 to 3.18)			
				Infant death within 1 year of birth (n = 434, 1 RCT)***	OR 1.93 (95% CI 0.35 to 10.63)			
				Infant death within 28 days of birth (n = 454, 1 RCT)	OR 1.94 (95% CI 0.17 to 21.54)			
				Incidence of stillbirth (n = 454, 1RCT)	OR 1.92 (95% CI 0.17 to 21.35)			
				Incidence of preterm delivery (n = 454, 1 RCT)	OR 0.47 (95% CI 0.16 to 1.39)			
				Incidence of low birthweight (n = 455, 1 RCT)	OR 0.84 (95% CI 0.47 to 1.49)			
				Any side effects in child (n = 451, 1 RCT)	OR 0.69 (95% CI 0.21 to 2.19)			
				Maternal death (n = 427, 1RCT)	OR 9.13 (95% CI 0.49 to 170.61)			

10.7.5 Does screening for HIV in pregnancy and instituting appropriate interventions lead to improved maternal and perinatal outcomes? (continued)

Study	Ref.	Population	Intervention	Outcomes	Results	Comments	Study type	EL
				Any side effect in mother (n = 466, 1 RCT)	OR 0.42 (95% CI 0.04 to 5.39)			
				Infant death within 1 year of birth (n = 718, 1 RCT)	OR 1.19 (95% CI 0.41 to 3.44)			
				Infant death within 28 days of birth (n = 748, 1 RCT)	OR 2.38 (95% CI 0.43 to 13.06)			
				Incidence of stillbirth (n = 754, 1 RCT)	OR 0.70 (95% CI 0.17 to 2.97)			
				Incidence of preterm delivery (n = 754, 1 RCT)	OR 0.42 (95% CI 0.13 to 1.34)			
				Incidence of low birthweight (n = 751, 1 RCT)	OR 0.87 (95% CI 0.56 to 1.35)			
				Any side effects in child (n = 740, 1 RCT)	OR 0.29 (95% CI 0.08 to 1.03)			
				Maternal death (n = 725, 1 RCT)	OR 2.38 (95% CI 0.21 to 26.32)			
				Any side effect in mother (n = 769, 1 RCT)	OR 1.20 (95% CI 0.34 to 4.18)			
				Infant death within 1 year of birth (n = 711, 1 RCT)	OR 0.87 (95% CI 0.27 to 2.75)			
				Infant death within 28 days of birth (n = 744, 1 RCT)	OR 0.60 (95% CI 0.05 to 6.60)			
				Incidence of stillbirth (n = 748, 1 RCT)	OR 0.48 (95% CI 0.09 to 2.47)			
				Incidence of preterm delivery (n = 748, 1 RCT)	OR 0.21 (95% CI 0.05 to 0.97)			
				Incidence of low birthweight (n = 745, 1 RCT)	OR 0.54 (95% CI 0.33 to 0.89)			
				Any side effects in child (n = 739, 1 RCT)	OR 0.69 (95% CI 0.27 to 1.76)			
				Maternal death (n = 717, 1 RCT)	OR 0.40 (95% CI 0.02 to 9.93)			
				Any side effect in mother (n = 764, 1 RCT)	OR 0.73 (95% CI 0.17 to 3.06)			
				Infant death within 1 year of birth (n = 616, 1 RCT)	OR 0.71 (95% CI 0.36 to 1.37)			
				Incidence of stillbirth (n = 631, 1 RCT)	OR 0.49 (95% CI 0.04 to 5.40)			
				Incidence of low birthweight (n = 601, 1 RCT)	OR 1.50 (95% CI 0.75 to 3.01)			
				Maternal death (n = 618, 1 RCT)	OR 0.33 (95% CI 0.01 to 8.14)			

10.7.5 Does screening for HIV in pregnancy and instituting appropriate interventions lead to improved maternal and perinatal outcomes? (continued)

Study	Ref.	Population	Intervention	Outcomes	Results	Comments	Study type	EL
Shey Wiysonge et al., 2002	618	2 RCTs, known HIV infected women who are pregnant Cochrane review Most recent update 2002	Vitamin A supplementation during pregnancy vs. placebo or micronutrient supplementation	Stillbirths (n = 1692, 2 RCTs) Very preterm births (n = 1578, 2 RCTs) All preterm births (n = 1577, 2 RCTs) Low birthweight (n = 1486, 2 RCTs) Very low birthweight (n = 1483, 2 RCTs) Postpartum CD4 levels (n = 727, 1 RCT) Maternal death (n = 728, 1 RCT)**	OR 1.07 (95% CI 0.63 to 1.80) OR 0.86 (95% CI 0.57 to 1.31) OR 0.88 (95% CI 0.68 to 1.13) OR 0.86 (95% CI 0.64 to 1.17) OR 0.71 (95% CI 0.40 to 1.28) Weighted mean difference −4.0, 95% CI −51.06 to 43.06 OR 0.49 (95% CI 0.04 to 5.40)**	No evidence of heterogeneity between the trials (p = 0.37) ** There were only 3 maternal deaths	SR	1a
Ricci and Parazzini, 2000	418	436 women between 34 to 38 weeks pregnancy with confirmed HIV-1 diagnosis without indication (or contraindication) for caesarean section delivery in various European countries, including the UK	Caesarean section delivery vs. vaginal delivery	Adverse effects of delivery in HIV-1 infected women (i.e., fever, wound infection, anaesthetic, anaemia, other)	Higher rates of fever in women who gave births by Caesarean section, but no significant differences in complication rates between women treated with zidovudine in pregnancy and those not treated	Analysis by actual mode of delivery	RCT	1b
Cunningham et al., 2002	419	242 from original PACTG (only US and French sites included) study with 25 excluded from final analysis (RCT substudy)	Emergence of nevirapine resistance mutations at 6 weeks postpartum in women receiving standard antiretroviral treatment	Detection of resistance mutations prior to receipt of study drug Detection of resistance mutations at 6 weeks postpartum among women who received the study drug (single dose oral 200 mg to mother and 2 mg/kg to infant)	Detection of resistance mutations prior to receipt of study drug: 5/217 women (2.3%) Detection of resistance mutations at 6 weeks postpartum among women who received the study drug: 14/95 (15%, 95% CI 8 to 23%)	International, multicentre substudy of PACTG 316 Risk for development of resistant mutations not correlated with CD4 cell counts or HIV-1 RNA viral load at delivery or with type of antiretroviral therapy	OB	3
Palumbo et al., 2001	420	220 HIV infected women and n24 of their HIV infected infants from 4 US cities from 1991 to 1997 who received zidovudine during pregnancy	Impact of antiretroviral resistance on vertical transmission rates	Detection of resistance mutations in mother Perinatal transmission and maternal presence of resistance mutations Detection of resistance mutation in neonate	38 women (17.3%) For zidovudine mutation: 15.8% yes, 15.1% no (NS) For nucleotide reverse-transcriptase inhibitor: 12.5% yes, 16% no (NS) 2 babies (8.3%) but mutation pattern not identical to mothers	All women received zidovudine treatment during pregnancy Phylogenetic and genotypic resistance testing	OB	3

Very preterm = ≤ 34 weeks of gestation   Preterm birth = < 37 weeks of gestation   Low birthweight = <2500 g   Very low birthweight = <2000 g

10.8 Rubella

10.8.1 What is the prevalence of rubella susceptibility in pregnant women in the UK?

Study	Ref.	Population	Intervention	Outcomes	Results	Comments	Study type	EL
Miller et al., 1997	423	Antenatal population in England and Wales	Impact of 1994 mumps and rubella vaccination campaign on future incidence of rubella in pregnant women	Antenatal susceptibility Incidence and risk of rubella infection in susceptible pregnant women	Susceptibility in antenatal population: 2% in nulliparous women (735/36509) and 1.2% (839/67615) in parous women for 1994/5 (p < 0.0001) Susceptibility in Asian (n = 5000) vs. non-Asian (n = 62,346) population was 4.4% compared with 1.3% In 1995, incidence in nulliparous 2/431 (risk/1000 = 4.6), in parous 0/547; overall risk 2/1005	Data on rubella monitored through serologically confirmed cases, terminated pregnancies because of rubella and notifications to NCRSP.	SV	3
Tookey et al., 2002	424	145,284 pregnant women from former North West Thames region from 1996-1999 from which antenatal rubella screening data were available for 137,398	Retrospective analysis of routinely collected data	Rubella susceptibility	2.5% overall Breakdown by ethnicity: 1.7% white were susceptible vs. 3.7% of women from Mediterranean region, 5.1% of Asian, 4.8% black and 8% Oriental	Database used for this analysis includes about 90% of the deliveries in the area	SV	3

10.8.2 What is the incidence of congenital rubella syndrome in babies in the UK?

Study	Ref.	Population	Intervention	Outcomes	Results	Comments	Study type	EL
Tookey, 2002	422				Annual average of 3 congenital rubella births and 4 rubella associated terminations for 1996 to 2000 Just over 60 terminations for rubella disease or contact in pregnancy for England and Wales for 1991 to 2000 (ONS 2001)	Data contained in a report provided by the UK National Screening Committee working group	SV	4
Miller et al., 1997	423	Registered congenital rubella births with NCRSP or terminations registered with ONS	To monitor impact of rubella immunisation on congenital rubella since 1971	Numbers of congenital rubella infection births, number of congenital rubella syndrome births and number of terminations for rubella disease or contact	From 1996 to 2000: congenital rubella infection: 1 case; congenital rubella syndrome: 16 cases; 17 terminations		SV	3

10.8.3 What are the diagnostic tests available for detection of rubella infection in pregnant women and how do they compare in terms of specificity, sensitivity, and cost-effectiveness?

Study	Ref.	Population	Intervention	Outcomes	Results	Comments	Study type	EL
Grageot-Keros and Enders, 1997	426	852 sera (575 negative for anti-rubella virus IgM antibodies, 98 previously reactive sera, 28 paired sera taken during the acute phase of the disease, 9 sera from follow-up of primary infections, 44 sera from follow-up of vaccinations, and 98 samples containing potentially interfering analytes)	Roche Rubella IgM eEIA recomb compared with Abbott IMx Rubella IgM test and Sorin ETI-RUBIK-M reverse test	Sensitivity and specificity	Sensitivity: Roche: 99.3% Abbott: 98.3% Sorin: 100% Specificity: Roche: 100% Abbott: 93.9% Sorin: 82.7%		EV	2a

10.8.4 Does screening pregnant women for rubella immunity lead to improved maternal and perinatal outcomes?

Study	Ref.	Population	Intervention	Outcomes	Results	Comments	Study type	EL
Miller et al., 1982	425	1016 pregnant women with confirmed rubella infection at different stages of pregnancy from January 1976 to September 1978 in England and Wales	Prospective follow-up up of infants to assess consequences of congenital infection	Pregnancy outcome; infection status of infant; rubella defects in seropositive (n = 102) vs. seronegative (n = 133) infants (congenital heart disease and deafness); frequency of congenital infection	Of 966 women, 523 (54%) had elective abortions, 36 (4%) had spontaneous miscarriages 9 women had stillbirths (4 of which had severe abnormalities); 5 infants died in neonatal period Of 269 infants tested (68% of surviving infants), 117 (43%) were infected Defects found in 20 children, all from seropositive group Incidence of other defects (delayed motor development, visual defects, speech delay, etc) were not found to be different among the two groups of infants Congenital infection in first 12 weeks of pregnancy among mothers with symptoms was over 80%, reduced to 25% at end of second trimester 100% of infants infected during first 11 weeks of pregnancy had rubella defects	Diagnosis of rubella (in mothers) based on 4-fold rise in antibody titre or the detection of specific IgM Infants defined as infected if IgM antibody present at birth or persistence of IgG after 1 year.	CH	2b

10.8.4 Does screening pregnant women for rubella immunity lead to improved maternal and perinatal outcomes? (continued)

Study	Ref.	Population	Intervention	Outcomes	Results	Comments	Study type	EL
Grillner et al., 1983	428	491 cases of rubella in pregnant women from 1978 to 1980 and 118 children followed up at age 20 months, 4 years or 7 years, in Sweden	Consequences of rubella during pregnancy with special reference to infection during 17th to 24th weeks of gestation Cases identified by surveillance and outcome determined by survey	Outcome of rubella infected pregnancies Intrauterine transmission of rubella Rubella defects	101 pregnancies infected from 17 to 24 weeks of gestation; all except one resulted in liveborn infant A decline in rate of infection from weeks 9 to 16 (57% to 70%) to weeks 17 to 20 (22%) and weeks 21 to 24 (17%) From 1 to 16 weeks of gestation, 10% to 40% of surviving children had rubella defects compared with 0% to 2% of children whose mothers were infected during 17 to 24 weeks of gestation		CH	2b
Morgan-Capner et al., 1985	429	7 pregnant women with asymptomatic rubella reinfection in early pregnancy	Reports of 7 cases	Identification of rubella specific antibody (IgM) in infants or products of conception	None detected		CST	3
CDC 2001	430	680 Live births from susceptible mothers in the UK, USA, Germany and Sweden	Inadvertent rubella vaccination with HPV-77, Cendehill or RA 27/3 at 3 months before or during pregnancy	Congenital rubella syndrome	No infant born with congenital rubella syndrome		SV	3

10.8.5 Is it cost effective to screen pregnant women for rubella immunity?

Study	Ref.	Population	Intervention	Outcomes	Results	Comments	Study type	EL
Stray-Pederson, 1982	619	Model based on annual pregnant population of 50,000 in Norway and prognosis of congenital rubella in unvaccinated population (n = 38 during epidemic period; n = 6 during nonepidemic period)	Modelling to assess cost benefit of rubella vaccination programmes (with goal of preventing rubella in pregnant women and subsequent congenital rubella syndrome)	Comparison of various vaccination programmes	All strategies were cost effective Based on cost/benefit ratios, net benefit came from vaccination offered to all women in puberty, supplemented with offering vaccination to nonimmunised women after delivery and women at high risk of exposure If participation in vaccination programme < 100%, vaccination offered at two ages (e.g. childhood and puberty) gives best results in prevention of congenital cases		EE	3 (?)

10.8.6 What are the interventions for a susceptible woman who is exposed to rubella infection during pregnancy?

Study	Ref.	Population	Intervention	Outcomes	Results	Comments	Study type	EL
Tookey, 2002	422				There is no treatment to prevent or reduce mother-to-child transmission of rubella once infection has been detected in pregnancy	Report provided by the UK National Screening Committee working group	REC	4

10.9 Streptococcus group B

10.9.1 What is the prevalence of streptococcus group B in pregnant women in the UK?

Study	Ref.	Population	Intervention	Outcomes	Results	Comments	Study type	EL
Merenstein et al., 1980	432	1218 cultures taken during routine antenatal care visits and 1441 maternal infant pairs evaluated at delivery in Colorado, USA	Swabs placed in selective broth and plated (modified Todd–Hewitt broth)	Colonisation rate within this population	Colonisation rate varied from 6.6% to 11.6% in pregnant mothers 3.8% of infants were colonised at birth	Site of swabs unspecified Todd–Hewitt broth selected for GBS isolation, because 'most effective' according to this study, but no false positive or false negative rates reported	CSS	3
Regan et al., 1991	433	7742 pregnant women from the USA (various states) from university clinical centres from Nov 1984 through Jun 1987	Vaginal and endocervical culture obtained between 23 and 26 weeks of gestation	Prevalence of GBS	18.6%		CSS	3
Hastings et al., 1986	434	1457 pregnant women in England	Low vaginal and rectal swabs from women at booking, 28 and 36 weeks	Overall GBS colonisation rate	28% with no association between maternal age, blood group or parity		CSS	3

10.9.2 What is the prevalence of GBS infection in the neonate and what are the consequences of infection?

Study	Ref.	Population	Intervention	Outcomes	Results	Comments	Study type	EL
Fey et al., 1999	437	Neonates in England and Wales between 1995 and 1997	Analysis of reports to CDSC and isolates submitted to laboratories	Rates of early onset (within first week of birth) disease Rates of late onset (between 1 week and 3 months of age) disease	0.4/1000 live births 0.2/1000 live births	Marked under-reporting suspected, as one region where all laboratories contributed reports had rates of 0.7/1000 and 0.3/1000 for early and late onset, respectively No actual numbers. Data from an abstract	SV	3
Oddie and Embleton, 2002	435	36 infants infected with GBS in the first week after birth out of 62,786 live births in the Northern health region of the UK from April 1998 to March 2000	Survey (cross-checked with surveillance by PHLS)	Isolation of GBS in infant during first week of life Effect of GBS isolated during pregnancy as risk factor for early onset disease	Prevalence of 0.57 per 1000 live births (36 of 62,786 live births). Adjusted OR 1.9 (95%CI 0.03, 142.7)		CCS	3
Health Protection Agency 2002	431	N = 537 confirmed cases of GBS in infants aged <90 days, reported by paediatricians and microbiologists from Feb 2000 to 28 Feb 2001 in the UK	Surveillance via the British Paediatric Surveillance Unit and cases reported by microbiologists to PHLS for typing	Isolation of GBS from a normally sterile site	From 537 cases, 67% aged under 7 days (early-onset disease); 33% aged between 7 and 90 days (late-onset disease) Overall mortality rate of 9.4% Incidence for England: 0.8/1000 live births (95% CI 0.7 to 0.9); early-onset disease 0.5 (0.5 to 0.6) Incidence for Wales: 0.6/1000 live births (0.4 to 0.9); early-onset disease 0.4 (0.2 to 0.7) Most common presentations of early-onset disease: sepsis in 62%; pneumonia in 26%		SV	3
Bignardi, 1999	438	15 confirmed cases of neonatal GBS infection from January 1995 through December 1997 from among 10,525 live births	Positive blood and CSF cultures that yielded GBS at Sunderland Royal Hospital from children under three months of age	Incidence of GBS	Neonatal infection 1.42/1000 live births (95% CI 0.8 to 2.04)		CSS	3

10.9.3 What are the diagnostic tests available for antenatal detection of GBS carriage and how do they compare in terms of specificity, sensitivity, and cost-effectiveness?

Study	Ref.	Population	Intervention	Outcomes	Results	Comments	Study type	EL
Schrag et al., 2002	443	A stratified random sample of 5144 live births were selected from 629,912 live births from 1998 and 1999 from 8 geographical areas in the USA. All births of infants with early-onset infection were included in the sample (n = 312)	Universal culture screening vs. screening by assessment of clinical risk factors to identify candidates for intrapartum antibiotics for GBS	Prevention of early onset GBS disease in infants less than 7 days old	Risk of early-onset disease lower in universally screened group: adjusted relative risk 0.46 (95% CI 0.36 to 0.60) After excluding all women with risk factors and adequate time for prophylaxis, adjusted relative risk was still similar: 0.48 (95% CI 0.37 to 0.63)		CH	2b
Spieker et al., 1999	442	240 pregnant women at 28 weeks of gestation in Florida, USA	Patients received written instructions on how to obtain rectovaginal swab and obtained own swab. Physician also obtained swab Reference standard was any culture obtained by physician or women found to be positive	Cultures positive for GBS	24% (24/240) cultures positive for GBS patient sensitivity 79%, physician sensitivity 83%, p = 0.365		CSS	3
Molnar et al., 1997	441	163 women presenting for their 26 to 28 week antenatal care visit at five family physician offices and eight obstetricians at a hospital in Toronto, Canada from November 1995 through March 1996	Patient survey about who women would prefer to do their swabs; vaginal/anorectal swab collected by patient on self and vaginal/anorectal swab collected by physician on same woman Any culture positive for GBS obtained by women or physician used as reference standard	Comparison of GBS detection rate	Overall prevalence of maternal GBS carriage: 24% (39/163) (95% CI 17% to 30%) Concordance between physician- and patient-collected swabs was 95% (95% CI 92% to 98%) Patients identified 38 cases for sensitivity of 97% (lower 95% CI 92%); physicians identified 32 cases for sensitivity of 82% (95% CI 70% to 94%) From 161 surveys, 54 (34%) of women preferred to do their own swab, 66 (41%) were indifferent and 41 (26%) preferred physician to do their swab		CSS	3

10.9.3 What are the diagnostic tests available for antenatal detection of GBS carriage and how do they compare in terms of specificity, sensitivity, and cost-effectiveness? (continued)

Study	Ref.	Population	Intervention	Outcomes	Results	Comments	Study type	EL
Boyer et al., 1983	440	5586 cultures from pregnant women at obstetric practices in Chicago, USA from April 1979 to Sept 1981	Cultures from vagina and rectum Colonies with suggestive haemolysis or morphology identified as GBS with CAMP test Women with positive prenatal cultures, cultures obtained again intrapartum and within three days of delivery 200 women with negative prenatal cultures also recultured	Value of prenatal culture for identifying GBS colonisation status at delivery	Overall, 22.8% (1272/5586) women were carriers of GBS In colonised women, rectal cultures were more frequently positive than vaginal cultures (82% vs. 65%) 575/1272 GBS carriers were restudied at delivery. Of 182 antenatal positive vaginal and rectal cultures, 132/182 (73%) were positive at delivery Of 67 antenatal positive vaginal cultures, 46/67 (69%) were positive at delivery Of 144 antenatal positive vaginal cultures, 86/144 (60%) were positive at delivery Of 200 antenatal negative vaginal and rectal cultures, 17/200 (9%) were positive at delivery Estimated sensitivity and specificity of prenatal culture: 70% and 90%, respectively	182/575 recultured women with incomplete or unquantified cultures were excluded	EV	3
Yancey et al., 1996	439	826 women attending antenatal clinics in the USA	Vaginal and rectal swabs at approx 35 to 36 weeks gestation and again at delivery	Overall colonisation rate Test performance by culture-delivery interval	GBS identified in 219/826 (26.5%) of women In cultures obtained 1 to 5 weeks before delivery, sensitivity 87% (95% CI 83% to 92%), specificity 96% (95% CI 95% to 98%) Among patients cultured 6 weeks or more before delivery, sensitivity 43% and specificity 85%		CSS	3

10.9.4 & 10.9.5 What are the available interventions for managing women who are GBS carriers and do these interventions improve maternal and perinatal outcomes?

Study	Ref.	Population	Intervention	Outcomes	Results	Comments	Study type	EL
Smaill, 1999	444	5 RCTs	Intrapartum antibiotics vs. no treatment	Infant colonisation with GBS Early-onset neonatal GBS sepsis Neonatal death from infection	4 trials (n = 624): Peto OR 0.10 (95% CI 0.07 to 0.14) 4 trials (n = 751): Peto OR 0.17 (95% CI 0.07 to 0.39) 2 trials (n = 427): Peto OR 0.12 (95% CI 0.01 to 2.0)	No studies used a placebo or blinded the observer to the treatment allocation	SR	1a
Gibbs and McNabb, 1996	446	15 patients admitted in labour who had GBS at 26 to 28 weeks of gestation from December 1993 to August 1994 in the USA	5ml of 2% clindamycin cream intravaginally vs. no treatment	GBS from swabs of distal vaginal and rectum in mother GBS in infant from 4 sites (throat, ear, umbilicus, and rectum)	5 of 15 were culture negative at admission Treatment group: 5/5 vaginal cultures were positive; 3/5 rectal cultures were positive 2/6 neonates positive at one or more sites No treatment group: 3/4 positive vaginally and rectally 1/4 neonates positive at all four sites RR (mothers) 1.33 (95% CI 0.76 to 2.35) RR (infants) 1.33 (95% CI 0.13 to 10.25)	Computer-generated randomisation	RCT	1b
Benitz et al., 1999	445	4 trials on antibiotics administered in antepartum period 5 trials on intrapartum prophylaxis RCTs and controlled trials	Treatment with broad-spectrum antibiotics to prevent early-onset infection and monotherapy to prevent transmission in antepartum period or intrapartum vs. no treatment	Reduced GBS colonisation in mother and infant at delivery Early onset GBS	2/4 studies on antepartum treatment reported reduction in maternal colonisation at delivery None of the antepartum treatment studies reported an effect on neonatal infections Reduction of 80% in early-onset GBS with intrapartum antibiotic treatment (pooled OR 0.188, 95% CI 0.07 to 0.53)	Literature review was conducted only on Medline and from references of other recent reviews	SR	2a
Schrag et al., 2000	447	7867 cases of invasive GBS disease in counties from 8 states in the USA from 1993 to 1998	Active surveillance of microbiology laboratories and analysis with census data	Incidence of early-onset disease from 1993 to 1998 and corresponding dates of guideline releases	Decline from 1.7/1000 live births in 1993 to 0.6/1000 live births in 1998 (65% decrease, p < 0.001)	Cases defined by isolation of GBS from normally sterile site (e.g. blood or cerebral spinal fluid), i.e., cases identified from amniotic fluid, placenta or urine alone were not included	SV	3

10.9.4 & 10.9.5 What are the available interventions for managing women who are GBS carriers and do these interventions improve maternal and perinatal outcomes? (continued)

Study	Ref.	Population	Intervention	Outcomes	Results	Comments	Study type	EL
Jeffrey and Moses, 1998	448	All neonates admitted to neonatal unit in Sydney, Australia. Background incidence determined from November 1986 to February 1988. Intervention from June 1988 to June 1996	Screening all women at 28 weeks (or 24 weeks with known risk factors for preterm birth) with low vaginal swab, cultured on to blood agar. Treatment of all carriers with intravenous ampicillin in labour (1 g/6 hour until delivery)	Incidence of early-onset GBS before and after intervention	Before: 5732 live births. Incidence 4.9/1000 live births After: 36,342 live births. Incidence 0.8/1000 live births (p < 0.0001)		CS	3

10.10 Syphilis

10.10.1 What is the prevalence of syphilis infection in pregnant women in the UK?

Study	Ref.	Population	Intervention	Outcomes	Results	Comments	Study type	EL
Hurtig et al., 1998	620	139 women treated for syphilis during pregnancy and 17 children meeting the case definition of congenital syphilis from 1994 to 1997, excluding Scotland (n = 136)	National survey of genitourinary medicine specialists and paediatricians; surveillance	Incidence of syphilis detected in pregnancy and congenital syphilis	121 women were detected through antenatal screening; 31 had confirmed or probably congenitally transmissible syphilis (30 excluding Scotland); NNT = 18,600 and 55,700 (maximum numbers) to detect one woman needing treatment and to prevent one case of congenital syphilis, respectively	Over the period 1994 to 1997, over 2 million women would have been screened as part of antenatal care	CSS	3
PHLS CDSC and PHLS Syphilis Working Group, 1998	453	139 women treated for syphilis during pregnancy and 17 children meeting the case definition of congenital syphilis from 1994 to 1997, excluding Scotland (n = 136)	National survey of genitourinary medicine specialists and paediatricians; surveillance	Minimum overall prevalence of women considered to need treatment for syphilis in pregnancy	For England and Wales: 0.068 (95% CI 0.057 to 0.080) per 1,000 live births	Denominators derived from routine ONS birth statistics.	CSS	3
Flowers and Camilleri-Ferrante, 1996	452	Pregnant women in East Anglia identified by screening	Surveillance	Positive screening test for syphilis	4-8 per million pregnancies	Estimated from 1991-1995 out of an estimated 130,000 pregnancies screened.	SV	3

10.10.2 What are the maternal and perinatal outcomes associated with syphilis infection in pregnancy?

Study	Ref.	Population	Intervention	Outcomes	Results	Comments	Study type	EL
Ingraham, 1951	455	1063 women with syphilis treated with penicillin and three control groups: 302 women with untreated syphilis, 594 women with arsenical treatment of syphilis and 10,323 women without syphilis in the USA in the 1940s	Comparison of pregnancy outcomes between the penicillin treated syphilis and control groups	Effect of untreated syphilis on pregnancy outcomes (n = 302) compared with nonsyphilitic pregnancy (n = 10,232)	Early syphilis (n = 220): 25% stillborn (vs. 2.6%) 14% died in neonatal period (vs. 2.2%) 41% live birth to infected infant (vs. 0%) 20% live birth without syphilis (vs. 95%) Late syphilis (n = 82): 12% stillborn (vs. 2.6%) 8.5% died in neonatal period (vs. 2.2%) 2% live birth to infected infant (vs. 0%) 77% chance of birth to healthy, uninfected infant (vs. 95%)	Because penicillin became widely available in 1950s, no prospective observational studies in developed countries All differences between the early untreated group and the treated group were reported to be significant but the level of significance was not reported	CS	3
Fiumara et al., 1952	458	1005 pregnant women admitted in labour in Boston, USA in 1951	Syphilis diagnosis occurred either before pregnancy, antenatally or after delivery	Pregnancy outcomes Preterm birth defined as gestational age less than 37 weeks	24 had syphilis, 13 of which were old and treated cases, 11 diagnosed antenatally or after delivery None resulted in congenital syphilis 6/24 preterm births (25%) compared with 113/981 (11.5%) among women without syphilis (NS)		CS	3
Rotchford et al., 2000	459	1783 pregnant women from 12 clinics in South Africa screened for syphilis at first antenatal care visit between June and Oct 1998	Adequate (n = 108) vs. inadequate (n = 50; includes n = 30 no treatment) with penicillin Inadequate = less than 2 doses Adequate = at least 2 doses	Perinatal outcome in mother (because data on how many live births were twin pregnancies not available)	Of 1783 women, 158 tested positive for syphilis, data on pregnancy outcome available for 142 women 17 perinatal deaths among 15 women; stillbirths among 6 women; 9 women had early neonatal deaths Of 43 inadequately treated women for whom pregnancy outcome was known, 11 experienced perinatal death compared to 4 among treated women (99 for whom pregnancy outcome was known); p < 0.0001 Risk reduction (adjusted for age and gravidity) for each additional dose of penicillin: 1 dose: 41% (95% CI 2% to 64%) 2 doses: 65% (95% CI 42% to 79%) 3 doses: 79% (95% CI 66% to 88%)	Baseline findings from RCT Treatment: 3 weekly intramuscular injections of 2.4 mega-units of benzathine penicillin (as per DoH South Africa) Perinatal death defined as stillbirth or early neonatal death	CS	3

10.10.3 What is the prevalence of congenitally acquired syphilis infection and what are the consequences of infection?

Study	Ref.	Population	Intervention	Outcomes	Results	Comments	Study type	EL
PHLS CDSC and PHLS Syphilis Working Group, 1998	453	Children under 2 years old in England and Wales between 1988 and 1995 Children identified through the British Paediatric Surveillance Unit	Surveillance of genitourinary medicine clinic data Surveillance programme from June 1993 to July 1997	Cases of syphilis in children Cases of syphilis in children as defined by US CDC Annual incidence	34 cases of early congenital syphilis reported from genitourinary medicine clinics; 2 more cases reported in 1996 9 reported with presumptive syphilis and 8 possible cases of congenital syphilis. No definite cases reported by paediatricians in the UK Rate of 0.06/1000 live births	Possible that some children with congenital syphilis were being treated outside genitourinary medicine clinic system; i.e., these estimates are conservative	SV	3

10.10.4 What are the diagnostic tests available for detection of syphilis infection and how do they compare in terms of specificity, sensitivity, and cost-effectiveness?

Study	Ref.	Population	Intervention	Outcomes	Results	Comments	Study type	EL
Egglestone and Turner, 2000	449	N/A	Algorithm for treponemal antibody screening and confirmatory testing		FTA-abs still generally considered to be the gold standard, but TPHA is more sensitive, except in the third and fourth weeks of infection. TPHA is also more specific. Therefore most appropriate for confirming reactive EIA results at present. If TPHA is used for screening, then EIA can be used as the confirmatory test Further evaluation of immunoblotting as confirmatory test is needed		SSW	4
PHLS CDSC and PHLS Syphilis Working Group, 1998	453	N/A	Treponemal tests: TPHA, FTA-Abs, EIAs Non-treponemal tests: RPR, VDRL		EIAs: over 98% sensitive, over 99% specific All treponemal tests sensitive at all stages of syphilis (except early primary syphilis) 98% and 98% to 99% specific May result in false negatives, particularly in very early or late syphilis, in patients with reinfection or who are HIV positive Predictive value of these tests is poor when used alone in low-prevalence populations	This information is from a report to the UK National Screening Committee (unpublished)	SR	4

10.10.5 What are the available interventions for managing women who are infected with syphilis?

Study	Ref.	Population	Intervention	Outcomes	Results	Comments	Study type	EL
Walker, 2001	462	Pregnant women with a confirmed diagnosis of syphilis, with and without concomitant HIV infection. Cochrane review, most recent update 2001	To determine the most effective antibiotic treatment regimen of syphilis	Maternal resolution of clinical symptoms, miscarriage, stillbirth, neonatal deaths, and congenital syphilis	No RCTs identified	Available evidence is insufficient to determine the optimal penicillin regimen	SR	1a
Hashisaki et al., 1983	465	Pregnant woman with history of allergy to penicillin diagnosed with primary syphilis	Two successive course of erythromycin therapy	Efficacy of erythromycin treatment	Failure to cure infection. Subsequent successful treatment with penicillin after desensitisation		CR	3

10.10.6 Do these interventions improve maternal and perinatal outcomes?

Study	Ref.	Population	Intervention	Outcomes	Results	Comments	Study type	EL
Alexander et al., 1999	463	448 were diagnosed with syphilis from 28,552 women who delivered at a hospital in Texas, USA, from September 1997 to August 1989	Treatment with 2.4 million units of intramuscular benzylpenicillin (penicillin G) for primary, secondary or early latent syphilis and 7.2 million units of intramuscular benzylpenicillin for women with late latent syphilis (over 3 weeks)	Syphilis status of child	340 diagnosed antenatally. Treatment prevented congenital syphilis in all 27 maternal primary and 136 maternal late infections. Congenital syphilis prevented in 100/102 in maternal early latent infection group. 4/75 treatment failures in maternal secondary syphilis group. 2 congenital syphilis cases stillborn. Overall, a 98.2% success rate for preventing congenital syphilis	108 were diagnosed postpartum and therefore not included in the study group. Women screened (RPR and VDRL) for syphilis at first prenatal visit, 28 to 32 weeks prenatal visit and at delivery (confirmed with microhaemagluttinin assay). Clinical stage assigned by clinical examination of dark field microscopy	CH	2b
Watson-Jones et al., 2002	464	1688 pregnant women at an antenatal clinic in Tanzania from September 1997 to November 1999 (556 RPR positive and 1132 RPR negative)	Treatment with single dose benzylpenicillin in women with a positive RPR. Screen for syphilis. Serum samples also tested at reference laboratory by TPHA. FTA assay performed on sera that gave conflicting results from RPR and TPHA	Pregnancy outcomes (stillbirth, IUGR or preterm birth and birthweight) in seronegative vs. women treated for syphilis	No significant differences in adverse pregnancy outcomes between the two groups: 17.3 vs. 15.2 for all outcomes (p=0.86). No significant difference in mean birthweight between the two groups (p=0.24)		CH	2a

10.10.7 Is it cost effective to undertake universal screening for syphilis infection in pregnant women in the UK?

Study	Ref.	Population	Intervention	Outcomes	Results	Comments	Study type	EL
Conner et al., 2000	602	Data provided by 8 laboratories that performed a total of 169,140 antenatal screening tests for syphilis in one year, approximately one-fifth of the number of antenatal tests conducted in the UK	Estimation of costs based on the assumption that 40 women a year are detected and treated through antenatal screening and that the number of screening tests performed equalled the number of live births in the UK (annual births 750,000)	Cost of screening in the UK based on the cost of screening tests, treatment, and follow-up of infected women and their infants	Costs of screening estimated to be £672,366 (£161,849 to £2,306,382), or £0.90 per pregnancy screened NNT = 18,602 women screened to detect one woman who needs treatment for syphilis and a maximum of 55,713 women need to be screened to prevent one case of congenital syphilis. This is the equivalent of £16,670 for each woman treated for syphilis, or £49,928 for each case of congenital syphilis prevented	Targeted screening of high-risk groups would detect 70% of cases but would be practically difficult. Costs for targeted screening strategies are also presented for women in the Thames region, pregnant women in nonwhite ethnic groups and women born outside the UK. Targeting or stopping screening would save relatively little money		

10.11 Toxoplasmosis

10.11.1 What is the prevalence of toxoplasmosis immunity in pregnant women in the UK?

Study	Ref.	Population	Intervention	Outcomes	Results	Comments	Study type	EL
Ades et al., 1993	467				Toxoplasmosis immunity in pregnant women in the UK has fallen from approx 22% to 8%			

10.11.2 What is the incidence of new toxoplasmosis infection in pregnant women in the UK?

Study	Ref.	Population	Intervention	Outcomes	Results	Comments	Study type	EL
Eskild, 1996	466	Pregnant women in Europe	Medline search from 1983 to 1996	Incidence of toxoplasmosis in pregnancy	Range of 2.4 (Finland) to 16 (France) per 1000 susceptible women USA: 2/1000 to 6/1000 susceptible women	No data for the UK were found	SR	3
Ryan et al., 1995[621]	621	All pregnant women in England and Wales from 1981 to 1992	Surveillance	Number of reports of toxoplasmosis related to pregnancy	423 cases reported		SV	3

10.11.3 What is the prevalence of neonatal toxoplasmosis infection and what are its consequences?

Study	Ref.	Population	Intervention	Outcomes	Results	Comments	Study type	EL
Pratlong et al., 1996	471	286 pregnant women infected with toxoplasmosis between 7 and 34 weeks of gestation in France from 1985 to 1993	Detection of fetal abnormalities by ultrasound and of toxoplasma in amniotic fluid and in fetal blood	Risk of congenital infection by time of maternal infection	18% (52/286) overall; 11% (17/155) at 7 to 15 weeks; 26% (28/109) at 16 to 28 weeks; 32% (7/22) at 29 to 34 weeks		CS	3
Dunn et al., 1999	472	603 confirmed maternal toxoplasmosis infections in France from 1987 to 1995	Data collected from routinely collected information in medical records	Pregnancy outcome Risk of congenital infection by time of maternal infection	Planned termination: 5 women; miscarriage: 3 women; stillbirth: 3 women; live birth: 591; unknown: 1 woman	Three women gave birth to twins; data reported on firstborn twin only	CS	3
			Diagnosis of fetal infection based on cordocentesis or amniocentesis with clinical examination after birth at 2, 5, 8 and 12 months and annually thereafter for a median of 4.5 years	Clinical outcome of liveborn infants with toxoplasmosis (n = 153) Risk of development of clinical signs in infant by time of maternal infection	Congenital infection confirmed in 153 infants; excluded in 396 infants; 42 infants lost to follow-up Overall transmission rate among liveborn infants: 26% (153/591); 6% (95% CI 3 to 9) at 13 weeks of gestation; 40% (95% CI 33 to 47) at 26 weeks of gestation; 72% (95% CI 60 to 81) at 36 weeks of gestation 27% (41/153) of infected infants had chorioretinal lesions (n = 33), intracranial calcification (n = 14) and/or hydrocephaly (n = 2) Risk of clinical sign at 13 weeks: 61% (95% CI 34% to 85%); at 26 weeks: 25% (95% CI 18% to 33%); at 36 weeks 9% (95% CI 4% to 17%)			
Foulon et al., 1999	473	144 women with confirmed toxoplasmosis infection from 5 European centres	Fetal infection detected by cordocentesis, amniocentesis or both Antibiotic treatment of 119/144 affected women Congenital toxoplasmosis determined by cord and neonatal blood samples. Infants followed-up to 1 year of age	Overall transmission Risk of congenital infection by time of maternal infection Clinical signs in infant	44% (64/144) gave birth to an infected infant (antibiotics made no difference in transmission rate, p = 0.7) At 6 to 10 weeks of gestation: 21%; 11 to 15 weeks: 19%; 16 to 20 weeks: 23%; 21 to 25 weeks: 60%; 26 to 30 weeks: 65%; 31 to 35 weeks: 93% 4 fetuses aborted; therefore, from 140 infants, 14% (19/140) either died in utero, had neurological abnormalities, hydroencephalus, cerebral calcifications, and/or choroidal scars with or without visual impairment	Analysis on infected (n = 64) vs. uninfected infant not presented	CS	3

10.11.3 What is the prevalence of neonatal toxoplasmosis infection and what are its consequences? (continued)

Study	Ref.	Population	Intervention	Outcomes	Results	Comments	Study type	EL
Lappalainen et al., 1995	622	16,733 pregnant women in Finland from 1988 to 1989	Screening for primary toxoplasmosis in mother Follow-up of 37 liveborn infected children	Mothers with toxoplasmosis infection Annual incidence of congenital toxoplasmosis	42 mothers with toxoplasmosis infection 4 infants with confirmed congenital toxoplasma infection; 0.3/1000 live born children per year		CS	3
Lebech et al., 1999	469	99,246 consecutive deliveries in Denmark from 1992 to 1996	Mothers screened at delivery for toxoplasma infection and infants of positive mothers followed for 12 months after delivery	Prevalence of toxoplasma infection in infants	0.3 per 1000	This study represented about one-third of all deliveries in Denmark	CS	3

10.11.4 What are the common sources of toxoplasmosis infection and how can pregnant women avoid infection?

Study	Ref.	Population	Intervention	Outcomes	Results	Comments	Study type	EL
Cook et al., 2000	470	252 pregnant women with acute toxoplasma infection and 858 controls from 5 centres in Europe from 1994 to 1995	Infection identified by antenatal screening Data collected by interview after diagnosis of infection	Associated risk with food and environmental factors for toxoplasmosis	Any cat in home: OR 1.0 (95% CI 0.7 to 1.5) Contact with soil: OR 1.8 (95% CI 1.2 to 2.7) Tasting meat while cooking: OR 1.5 (95% CI 1.0 to 2.4) Raw or undercooked beef: OR 1.7 (95% CI 1.1 to 7.2) Raw or undercooked lamb: OR 3.1 (95% CI 1.4 to 7.2) Raw or undercooked pork: OR 1.4 (95% CI 0.7 to 2.8)		CS	3

10.11.5 What are the diagnostic tests available for detection of toxoplasmosis infection and how do they compare in terms of specificity, sensitivity and cost effectiveness?

Study	Ref.	Population	Intervention	Outcomes	Results	Comments	Study type	EL
Cubitt et al., 1992	474	Sera from 1000 pregnant women booking for antenatal care at a London hospital	Serological screening for antibodies to toxoplasmosis with gold standard based on repeat testing results	Comparison of DA, LA and EIAs	49/1000 discordant results among all assays and required repeat testing; 9 remained undetermined EIAs: 0/773 false positives, 2/218 false negatives LA: 0/218 false negatives, 1/773 false positives DA: 0/218 false negative, 23/773 false positives		TES	3

10.11.6 What are the available interventions for managing women who are infected with toxoplasmosis?

Study	Ref.	Population	Intervention	Outcomes	Results	Comments	Study type	EL
Peyron et al., 2002	476	0 RCTs	Treatment vs. no treatment of toxoplasmosis in pregnancy to reduce the risk of congenital toxoplasma infection	Congenital infection and clinical congenital infection	No RCTs identified		SR	1a
Wallon et al., 1999	477	9 studies identified	Treatment (spiramycin alone, pyrimethamine-sulphonamides, or a combination of the two) vs. no treatment of toxoplasmosis in pregnancy to reduce the risk of congenital toxoplasma infection	Congenital toxoplasmosis infection vs. no infection	5 studies showed effectiveness of treatment (p < 0.001): 22% vs. 52% 13% vs. 100% 21% vs. 47% 0% vs. 100% 4% vs. 83% 4 showed treatment was not effective: 5% vs. 17% 0% vs. 10% 10% vs. 10% 24% vs. 21%		SR	2a

10.11.7 Does screening pregnant women for toxoplasmosis infection lead to improved maternal and perinatal outcomes?

Study	Ref.	Population	Intervention	Outcomes	Results	Comments	Study type	EL
Bader et al., 1997	479	N/A	Decision analysis to compare no testing for congenital toxoplasmosis, targeted screening in cases of abnormalities noted on ultrasound and universal serological screening of pregnant women followed by amniocentesis to diagnose fetal infection in cases of maternal seroconversion	Pregnancy loss avoided	By medical treatment: universal screening reduced the number of cases of congenital toxoplasmosis at the 'cost' of 18.5 additional pregnancy losses for each case avoided By pregnancy termination: additional 12.1 pregnancy losses for each case avoided		ME	3

11.1 Gestational diabetes

11.11.1 What are the maternal and perinatal outcomes associated with gestational diabetes?

Study	Ref.	Population	Intervention	Outcomes	Results	Comments	Study type	EL
Mestman et al., 1972	485	360 pregnant women in the USA	All had GTT and prednisolone GTT. All women followed up for 5 years	Abnormal GTT at pregnancy Abnormal GTT five year after pregnancy	During pregnancy: 51/360 with elevated fasting blood sugar; 181/360 abnormal GTT; 90/360 positive PGTT; 38/360 normal 5 years later: with elevated fasting blood sugar, 17/51 had abnormal GTT; with abnormal GTT, 59/181 still had abnormal GTT; with positive PGTT, 12/90 had abnormal GTT; 0/38 normal had abnormal GTT		CH	2a
Jensen et al., 2000	486	143 women diagnosed with gestational diabetes and 143 controls (with at least one risk factor, but normal OGTT) in Denmark from 1989 to 1996	Retrospective study of case notes. Women screened by risk factors, urinanalysis, and FPG. Diagnosis established if FPG or 75 OGTT met WHO criteria for diabetes mellitus in nonpregnant state Women with GDM were treated with diet and/or insulin	Maternal outcomes in cases vs. controls Fetal outcomes in cases vs. controls	Hypertensive disorders: 28 (20%) vs. 15 (11%), p=0.046 Caesarean section: 47 (33% vs. 30 (21%), p=0.033 Induced labour: 88 (62%) vs. 34 (24%), p < 0.0001 Preterm delivery: 15 (11%) vs. 7 (5%), p=0.12 Gestational age: 39.0 ± 2 weeks vs. 39.9 ± 1.8, p < 0.0001 Ponderal index (kg/m³): 25.5 ± 2.8 vs. 24.9 ± 2.2, p=0.05 Macrosomia (birthweight ≥ 4500 g): 20 (14%) vs. 9 (6.3%), p=0.049 Admission to neonatal unit: 66 (46.2%) vs. 17 (11.9%), p < 0.0001 Birthweight (corrected for gestational age), length at birth, Apgar score at 5 minutes, jaundice, congenital malformations and perinatal deaths were not significantly different		CCS	3
O'Sullivan et al., 1973	487	187 GDM patients and 259 negative control patients in Boston, USA from 1962 to 1970	GDM diagnosed with GTT	Perinatal mortality (28th week of gestation to 14 days postpartum)	GDM: 12/187 (6.4%) babies died; normal GTT: 4/259 (1.5%) babies died, p < 0.05		CCS	3

11.1.2 How do the following tests for the detection of GDM (risk factor screening, urinalysis, timed random blood glucose, Mini GTT, Full GTT) compare in terms of specificity, sensitivity, likelihood ratios and cost-effectiveness?

Study	Ref.	Population	Intervention	Outcomes	Results	Comments	Study type	EL
Marquette et al., 1985	490	434 pregnant women from an obstetric clinic in the USA	Glucose screen at 28 weeks of gestation with 50 g GCT after fasting. All positive women tested again within 2 weeks with 3hour OGTT. Maternal risk factors included obesity, excessive weight gain, glycosuria, family history of diabetes, and poor obstetric history	Comparison of 182 women with maternal risk factors vs. 252 women without risk factors / Analysis by number of risk factors present	Number of positive screens: 56 (30.8%) vs. 56 (22.2%), p=0.06 / Number with GDM: 6 (3.2%) vs. 6 (2.4%), p=0.57 / 6/252 (2.4%) had no risk factors present; 5/144 (3.5%) had one risk factor present; 1/31 (3.2%) had two risk factors present; 0/7 had more than two risk factors. NS difference in rates of diabetes among these groups. / Sensitivity 50% / Specificity 58%		CH	2b
O'Sullivan et al., 1973	491	18,812 antenatal patients from 1954 to 1959 from Boston, USA and 752 pregnant women from 1956 to 1957 (i.e., the entire antenatal care population from Boston City hospital during this period)	For 18,812: a venous blood sugar was obtained at 1 hour after 50-g GCT from all women and risk factors were obtained from clinical histories / Those with high blood sugar levels or risk factors were scheduled for GTT / For 986: 1-hour, 50-g GCT compared with 3 hour, 100-g GTT	For 18,812: proportion of general antenatal population found to have one or more risk factors (i.e., excluding those with diagnosed GDM) to have one or more risk factors / Risk factors included birth of baby > 9 lb, history of adverse pregnancy outcome, and family history of diabetes / For 986: sensitivity and specificity of 1-hour, 50-g GCT	56.2% were negative to all factors; 43.8% had at least one risk factor / Sensitivity of GCT 79% / Specificity of GCT 87%		CH	2a
Gribble et al., 1995	494	2745 pregnant women in Wisconsin, USA from 1991 to 1993	Retrospective analysis of urinanalysis compared with 24- and 28-week blood glucose screening after 50-g GCT followed by 100-g OGTT for glucose levels > 140 mg/dl from 50-g test	Sensitivity and specificity	Sensitivity 7% / Specificity 98%		CS	3

11.1.2 How do the following tests for the detection of GDM (risk factor screening, urinalysis, timed random blood glucose, Mini GTT, Full GTT) compare in terms of specificity, sensitivity, likelihood ratios and cost-effectiveness? (continued)

Study	Ref.	Population	Intervention	Outcomes	Results	Comments	Study type	EL
Hooper, 1996	495	610 pregnant women in Baltimore, USA	Retrospective analysis of urinanalysis compared with 50-g GCT between 24 and 28 weeks of gestation followed by 100-g, 3-hour, GTT for glucose levels >135 mg/dl from 50-g test	Glycosuria Sensitivity and specificity	Glycosuria: 6 women with GDM and 9 without GDM No glycosuria: 7 with GDM and 588 without GDM Sensitivity 46.2% Specificity 98.5%		CS	3
Watson, 1990	493	500 consecutive patients at an antenatal clinic in Germany	Urinanalysis compared with 50g, 1 hour, GCT at 28 weeks gestation followed by 100 g, 3 hour, OGTT for glucose levels >140 mg/dl from 50g test	GDM Glycosuria Sensitivity and specificity	22/500 (4.4%) diagnosed with GDM 85/500 (17%) showed some degree of glycosuria (defined as present at at least two antenatal visits) 6/22 (27%) of women with GDM showed glycosuria Sensitivity 27.3% Specificity 83.5%		CH	2b
McElduff et al., 1994	496	714 women attending antenatal clinic in New South Wales, Australia	RPG measured within two hours of a meal (≥ 6.1 mmol/l considered positive) compared with 1-hour, 50-g GCT at 28 weeks GDM diagnoses confirmed by 100-g GTT	GDM Sensitivity and specificity of RPG	28/714 (3.9%) with GDM Sensitivity 46% Specificity 86%		CH	2b
Jowett et al., 1987	497	110 pregnant women with suspected GDM in England	RPG levels tested over 24-hour period (0800, 1200, 1500, 1700, 2200 hours) and 75-g GTT administered	Sensitivities and specificities at various thresholds and at various times of day of RPG test	At threshold 5.6 mmol/l: sensitivity range 29% to 80%; specificity range 74% to 80% At threshold 6.1 mmol/l: sensitivity range 41% to 58%, specificity range 74% to 96% Highest sensitivities reported at 1500 hours		TES	3
Reichelt et al., 1998	498	5010 pregnant women in Brazil from 1991 to 1995 with no prior diagnosis of diabetes	FPG at 24 to 28 weeks of gestation was compared with 2-hour, 75-g GTT (used for diagnosis)	GDM Optimal threshold for maximising sensitivity and specificity of FPG	379/5010 (7.6%, 95% CI 6.8 to 8.3) women with GDM At 89 mg/dl (4.9 mmol/l), sensitivity and specificity maximised at 88% and 78%, respectively	Period of fasting not specified	2	IIa

11.1.2 How do the following tests for the detection of GDM (risk factor screening, urinalysis, timed random blood glucose, Mini GTT, Full GTT) compare in terms of specificity, sensitivity, likelihood ratios and cost-effectiveness? (continued)

Study	Ref.	Population	Intervention	Outcomes	Results	Comments	Study type	EL
Perucchini et al., 1999	499	520 women in Switzerland from 1995 to 1997	FPG compared with 1-hour, 50-g GCT between 24 and 28 weeks of gestation. One week later, all patients also took 3-hour, 100-g GTT	GDM. Optimal threshold for maximising sensitivity and specificity of FPG and 1-hour, 50-g GCT	53/520 (10.2%) women with GDM. At 4.8 mmol/l, sensitivity and specificity for FPG maximised at 81% and 76%, respectively, (155/520 (30%) of women would have had to proceed to GTT for diagnosis). At 7.0 mmol/l, sensitivity and specificity maximised at 68% and 82%, respectively	Results were irrespective of last time women had eaten	CH	2a
Lewis et al., 1993	500	10 women with GDM and 12 controls from Chicago, USA	Between 26 and 32 weeks of gestation, each person underwent 3 GCT tests within a 2-week period (order of tests was randomised for each person). Test 1: 50-g GCT in fasting state. Test 2: 50-g GCT 1 hour after a meal. Test 3: 50-g GCT 2 hours after a meal	Plasma glucose levels after each test for women with GDM vs. controls	Cases: fasting = 10.5 mM plasma glucose, 1-hour = 11.0 mM plasma glucose, 2-hour = 9.3 mM plasma glucose (p < 0.03). Controls: fasting = 7.8 mM plasma glucose, 1-hour = 6.7 mM plasma glucose (p < 0.01), 2-hour = 6.4 mM plasma glucose. 7/12 (58%) controls with glucose ≥ 7.8 mM in fasting state		TESC	3

11.1.3 Does screening for and instituting interventions for GDM result in improved maternal and perinatal outcomes?

Study	Ref.	Population	Intervention	Outcomes	Results	Comments	Study type	EL
Walkinshaw, 2000	504	4 RCTs (612 women with impaired glucose tolerance or gestational diabetes)	Diet therapy vs. no specific treatment	Maternal and fetal complications associated with diabetes	Caesarean section (4 RCTs, n = 612): Peto OR 0.97 (95% CI 0.65 to 1.44) Preterm birth (1 RCT, n = 158): Peto OR 0.57 (95% CI 0.10 to 3.36) Birthweight > 4000 g (2 RCTs, n = 457): Peto OR 0.78 (95% CI 0.45 to 1.35) Birthweight > 4500 g (2 RCTs, n = 457): Peto OR 0.85 (95% CI 0.28 to 2.56) Birth trauma (2 RCTs, n = 457): Peto OR 0.13 (95% CI 0.02 to 0.96) Perinatal death: not estimable Admission to NICU (1 RCT, n = 126): Peto OR 0.55 (95% CI 0.16 to 1.90) Maternal hypertensive disorder (1 RCT, n = 126): Peto OR 0.66 (95% CI 0.11 to 3.93)		SR	1a
Persson, 1985	505	202 pregnant women with impaired glucose tolerance from 1981 to 1984 in Sweden	Treatment by diet (n = 105) vs. diet and insulin (n = 97) (insulin doses adjusted according to blood glucose values)	Obstetric complications Fetal complications	Proteinuria, hypertension, pre-eclampsia, and polyhydramnios not significantly different No perinatal deaths. Birthweight, gestational age, and skinfold thickness not significantly different 30 in diet group and 40 in insulin group showed one or more episodes of neonatal morbidity	Insulin was instituted in 15/105 (14%) of women whose control exceeded 7 mmol/l (fasting) or 9 mmol/l (postprandial) who were originally randomised to the diet only group	RCT	1b
Avery et al., 1997	507	33 women at less than 34 weeks of gestation selected from a health maintenance organisation in the USA	30 minutes of exercise 3 to 4 times weekly (n = 15) vs. control group (n = 14)	Mean haemoglobin A1c Caesarean section Neonatal outcomes	Mean haemoglobin A1c (5.2% vs. 5.2%, NS) Caesarean section: 3 (20%) vs. 3 (21.4%), p = 1.0 Birthweight: 3419 ± 528g vs. 3609 ± 428 g, p = 0.30 Neonatal hypoglycaemia (NS) Gestational age: 39.4 ± 1.2 weeks vs. 39.7 ± 0.9 weeks, p = 0.7 No preterm births	144 women were approached for the study, 43 did not meet inclusion criteria and 68 declined From the original 33, 1 from the experimental and 3 from the control group dropped out	RCT	1b

11.1.3 Does screening for and instituting interventions for GDM result in improved maternal and perinatal outcomes? (continued)

Study	Ref.	Population	Intervention	Outcomes	Results	Comments	Study type	EL

Naylor et al., 1996	506	3778 women presenting for antenatal care in Toronto, Canada, from 1989 to 1992	50-g, 1-hour GCT screening at 26 weeks of gestation and diagnostic 100-g, 3-hour OGTT at 28 weeks of gestation (for all women)
			
			Group 1: known and treated GDM (n = 143)
			
			Group 2: untreated borderline GDM (n = 115)
			
			Group 3: false positive group (positive result on GCT, normal result on OGTT) (n = 580)
			
			Group 4: negative screenees (less than 7.8 mmol/l on GCT and normal result on OGTT) (n = 2940)
				Macrosomia
				
				Pre-eclampsia
				
				Caesarean delivery
					Macrosomia (> 4000 g):
					  Group 1 15 (10.5%)
					  Group 2 33 (28.7%)
					  Group 3 14 (80%)
					  Group 4 395 (13.7%)
					
					Macrosomia (> 4500 g):
					  Group 1 5 (3.5%)
					  Group 2 7 (6.1%)
					  Group 3 12 (2.1%)
					  Group 4 56 (1.9%)
					
					Pre-eclampsia:
					  Group 1 12 (8.4%)
					  Group 2 10 (8.7%)
					  Group 3 31 (5.4%)
					  Group 4 144 (4.9%)
					
					Caesarean:
					  Group 1 48 (33.6%)
					  Group 2 34 (29.6 %)
					  Group 3 136 (23.9%)
					  Group 4 585 (20.2%)(
					
					In multivariate model, caesarean vs. spontaneous vaginal delivery in Group 4 vs. Group 1: OR 2.2 (95% CI 1.3 to 3.7)
							CH	2a

Wu Wen et al., 2000	492	1,729,225 pregnant women and 1,738,863 infants from 1984 to 1997 in Canada	Universal screening after guidelines introduced in 1985 vs. one area where no universal screening was implemented and retrospective analysis of medical records by ICD-9 codes	Number of women diagnosed with GDM Pregnancy complications in areas of universal screening vs. no universal screening	Overall: 38,274 women with GDM; an increase of 0.3% in 1984 to 2.7% in 1996; universal screening: 1.6% in 1990 to 2.2% in 1996 vs. 1.4% to 1.0 in no screening area Caesarean section: 18.8% vs. 18.9% Pre-eclampsia: 2.9% vs. 3.5% Polyhydramnios: 0.3 vs. 0.5 Amniotic infection: 0.9 vs. 0.5 Fetal macrosomia: 12.5% vs. 12.7% of newborn in each region		CS	3

11.1.3 Does screening for and instituting interventions for GDM result in improved maternal and perinatal outcomes? (continued)

Study	Ref.	Population	Intervention	Outcomes	Results	Comments	Study type	EL
Goldberg et al., 1986	508	58 pregnant women and 58 controls from an antenatal diabetes clinic in the USA from 1979 to 1984	Home glucose monitoring vs. controls Insulin therapy begun in subjects of either group if glucose values were >95 mg/dl or if postprandial values were >120 mg/dl	Use of insulin Neonatal outcomes Caesarean section	Use of insulin: 29 (50%) vs. 12 (21%), p < 0.01 Birthweight: 3231 ± 561 vs. 3597 ± 721, p < 0.002 Macrosomia (≥4000 g): 5 (9%) vs. 14 (24%), p < 0.05 Large for gestational age: 7 (12%) vs. 24 (41%), p < 0.005 Caesarean section: 32% vs. 25%, NS		CCS	3

11.2 Pre-eclampsia

Study	Ref.	Population	Intervention	Outcomes	Results	Comments	Study type	EL
Barton et al., 2001	515	748 women with a singleton pregnancy with hypertension in the USA from 1995 to 1998	Women from 24 to 35 weeks of gestation with no proteinuria by dipstick (0 or trace) at admission to study monitored for progression to proteinuria	Progression to proteinuria Progression to severe pre-eclampsia Rate of progression to proteinuria by gestational age at enrolment Incidence of SGA babies	Proteinuria developed in 343/748 (46%) women Severe pre-eclampsia developed in 72/748 (9.6%) women Rate of progression greater in women enrolled at less than 30 weeks compared with 34 to 35 weeks, p = 0.008 SGA in women with proteinuria versus hypertension alone: 24.8% vs. 13.8%, p < 0.001	Gestational hypertension defined as maternal blood pressure greater than or equal to 140 mmHg systolic or 90 mmHg diastolic. Proteinuria defined as greater than or equal to 1+ (by dipstick) on at least two occasions. Severe pre-eclampsia defined as either 1) severe hypertension (160/110 mmHg on 2 occasions), 2) mild hypertension with severe proteinuria (greater than or equal to 3+) or 3) development of thrombocytopenia	CSS	3
Page and Christianson, 1976	516a	14,833 singleton pregnancies in California, USA from 1959 to 1967	Levels of mean arterial pressure in the middle trimester (121 to 180 days) assessed in relation to pregnancy outcomes	Stillbirth rate Neonatal mortality rate Incidence of SGA babies (weighing less than 2500 g at gestations greater than or equal to 37 weeks)	Middle trimester: progressive rise in stillbirth and neonatal death rate above 85 mmHg, with sharp rise after 90 mmHg An increase in frequency of SGA babies above 85 mmHg		CH	2a

11.2 Pre-eclampsia (continued)

Study	Ref.	Population	Intervention	Outcomes	Results	Comments	Study type	EL
Page and Christianson, 1976	516b	12,954 singleton pregnancies in California, USA from 1959 to 1967	Levels of mean arterial pressure in the middle (121 to 180 days) and third (after 180 days) trimester assessed in relation to pregnancy outcomes in women with or without proteinuria	Fetal mortality and morbidity Stillbirth rate/1000 Perinatal death/1000	In third trimester: increase in fetal deaths and morbidity above 95 mmHg Middle trimester, stillbirth rate: In white women (n = 10,074): – without proteinuria and < 90 mmHg = 8.4 – without proteinuria and ≥ 90 mmHg = 14.8 – with proteinuria and < 90 mmHg = 15.4 – with proteinuria and ≥ 90 mmHg = 47.6 In black women (n = 2880): – without proteinuria and < 90 mmHg = 10.8 – without proteinuria and ≥ 90 mmHg = 28.5 – with proteinuria and < 90 mmHg = 37.7 – with proteinuria and ≥ 90 mmHg = 142.9 Middle trimester, perinatal death rate: In white women (n = 10,074): – without proteinuria and < 90 mmHg = 15.2 – without proteinuria and ≥ 90 mmHg = 25.8 – with proteinuria and < 90 mmHg = 38.5 – with proteinuria and ≥ 90 mmHg = 17.0 In black women (n = 2880): – without proteinuria and < 90 mmHg = 20.3 – without proteinuria and ≥ 90 mmHg = 34.6 – with proteinuria and 90 mmHg = 56.6 – with proteinuria and ≥ 90 mmHg = 142.9		CH	2a

11.2 Pre-eclampsia (continued)

Study	Ref.	Population	Intervention	Outcomes	Results	Comments	Study type	EL
Cuckson et al., 2002	525	11 devices for blood pressure monitoring from 15 studies	Meta-analysis of accuracy of devices in pregnancy and pre-eclampsia. Mean pressure differences of mercury devices compared with mean pressure differences of automated devices	Mean pressure differences (MPD) and standard deviation (SD)	MPD of mercury devices in pregnancy (SD): systolic 1.0 (6), diastolic 1.7 (7) MPD of mercury devices in pre-eclampsia (SD): systolic 5.5 (9), diastolic 7.9 (8) MPD of automated devices in pregnancy (SD): systolic –3.0 (12), diastolic –4.0 (8) MPD of automated devices in pre-eclampsia (SD): systolic 18.7 (11), diastolic 8.2 (7)		TES	3
Brown et al., 1998	527	220 woman with diastolic hypertension after 20th week of pregnancy in Australia	Management with K4 (n = 103) vs. management with K5 (n = 117)	Severe hypertension Prolonged pregnancy Requirements for antihypertensive treatment Laboratory data (including serum creatinine, uric acid, aspartate aminotransferase, platelet count and haemoglobin) Birthweight Fetal growth restriction Perinatal mortality Eclampsia Maternal death	No significant difference in number of episodes of severe hypertension, however more women were found to have severe diastolic hypertension with K4: 34 (33%) vs. 20 (17%), p = 0.006) No significant difference in proportion of women who needed antihypertensive treatment or in laboratory data No significant difference in birthweight, fetal growth restriction, prolonged pregnancy, or perinatal mortality No cases of eclampsia or maternal death	Analysis was by intention to treat Blinded endpoint analysis, but patients, doctors and midwives were aware of random allocation Severe hypertension defined as systolic greater than or equal to 170mm Hg, diastolic greater than or equal to 110mm Hg	RCT	1b

11.2 Pre-eclampsia (continued)

Study	Ref.	Population	Intervention	Outcomes	Results	Comments	Study type	EL
Duckitt, 2003	512	Pregnant women	Systematic review of studies on risk factors for pre-eclampsia to July 2002	Parity	Nulliparity OR 2.71, 95% CI 1.16 to 6.34 (14 studies)		CH & CCS	2b and 3
				Age	Maternal age over 40 years and primiparous OR 2.17, 95% CI 1.36 to 3.47; maternal age over 40 years and multiparous OR 2.05, 95% CI 1.47 to 2.87 (15 studies)			
				History of previous pre-eclampsia	Pre-eclampsia in first pregnancy OR 8.23, 95% CI 6.49 to 10.45; pre-eclampsia in second pregnancy OR 11.51, 95% CI 5.76 to 22.98 (10 studies)			
				Family history of pre-eclampsia	Positive family history of pre-eclampsia OR 5.27, 95% CI 1.57 to 17.64 (1 cohort study)			
				Underlying medical conditions	Pre-existing diabetes (type 1) OR 4.53, 95% CI 3.30 to 6.23 (5 studies)			
				Multiple pregnancy	Multiple pregnancy (regardless of parity) OR 2.76, 95% CI 1.99 to 3.82 (9 studies)			
				BMI	BMI over 35 at booking OR 2.29, 95% CI 1.61 to 3.24 (2 studies)			
Villar and Khan-Neelofur, 2001	32	3 RCTs, 3041 women	Midwife and GP-managed care vs. obstetrician and gynaecologist-led shared care	Pre-eclampsia	Pre-eclampsia (2 RCTs, n = 2952): Peto OR 0.37, 95% CI 0.22 to 0.64	Please refer to section 4.1 for other outcomes and results of this study.	SR	1a

11.3 Preterm birth

Study	Ref.	Population	Intervention	Outcomes	Results	Comments	Study type	EL
Buekens et al., 1994	542	5440 women from antenatal clinics in Belgium, Denmark, Hungary, Ireland, Italy, Portugal and Spain from 1988 to 1990	Routine cervical examination at every antenatal appointment (n = 2719) vs. avoidance of cervical examination if possible (n = 2721)	Median number of appointments Preterm birth (< 37 weeks) Low birthweight (< 2500g) Premature rupture of the membranes (PROM) Stillbirth	Median number of appointments for women in both groups: 8 Preterm birth: 5.7% vs. 6.4%, RR 0.88, 95% CI 0.72 to 1.09 Low birthweight: 6.6% vs. 7.7%, RR 0.86, 95% CI 0.71 to 1.04 PROM: 27.1% vs. 26.5%, RR 1.02, 95% CI 0.94 to 1.12 Stillbirth: 8.7% vs. 8.0%, RR 1.09, 95% CI 0.61 to 1.94	Computer generated randomisation in sealed envelopes	RCT	1b
Iams et al., 1996	543	2915 women from 10 university affiliated antenatal clinics in the USA from 1992 to 1994	Vaginal ultrasonography at approximately 24 and again at 28 weeks of gestation (2531/2915)	Preterm birth (< 35 weeks) Sensitivity and specificity	At 24 weeks, compared with women with cervical lengths (CL) above the 75th percentile: – women at or below 75% (CL 40 mm) had RR 1.98, 95% CI 1.2 to 3.27 – women at or below 50% (CL 35 mm) had RR 2.35, 95% CI 1.42 to 3.89 – women at or below 25% (CL 30 mm) had RR 3.79, 95% CI 2.32 to 6.19 – women at or below 10% (CL 26 mm) had RR 6.19, 95% CI 3.84 to 9.97 – women at or below 5% (CL 22 mm) had RR 9.49, 95% CI 5.95 to 15.15 – women at or below 1% (CL 13 mm) had RR 13.99, 95% CI 7.89 to 24.78 At 28 weeks, compared with women with cervical lengths above the 75th percentile: – women at or below 75% (CL 40 mm) had RR 2.8, 95% CI 1.41 to 5.56 women at or below 5o% (CL 35 mm) had RR 3.52, 95% CI 1.79 to 6.92 – women at or below 25% (CL 30 mm) had RR 5.39, 95% CI 2.82 to 10.28 – women at or below 10% (CL 26 mm) had RR 9.57, 95% CI 5.24 to 17.48 – women at or below 5% (CL 22 mm) had RR 13.88, 95% CI 7.68 to 25.10 – women at or below 1% (CL 13 mm) had RR 24.94, 95% CI 13.81 to 45.04 Sensitivity for at 24 and 28 weeks for less than or equal to 30 mm CL: 54% and 70% Specificity for at 24 and 28 weeks for less than or equal to 30 mm CL: 76% and 69%		CH	2a

11.3 Preterm birth (continued)

Study	Ref.	Population	Intervention	Outcomes	Results	Comments	Study type	EL
Goldenberg et al., 2000	544	10456 women with singleton pregnancies in the USA from 1995 to 1998	Measurement of fetal fibronectin values at 8 to 22 weeks	Preterm birth (greater than or equal to 13 weeks and less than 35 weeks)	Comparing fetal fibronectin level in greater than or equal to 90th percentile with less than 90th percentile: – at 13 to 14 weeks, 12.1% vs. 5.5%, RR 2.19, 95% CI 1.27 to 3.80 – at 15 to 16 weeks, 13.5% vs. 4.4%, RR 3.06, 95% CI 1.73 to 5.41 – at 17 to 18 weeks, 5.9% vs. 3.8%, RR 1.54, 95% CI 0.74 to 3.17 – at 19 weeks or more, 9.7% vs. 3.7%, RR 2.63, 95% CI 1.75 to 3.94		CH	2a
Goldenberg et al., 1996	545	2929 women from 10 centres in the USA from 1992 to 1994	Measurement of fetal fibronectin in the cervix and vagina every two weeks from 22 to 24 weeks of gestation to 30 weeks of gestation as a screening test for preterm birth	Sensitivity and specificity (positive test defined as fetal fibronectin greater than or equal to 50 ng/mL)	Sensitivity and specificity for birth at 34 weeks or earlier for fetal fibronection measurement at: 24 weeks, 23% (95% CI 16 to 31) and 97% 26 weeks, 22% (95% CI 14 to 32) and 97% 28 weeks 20% (95% CI 11 to 30) and 97% 30 weeks, 29% (95% CI 18 to 41) and 96% Sensitivity of fibronectin at 22 to 24 weeks for preterm birth occurring at: 24 to 27 weeks, 63% (95% CI 38 to 84) 24 to 29 weeks, 54% (95% CI 28 to 66) 24 to 31 weeks, 38% (95% CI 25 to 53) 24 to 34 weeks, 21% (95% CI 14 to 29) 24 to 36 weeks, 10% (95% CI 7 to 14)		CH	2a
Mercer et al., 1996	546	2929 women from 10 centres in the USA from 1992 to 1994	Risk assessment for the prediction of preterm birth using clinical information collected at 23 to 24 weeks	Sensitivity and specificity	For a predicted probability of 20% or greater for preterm birth, sensitivity and specificity for multiparous women was 24.2% and 92.1% For a predicted probability of 20% or greater for preterm birth, sensitivity and specificity for nulliparous women was 18.2% and 95.4%	Factors assessed included demographics, socioeconomic status, home and work environment, drug or alcohol use, medical history, height, weight, body mass index, speculum examination, and pelvic examination	CH	2a

11.4 Placenta praevia

Study	Ref.	Population	Intervention	Outcomes	Results	Comments	Study type	EL
Leerentveld et al., 1990	549	100 women with second or third trimester haemorrhage, suspected placenta praevia, fetal malpresentaion or nonengaged presenting part from 1988 to 1990	In group with suspected placenta praevia (n = 15), transvaginal scan performed at 31 weeks (median). In the rest of the women (n = 85), transvaginal ultrasound performed at 29 weeks (median) Findings at delivery used as gold standard	Sensitivity and specificity of transvaginal placental localisation Cases of vaginal bleeding	Sensitivity: 87.5%, 95% CI 61.7 to 98.4 Specificity: 98.8%, 95% CI 93.4 to 100 No cases of vaginal bleeding and no woman who presented with vaginal haemorrhage (n = 76) displayed aggravated bleeding after sonography.		CS	3
Oppenheimer et al., 2001	550	36 pregnant women with a placenta lying within 30mm of the internal cervical os or overlapping it at or after 26 weeks	Eligible women identified by transvaginal ultrasound and repeated every 4 weeks until leading edge migrated beyond 30 mm or delivery	Cases of vaginal bleeding from transvaginal ultrasound	No case of vaginal bleeding Procedure also reported to be well tolerated by all women		CS	3
Sherman et al., 1991	551	38 women with suspected placenta praevia at 26 weeks or more	Group 1 (n = 20): abdominal ultrasound Group 2 (n = 18): abdominal ultrasound followed by vaginal ultrasound All women rescanned at 4 week intervals	Diagnosis of placenta praevia Cases of vaginal bleeding	Group 1, on initial transabdominal scan: 9 complete praevias, 3 partial praevias, 4 marginal praevias, and 4 low lying Group 2, on initial transabdominal scan: 5 complete praevias, 5 partial praevias, 2 marginal praevias, and 6 low lying Group 2, on transvaginal scan: 4 complete praevias, 3 partial praevias, 5 marginal praevias, and 6 low lying In subset of women who gave birth within two weeks of last scan (n = 19), in both groups, transabdominal and transvaginal scans correctly identified all cases of complete praevia. For partial praevia, 2 women in group 1 were identified at delivery but the transabdominal scan had identified 3 women. In group 2, 2 women with partial praevia at delivery were identified, concording with results from the tranvaginal scan, but not with the transabdominal scan which identified only 1 woman. No patient experienced increased vaginal bleeding within 24 hours after transvaginal scan	Method of randomisation not specified	RCT	1b

11.4 Placenta praevia (continued)

Study	Ref.	Population	Intervention	Outcomes	Results	Comments	Study type	EL
Farine et al., 1990	552	77 women with second or third trimester bleeding or previous diagnosis of placenta praevia	Transabdominal ultrasound followed by transvaginal ultrasound within 24 hours. Findings at delivery used as 'gold standard'	Sensitivity and specificity. False positives and false negatives. Cases of vaginal bleeding	Transvaginal sensitivity and specificity: 100% and 81%. Transabdominal sensitivity and specificity: 79% and 39%. Transvaginal false positive and false negative rate: 29% and 0% (all false positive cases were marginal placenta praevia). Transabdominal false positive and false negative rate: 62% and 20%. None had vaginal bleeding in 12 hours following scan		CS	3
Taipale et al., 1997	553	6428 women with singleton pregnancies from an obstetric clinic in Finland from 1993 to 1994	Transvaginal ultrasound performed at 12 to 16 weeks. Placenta that extended over the internal cervical os was measured with electronic calipers	Number of women with placenta at or over internal cervical os at 12 to 16 weeks. Number of women with placenta praevia at birth. Sensitivity	287/6428 (4.5%) had placenta at or over internal os. 10/6428 (0.16%) had placenta praevia at time of birth. 8/10 women with placenta praevia were identified with transvaginal scan: sensitivity 80%, 95% CI 44 to 98. In all 8 of these women, the placenta extended 15mm or more over the internal os at 12 to 16 weeks		CH	2b
Taipale et al., 1998	554	3696 women with singleton pregnancies in Finland from 1995 to 1996	Transvaginal ultrasound performed at 18 to 23 weeks. Distance from edge of placenta to internal cervical os was measured with electronic calipers	Number of women with placenta at or over internal cervical os at 18 to 23 weeks. Number of women with placenta praevia at birth. Sensitivity and specificity. Positive predictive value (PPV) with 15-mm cutoff	57/3696 (1.5%) had placenta at or over internal os. 5/3696 (0.14%) had placenta praevia at time of birth. Sensitivity: 100%, 95% CI 48 to 100. Specificity: 99.4%, 95% CI 99.1 to 99.6. In all 5 women, placenta extended 15mm or more over the internal os at 18 to 23 weeks. PPV: 19%, 95% CI 6 to 38		CH	2b

11.4 Placenta praevia (continued)

Study	Ref.	Population	Intervention	Outcomes	Results	Comments	Study type	EL
Hill et al., 1995	555	1252 pregnant women from a women's hospital in the USA	Transvaginal ultrasound performed between 9 and 13 weeks of gestation. The distance from the edge of the placenta to the internal cervical os was measured with electronic calipers	Number of women with placenta at or over internal cervical os between 9 and 13 weeks Number of women with placenta praevia at birth	77/1252 (6.2%) had placenta at or over internal os 4/1252 (0.32%) had placenta praevia at time of birth In all 4 women, the placenta extended more than 1.6 cm over the internal os by transvaginal ultrasound at 9 to 13 weeks.		CSS	3
Dasche et al., 2002	556	714 women with singleton pregnancies and suspected placenta praevia from 1991 to 2000	Retrospective analysis of women who had transvaginal or transabdominal ultrasound between 15 and 36 weeks of gestation	Persistence of placenta praevia to delivery from gestational age at detection	From 15 to 19 weeks: 12% From 20 to 23 weeks: 34% From 24 to 27 weeks: 49% From 28 to 31 weeks: 62% From 32 to 35 weeks: 73%		CS	3

12.2 Measurement of symphysis–fundal distance

Study	Ref.	Population	Intervention	Outcomes	Results	Comments	Study type	EL
Gardosi and Francis, 1999	567	1272 consecutive women with singleton pregnancies booked before 22 weeks from 1995 to 1995	Fundal height measurement plotted on customised charts (n = 734) vs. fundal height assessment by abdominal palpation and recorded on standard co-operation card (n = 605)	Detection of small- and large-for-gestational-age babies (SGA and LGA) Number of referrals for investigations	SGA: 47.9% vs. 29.2%, OR 2.23, 95% CI 1.12 to 4.45 LGA: 45.7% vs. 24.2%, OR 2.63, 95% CI 1.27 to 5.45 Referrals for investigations in pregnancy assessment centre: 0.33 vs. 0.56 visits per pregnancy, p < 0.005		CT	2a

12.5 Cardiotocography

Study	Ref.	Population	Intervention	Outcomes	Results	Comments	Study type	EL
Pattison and McCowan, 2001	573	4 RCTs, 1588 pregnancies	Antenatal cardiotocography vs. control for fetal assessment	Perinatal outcomes Methods of delivery Hospital admissions	Perinatal deaths: 3 RCTs, n = 127, Peto OR 2.85, 95% CI 0.99 to 7.12 Neonatal admissions: 2 RCTs, n = 883, Peto OR 1.11, 95% CI 0.80 to 1.54 Elective caesarean section: 3 RCTs, n = 1047, Peto OR 1.01, 95% CI 0.68 to 1.51 Emergency caesarean section: 3 RCTs, n = 1049, Peto OR 1.27 95% CI 0.83 to 1.92 Induction of labour: 3 RCTs, n = 1049, Peto OR 1.09 95% CI 0.85 to 1.40 Hospital admissions: 1 RCT, n = 300, Peto OR 0.37 95% CI 0.17 to 0.83		SR	1a

12.7 Umbilical and uterine artery Doppler ultrasound

Study	Ref.	Population	Intervention	Outcomes	Results	Comments	Study type	EL
Bricker and Neilson, 2001	575	5 RCTs, 14,388 pregnant women	Routine Doppler ultrasound vs. no/concealed/selective Doppler ultrasound	Antenatal admission	Antenatal admission: (3 RCTs, n = 9359) Peto OR 1.05, 95% CI 0.95 to 1.15		SR	1a
				Further Doppler ultrasound	Further Doppler ultrasound: (1 RCT, n = 3898) Peto OR 1.57 95% CI 1.30 to 1.90			
				Birthweight	Birthweight: (mean, SD) (1 RCT, n = 2016) WMD −27.000 95% CI −74.235 to 20.235			
				Apgar score	Apgar score < 7 at 5 minutes: (4 RCTs, n = 11375) Peto OR 0.88 95% CI 0.56 to 1.40			
				Admission to special care baby unit	Special care admission: (3 RCTs, n = 7477) Peto OR 0.99 95% CI 0.82 to 1.19			
				Preterm delivery	Preterm delivery < 37 weeks of gestation: (3 RCTs, n = 9359) Peto OR 1.09, 95% CI 0.89 to 1.33			
				Perinatal mortality	Perinatal mortality (excluding congenital abnormalities): (3 RCTs, n = 9359) Peto OR 1.10 95% CI 0.59 to 2.07			
				Caesarean section	Emergency caesarean section: (2 RCTs, n = 5461) Peto OR 1.02, 95% CI 0.84 to 1.23			
			Serial ultrasound and Doppler ultrasound vs. selective ultrasound	Caesarean section	Emergency caesarean section: (1 RCT, n = 2834) Peto OR 0.80 95% CI 0.62 to 1.05			
				Gestation at delivery	Gestation at delivery: (mean, SD) (1 RCT, n = 2834) −WMD 0.100, 95% CI −1.205 to 1.005			
				Birthweight	Birthweight (mean, SD) (1 RCT, n = 2834): −WMD −25.000 95% CI −67.526 to 17.526			
				Apgar score	Apgar score < 5 at 7 minutes (1 RCT, n = 2834) Peto OR 0.76 95% CI 0.46 to 1.27			
				Admission to neonatal unit	Admission to neonatal unit (1 RCT, n = 2834) Peto OR 0.94 95% CI 0.67 to 1.33			
				Perinatal mortality	Perinatal mortality: (1 RCT, n = 2834) Peto OR 0.60, 95% CI 0.31 to 1.16			

13.1 Pregnancy after 41 weeks

13.1.1 How is pregnancy after 41 weeks determined and what is it its incidence in the UK?

Study	Ref.	Population	Intervention	Outcomes	Results	Comments	Study type	EL
Hilder et al., 1998	577	171,527 births from maternity units in North East Thames region, London, in 1989 to 1991	Retrospective analysis of regional database of birth notifications	Number of deliveries by week of gestation	At 40 weeks, 58% of women delivered At 41 weeks, 74% of women delivered At 42 weeks, 82% of women delivered	Gestational age based on maternal history or ultrasound data Gestations of more than 45 weeks were excluded	CH	2a

13.1.2 What are the maternal and perinatal outcomes associated with pregnancy after 41 weeks?

Study	Ref.	Population	Intervention	Outcomes	Results	Comments	Study type	EL
Hilder et al., 1998	577	171,527 notified births from maternity units in North East Thames region, London, in 1989 to 1991	Retrospective analysis of regional database of birth notifications linked to stillbirth and infant death registration	Rates of stillbirth and neonatal mortality/1000 ongoing pregnancies	At 37 weeks, risk of stillbirth was 0.35/1000 and risk of neonatal death was 0.14/1000 ongoing pregnancies At 42 weeks, risk of stillbirth was 1.5/1000 and risk of neonatal death was 1.45/1000 ongoing pregnancies At 43 weeks, risk of stillbirth was 2.12/1000 and risk of neonatal death was 1.59/1000 ongoing pregnancies	Gestational age based on maternal history or ultrasound data Post-term deliveries were defined as those occurring at 42 weeks (294 days) of gestation or later Term deliveries defined as those born at 37 to 41 completed weeks of gestation Gestations of more than 45 weeks were excluded	CH	2a

13.1.3 & 13.1.4 Does induction of labour versus conservative management decrease the risk of adverse perinatal and maternal outcomes and do these interventions improve maternal and perinatal outcomes?

Study	Ref.	Population	Intervention	Outcomes	Results	Comments	Study type	EL
Crowley, 2003	578	26 RCTs	Routine versus selective induction of labour for post-term pregnancy (after 41 weeks)	Induction of labour for post-term pregnancy (after 41 weeks gestation)	Induction of labour: (4 trials) Peto OR 0.68 (95% CI 0.57 to 0.82)		SR	1a
				Perinatal death	Perinatal death: (13 trials, n = 6073): Peto OR 0.23 (95% CI 0.06 to 0.90)			
				Caesarean section	Caesarean section: (12 trials, n = 5954): Peto OR 0.87 (95% CI 0.77, 0.99)			
				Instrumental delivery (overall)	Instrumental delivery: (14 trials, n = 6591): Peto OR 0.96 (95% CI 0.85 to 1.08)			
				Use of epidural analgesia (overall)	Use of epidural: (5 trials, n = 1543): Peto OR 1.15 (95% CI 0.91 to 1.45)			
				Meconium-stained amniotic fluid	Meconium-stained amniotic fluid: (9 trials, n = 5662): Peto OR 0.74 (95% CI 0.65 to 0.84)			
				Fetal heart rate abnormalities	Fetal heart rate abnormalities: (6 trials, n = 1745): Peto OR 0.91 (95% CI 0.66 to 1.24)			
				Maternal satisfaction with birth (overall)	Maternal satisfaction: (1 trial, n = 402): Peto OR 0.84 (95% CI 0.57 to 1.24)			

13.1.5 In women with an uncomplicated singleton pregnancy whose pregnancies progress beyond 41 weeks, does serial antenatal monitoring result in worse maternal and perinatal outcomes than induction of labour?

Study	Ref.	Population	Intervention	Outcomes	Results	Comments	Study type	EL
Crowley, 2003	578	26 RCTs	Complex versus simple fetal monitoring of post-term pregnancy (from 42 weeks)	Induction of labour	Induction of labour: (1 trial, n = 145): Peto OR 2.10 (95% CI 1.10 to 4.01)		SR	1a
				Perinatal death	Perinatal death: Peto OR 7.49 (95% CI 0.15 to 377.66)			
				Caesarean section	Caesarean section: Peto OR 2.03 (95% CI 0.79 to 5.20)			

13.2 Breech presentation at term

13.2.1 What is the prevalence of breech presentation at term and what are the outcomes associated with it?

Study	Ref.	Population	Intervention	Outcomes	Results	Comments	Study type	EL
Danielian et al., 1996	623	1645 infants delivered alive at term > 37 weeks after breech presentation in a Scottish region from 1981 to 1990 269 had handicap	Observational study	Long-term outcome of infants delivered in breech presentation at term by intended mode of delivery Included: handicap, developmental delay, neurological deficit, psychiatric referral	Handicap occurred in 269/1387 (16.9%) of infants Handicap by mode of delivery: Elective CS: 100/482 (20.7%) Planned vaginal delivery: 169/905 (18.7%)	There were no significant differences in the frequency of handicap by intended mode of delivery	CH	2b
Krebs et al., 1999	624	345 infants with cerebral palsy born in East Denmark from 1979 and 1986 Total of 233,764 infants	Observational study	Presentation	Rates of cerebral palsy in term infants according to presentation at birth: CP All OR (95% CI) Breech 5.2% 3.5% 1.56 (0.9 to 2.4) Vertex 90.7% 93.4% 0.7 (0.5 to 1.0) Other 14% 3.1% 1.3 (0.7 to 2.2)		CCS	3
Milsom et al., 2002	625	225 deliveries at 37 weeks in 3 hospitals in Sweden from 1985 to 1991	Observational study	Birth asphyxia defined as Apgar score < 7 at 5 minutes	Association of breech delivery with birth asphyxia: OR (95% CI) 20.3 (3.0 to 416.5) (adjusted)		CCS	3

13.2.2 Does external cephalic version (ECV) at term reduce the likelihood of breech presentation?

Study	Ref.	Population	Intervention	Outcomes	Results	Comments	Study type	EL
Hofmeyr and Kulier, 1999	597	6 RCTs, 612 women with a breech presentation at term (36 or more weeks) and no contraindication to external cephalic version: 1in South Africa, 1 in Zimbabwe, 2 in the Netherlands, 1 in Denmark, 1 in the USA Cochrane review, updated 1999	ECV at term (36 or more weeks) (with or without the use of tocolysis) vs. no ECV	Noncephalic births	ECV: 99/303 (32.7%) No ECV: 242/309 (78.3%) RR: 0.42 (95% CI 0.35 to 0.50)	Results were consistent from study to study	SR	1a

13.2.3 When should ECV be performed?

Study	Ref.	Population	Intervention	Outcomes	Results	Comments	Study type	EL
Hofmeyr, 1994	589	3 RCTs, 889 women with singleton breech presentation in Sweden, Zimbabwe and the Netherlands Cochrane systematic review, updated 1994	ECV before 37 weeks of gestation vs. no ECV attempt	Noncephalic births	ECV: 197/434 (38.5%) No ECV: 204/455 (44.8%) RR: 1.02 (95% CI 0.89 to 1.17)	Results were consistent from study to study	SR	1a

13.2.4 Does tocolysis increase the chance of successful version?

Study	Ref.	Population	Intervention	Outcomes	Results	Comments	Study type	EL
Hofmeyr, 2002	594	6 RCTs, 617 women with breech presentation at term and no contraindication to ECV Cochrane review, updated 2001	Routine betamimetic tocolysis for ECV at term vs. no tocolysis	Failed ECV	Tocolysis: 136/317 (42.9%) No tocolysis: 176/300 (58.7%) RR: 0.74 (95% CI 0.64 to 0.87)	Results were consistent from study to study	SR of RCT & QR	1a

13.2.5 Does pelvimetry predict who will deliver vaginally compared with clinical examination?

Study	Ref.	Population	Intervention	Outcomes	Results	Comments	Study type	EL
van Loon et al., 1990	626	235 women with singleton breech presentation at term Term defined as duration 37 weeks of gestation or more Randomised between January 1993 and April 1996 US hospital	Pelvimetry results revealed to obstetricians vs. pelvimetry results not disclosed to obstetricians (mode of delivery decided clinically)	Vaginal delivery Overall caesarean section rate Emergency caesarean section rate	Vaginal delivery: Pelvimetry results revealed: 68/118 (57.6% caesarean) Pelvimetry results not disclosed: 58/117 (49.6% caesarean) Absolute risk reduction: 8.0% (95% CI −3.8% to −19.8%) Overall caesarean section rate: Pelvimetry results revealed: 50/118 (42.2% caesarean) Pelvimetry results not disclosed: 59/117 (50.4% caesarean) Absolute risk reduction: 8.2% (95% CI −3.8% to −19.8%) Emergency caesarean section rate: Pelvimetry results revealed: 22/118 (18.6% caesarean) Pelvimetry results not disclosed: 41/117 (35.0% caesarean) Risk reduction: 16.4 % (95% CI 6.6% to 22.6%) NNT: 6	Computer-generated randomisation No description of allocation concealment Women were analysed by intention to treat	RCT	1b

13.2.6 What is the effect of planned caesarean section compared with planned vaginal birth for mother and baby outcomes or singleton term breech presentation?

Study	Ref.	Population	Intervention	Outcomes	Results	Comments	Study type	EL
Mother outcomes								
Hofmeyr and Hannah, 2000	627	3 RCTs, 2396 women with a breech presentation at term suitable for vaginal delivery Cochrane systematic review, updated 2000	Planned caesarean section vs. planned vaginal delivery	Maternal morbidity (pooled) Maternal morbidity measures included: postpartum bleeding (including blood transfusion), genital tract injury, wound infection, dehiscence or breakdown, maternal systemic infection, early postpartum depression, time in hospital after delivery	Planned caesarean section: 107/1169 (9.2%) Planned vaginal delivery: 106/1227 (8.6%) RR: 1.29 (95% CI 1.03 to 1.61)	Results generally consistent from study to study	SR of RCT	1b
Hannah et al., 2000	628	2088 women with a singleton fetus in a frank or complete breech presentation at term International randomised trial at 121 centres in 26 countries (high and low perinatal mortality rates)	Planned caesarean section vs. planned vaginal delivery	Maternal mortality	Planned caesarean section: 0/1041 Planned vaginal delivery: 1/1041	Centrally-controlled randomisation Analysis was by intention to treat	RCT	1b
Gimovsky et al., 1983	629	105 women with non-frank breech presentations at term US hospital	Trial of labour vs. elective caesarean section	Maternal mortality	No report of maternal deaths	Method of randomisation not indicated	RCT	1b
Collea et al., 1980	630	208 women with frank breech presentation at term US hospital	Trial of labour vs. elective caesarean section	Maternal mortality	No report of maternal deaths	Method of randomisation not indicated	RCT	1b

13.2.6 What is the effect of planned caesarean section compared with planned vaginal birth for mother and baby outcomes or singleton term breech presentation? (continued)

Study	Ref.	Population	Intervention	Outcomes	Results	Comments	Study type	EL
Baby outcomes								
Hofmeyr and Hannah, 2000	627	3 RCTs, 2396 women with a breech presentation at term suitable for vaginal delivery Cochrane systematic review, updated 2000	Planned caesarean section vs. planned vaginal delivery	Perinatal and neonatal death (excluding fatal anomalies)	Planned caesarean section: 3/1166 (0.26%) Planned vaginal delivery: 14/1222 (1.15%) RR: 0.29 (95% CI 0.10 to 0.86) Countries with low (20/1000 or less) perinatal mortality rate was 0.26 (95% CI 0.03 to 2.00)	Planned caesarean section is associated with a 70% decrease in mortality compared with planned vaginal delivery for breech delivery at term	SR of RCT	1a
Hofmeyr and Hannah, 2000	627	3 RCTs involving 2396 women with a breech presentation at term suitable for vaginal delivery Cochrane systematic review, updated 2000	Planned caesarean section vs. planned vaginal delivery	Perinatal death or neonatal morbidity Events included: birth trauma, seizures occurring at less than 24 hours of age or requiring two or more drugs to control them, Apgar score of < 4 at 5 minutes, cord blood base deficit of at least 15, hypotonia for at least 2 hours, stupor (decreased response to pain or coma), intubation and ventilation for at least 24 hours, tube feeding for 4 days or more, admission to neonatal unit for longer than 4 days	Planned caesarean section: 20/1132 (0.18%) Planned vaginal delivery: 66/1152 (5.73%) RR: 0.31 (95% CI 0.19 to 0.52) Countries with low (20/1000 or less) perinatal mortality rate was 0.13 (95%CI 0.05 to 0.31)	Planned caesarean section is associated with a 70% decrease in death or morbidity compared to planned vaginal delivery for breech delivery at term	SR of RCT	1a
Hofmeyr and Hannah, 2000	627	3 RCTs involving 2396 women with a breech presentation at term suitable for vaginal delivery Cochrane systematic review, updated 2000	Planned caesarean section vs. planned vaginal delivery	5-minute Apgar < 7	Planned caesarean section: 11/1164 (0.94%) Planned vaginal delivery: 38/1211 (3.14%) RR: 0.32 (95% CI 0.17 to 0.61)		SR of RCT	1a

References

1. Expert Maternity Group. Woman centred care. In: Department of Health. *Changing Childbirth. Report of the Expert Maternity Group.* London: HMSO; 1993. p.5–8.

2. Garcia J, Loftus-Hills A (National Perinatal Epidemiology Unit: Oxford University). An overview of research on women's views of antenatal care. Personal communication 2001.

3. Singh D, Newburn M, editors. *Access to Maternity Information and Support; the Experiences and Needs of Women Before and After Giving Support.* London: National Childbirth Trust; 2000.

4. Cochrane AL. *Effectiveness and efficiency. Random reflections on health services.* London: Nuffield Provincial Hospitals Trust; 1972.

5. Department of Health. Screening for infectious diseases in pregnancy: standards to support the UK antenatal screening programme. [In preparation]. 2003.

6. National Institute for Clinical Excellence. *Information for national collaborating centres and guideline development groups.* Guideline development process series 3. London: Oaktree Press; 2001.

7. Henderson J, McCandlish R, Kumiega L, Petrou S. Systematic review of economic aspects of alternative modes of delivery. *BJOG* 2001;108:149–57.

8. Bekker H, Thornton JG, Airey CM, Connelly JB, Hewison J, Robinson MB, *et al.* Informed decision making: An annotated bibliography and systematic review. *Health Technology Assessment* 1999;3(1):1–156.

9. Department of Health. *Changing childbirth. Report of the Expert Maternity Group.* London: HMSO; 1993.

10. Audit Commission for Local Authorities, NHS in England and Wales. *First class delivery: improving maternity services in England and Wales.* London: Audit Commission Publications; 1997. p. 1–98.

11. Murray J, Cuckle H, Sehmi I, Wilson C, Ellis A. Quality of written information used in Down syndrome screening. *Prenatal Diagnosis* 2001;21:138–42.

12. Thornton JG, Hewison J, Lilford RJ, Vail A. A randomised trial of three methods of giving information about prenatal testing. *British Medical Journal* 1995;311:1127–30.

13. O'Cathain A, Walters SJ, Nicholl JP, Thomas KJ, Kirkham M. Use of evidence based leaflets to promote informed choice in maternity care: randomised controlled trial in everyday practice. [comment]. *British Medical Journal* 2002;324:643.

14. Stapleton H. Qualitative study of evidence based leaflets in maternity care. *British Medical Journal* 2002;324:639.

15. Dodds R, Newburn M. Support during screening: an NCT report. *Modern Midwife* 1997;7:23–6.

16. Carroll JC, Brown JB, Reid AJ, Pugh P. Women's experience of maternal serum screening. *Canadian Family Physician* 2000;46:614–20.

17. Marteau TM, Slack J, Kidd J, Shaw, RW. Presenting a routine screening test in antenatal care: practice observed. *Public Health* 1992;106(2):131–41.

18. Smith D, Shaw RW, Marteau T. Lack of knowledge in health professionals: a barrier to providing information to patients. *Quality in Health Care* 1994;3:75–8.

19. Smith DK, Shaw RW, Slack J, Marteau TM. Training obstetricians and midwives to present screening tests: evaluation of two brief interventions. *Prenatal Diagnosis* 1995;15:317–24.

20. Green JM. Serum screening for Down's syndrome: experiences of obstetricians in England and Wales. *British Medical Journal* 1994;309:769–72.

21. Michie S, Marteau TM. Non-response bias in prospective studies of patients and health care professionals. *International Journal of Social Research Methodology* 1999;2:203–12.

22. Marteau TM. Towards informed decisions about prenatal testing: a review. *Prenatal Diagnosis* 1995;15(13):1215–26.

23. National Health Service. *The Pregnancy Book.* London: Health Promotion England; 2001.

24. Bro Taf Health Authority. *Tests for you and your baby during pregnancy.* Cardiff, Wales: Bro Taf Health Authority; 2000.

25. Nolan ML, Hicks C. Aims, processes and problems of antenatal education as identified by three groups of childbirth teachers. *Midwifery* 1997;13:179–88.

26. Johnson R, Slade P. Does fear of childbirth during pregnancy predict emergency caesarean section? *BJOG* 2002;109:1213–21.

27. Gagnon AJ. Individual or group antenatal education for childbirth/parenthood. *Cochrane Database of Systematic Reviews* 2001;(3).

28. Hibbard BM, Robinson JO, Pearson JF, Rosen M, Taylor A. The effectiveness of antenatal education. *Health Education Journal* 1979;38:39–46.

29. Rautauva P, Erkkola R, Sillanpaa M. The outcome and experiences of first pregnancy in relation to the mother's childbirth knowledge: The Finnish Family Competence Study. *Journal of Advanced Nursing* 1991;16:1226–32.

30. Lumley J, Brown S. Attenders and nonattenders at childbirth education classes in Australia: how do they and their births differ? *Birth* 1993;20:123–30.

31. Sullivan P. Felt learning needs of pregnant women. *Canadian Nurse* 1993;89:42.

32. Villar J, Khan-Neelofur D. Patterns of routine antenatal care for low – risk pregnancy. *Cochrane Database of Systematic Reviews* 2003;(1).

33.   Hodnett ED. Continuity of caregivers for care during pregnancy and childbirth. *Cochrane Database of Systematic Reviews* 2001;(3).

34.   Waldenstrom U, Turnbull D. A systematic review comparing continuity of midwifery care with standard maternity services. *British Journal of Obstetrics and Gynaecology* 1998;105:1160–70.

35.   North Staffordshire Changing Childbirth Research Team. A randomised study of midwifery caseload care and traditional 'shared care'. *Midwifery* 2000;16:295–302.

36.   Homer CS, Davis GK, Brodie PM, Sheehan A, Barclay LM, Wills J, *et al.* Collaboration in maternity care: a randomised controlled trial comparing community-based continuity of care with standard hospital care. *BJOG* 2001;108:16–22.

37.   Homer CS, Davis GK, Brodie PM. What do women feel about community-based antenatal care? *Australian and New Zealand Journal of Public Health* 2000;24:590–5.

38.   Biro MA, Waldenstrom U. Team midwifery care in a tertiary level obstetric service: a randomized controlled trial. *Birth* 2000;27:168–73.

39.   Waldenstrom U. Does team midwife care increase satisfaction with antenatal, intrapartum, and postpartum care? A randomized controlled trial. [see comments.]. *Birth* 2000;27:156–67.

40.   Blondel B, Breart G. Home visits for pregnancy complications and management of antenatal care: an overview of three randomized controlled trials. *British Journal of Obstetrics and Gynaecology* 1992;99:283–6.

41.   Lilford RJ, Kelly M, Baines A, Cameron S, Cave M, Guthrie K, *et al.* Effect of using protocols on medical care: randomised trial of three methods of taking an antenatal history. *British Medical Journal* 1992;305:1181–4.

42.   Elbourne D, Richardson M, Chalmers I, Waterhouse I, Holt E. The Newbury Maternity Care Study: a randomized controlled trial to assess a policy of women holding their own obstetric records. *British Journal of Obstetrics and Gynaecology* 1987;94:612–19.

43.   Homer CS, Davis GK, Everitt LS. The introduction of a woman-held record into a hospital antenatal clinic: the bring your own records study. *Australian and New Zealand Journal of Public Health* 1999;39:54–7.

44.   Lovell A, Zander LI, James CE, Foot S, Swan AV, Reynolds A. The St. Thomas's Hospital maternity case notes study: a randomised controlled trial to assess the effects of giving expectant mothers their own maternity case notes. *Paediatric and Perinatal Epidemiology* 1987;1:57–66.

45.   Petrou S, Kupek E, Vause S, Maresh M. Antenatal visits and adverse perinatal outcomes: results from a British population-based study. *European Journal of Obstetrics Gynecology and Reproductive Biology* 2003;106:40–9.

46.   Carroli G, Villar J, Piaggio G, Khan-Neelofur D, Gulmezoglu M, Mugford M, *et al.* WHO systematic review of randomised controlled trials of routine antenatal care. *Lancet* 2001;357:1565–70.

47.   Clement S, Sikorski J, Wilson J, Das S, Smeeton N. Women's satisfaction with traditional and reduced antenatal visit schedules. *Midwifery* 1996;12:120–8.

48.   Hildingsson I, Waldenstrom U, Radestad I. Women's expectations on antenatal care as assessed in early pregnancy: Number of visits, continuity of caregiver and general content. *Acta Obstetricia et Gynecologica Scandinavica* 2002;81:118–25.

49.   Henderson J, Roberts T, Sikorski J, Wilson J, Clement S. An economic evaluation comparing two schedules of antenatal visits. *Journal of Health Services and Research Policy* 2000;5:69–75.

50.   Kaminski M, Blondel B, Breart G. Management of pregnancy and childbirth in England and Wales and in France. *Paediatric and Perinatal Epidemiology* 1988;2:13–24.

51.   Ryan, M, Ratcliffe, J, Tucker, J. Using willingness to pay to value alternative models of antenatal care. *Social Science and Medicine* 1997;44(3):371–80.

52.   Crowther CA, Kornman L, O'Callaghan S, George K, Furness M, Willson K. Is an ultrasound assessment of gestational age at the first antenatal visit of value? A randomised clinical trial. [see comments]. *British Journal of Obstetrics and Gynaecology* 1999;106:1273–9.

53.   Savitz DA, Terry JW Jr, Dole N, Thorp JM Jr, Siega-Riz AM, Herring AH. Comparison of pregnancy dating by last menstrual period, ultrasound scanning, and their combination. *American Journal of Obstetrics and Gynecology* 2002;187:1660–6.

54.   Backe B, Nakling J. Term prediction in routine ultrasound practice. *Acta Obstetricia et Gynecologica Scandinavica* 1994;73:113–8.

55.   Tunon K, Eik-Nes SH, Grottum P. A comparison between ultrasound and a reliable last menstrual period as predictors of the day of delivery in 15000 examinations. *Ultrasound in Obstetrics and Gynecology* 1996;8:178–85.

56.   Blondel B, Morin I, Platt RW, Kramer MS, Usher R, Breart G. Algorithms for combining menstrual and ultrasound estimates of gestational age: consequences for rates of preterm and post-term birth. *BJOG* 2002;109:718–20.

57.   Neilson JP. Ultrasound for fetal assessment in early pregnancy. *Cochrane Database of Systematic Reviews* 1999;(2).

58.   Moutquin J-M, Gagnon R, Rainville C, Giroux L, Amyot G, Bilodeau R, *et al.* Maternal and neonatal outcome in pregnancies with no risk factors. *Canadian Medical Association Journal* 1987;137:728–32.

59.   Mohamed H, Martin C, Haloob R. Can the New Zealand antenatal scoring system be applied in the United Kingdom? *Journal of Obstetrics and Gynaecology* 2002;22:389–91.

60.   Doyle P, Roman E, Beral V, Brookes M. Spontaneous abortion in dry cleaning workers potentially exposed to perchloroethylene. *Occupational and Environmental Medicine* 1997;54:848–53.

61.   Kolstad HA, Brandt LP, Rasmussen K. [Chlorinated solvents and fetal damage. Spontaneous abortions, low birth weight and malformations among women employed in the dry – cleaning industry]. [Danish]. *Ugeskrift for Laeger* 1990;152:2481–2.

62.   Kyyronen P, Taskinen H, Lindbohm ML, Hemminki K, Heinonen OP. Spontaneous abortions and congenital malformations among women exposed to tetrachloroethylene in dry cleaning. *Journal of Epidemiology and Community Health* 1989;43:346–51.

63.   Mozurkewich EL, Luke B, Avni M, Wolf FM. Working conditions and adverse pregnancy outcome: A meta-analysis. *Obstetrics and Gynecology* 2000;95:623–35.

64.   Hanke W, Kalinka J, Makowiec-Dabrowska T, Sobala W. Heavy physical work during pregnancy: a risk factor for small-for-gestational-age babies in Poland. *American Journal of Industrial Medicine* 1999;36:200–5.

65. Kramer, MS. Nutritional advice in pregnancy. *Cochrane Database of Systematic Reviews* 2003;(1):1–10.

66. Abramsky L, Botting B, Chapple J, Stone D. Has advice on periconceptional folate supplementation reduced neural-tube defects? *Lancet* 1999;354:998–9.

67. Lumley J, Watson L, Watson M, Bower C. Periconceptional supplementation with folate and/or multivitamins for preventing neural tube defects. *Cochrane Database of Systematic Reviews* 2002;(1).

68. Li Z, Gindler J, Wang H, Berry RJ, Li S, Correa A, *et al.* Folic acid supplements during early pregnancy and likelihood of multiple births: a population-based cohort study. *Lancet* 2003;361:380–4.

69. Royal College of Obstetricians and Gynaecologists. *Periconceptual folic acid and food fortification in the prevention of neural tube defects.* Scientific Advisory Committee Opinion Paper No. 4, London: RCOG; 2003.

70. Daly LE, Kirke PN, Molloy A, Weir DG, Scott JM. Folate levels and neural tube defects. Implications for prevention. *JAMA* 1995;274:1698–702.

71. Expert Advisory Group. Department of Health, Scottish office Home and Health Department, Welsh Office, and Department of Health and Social Services, Northern Ireland. *Folic acid and the prevention of neural tube defects.* London: HMSO; 1992.

72. Prevention of neural tube defects: results of the Medical Research Council Vitamin Study. MRC Vitamin Study Research Group [see comments]. *Lancet* 1991;338:131–7.

73. Wald NJ, Law MR, Morris JK, Wald DS. Quantifying the effect of folic acid. *Lancet* 2001;358:2069–73.

74. Mahomed K. Iron and folate supplementation in pregnancy. *Cochrane Database of Systematic Reviews* 2001;(2).

75. Hemminki E, Rimpela U. A randomized comparison of routine versus selective iron supplementation during pregnancy. *Journal of the American College of Nutrition* 1991;10:3–10.

76. Mahomed K. Iron supplementation in pregnancy. *Cochrane Database of Systematic Reviews* 2001;(2).

77. British Medical Association, Royal Pharmaceutical Society of Great Britain. *British National Formulary.* London: March 2003. p. 439–40.

78. van den Broek N, Kulier R, Gulmezoglu AM, Villar J. Vitamin A supplementation during pregnancy. *Cochrane Database of Systematic Reviews* 2003;(1):1–21.

79. Dolk HM, Nau H, Hummler H, Barlow SM. Dietary vitamin A and teratogenic risk: European Teratology Society discussion paper. *European Journal Obstetrics and Gynecology Reproductive Biology* 1999;83:31–6.

80. Oakley GP Jr, Erickson JD. Vitamin A and birth defects. Continuing caution is needed. *New England Journal of Medicine* 1995;333:1414–15.

81. Rothman KJ, Moore LL, Singer MR, Nguyen US, Mannino S, Milunsky A. Teratogenicity of high vitamin A intake. *New England Journal of Medicine* 1995;333:1369–73.

82. Mahomed K, Gulmezoglu, A. M. Vitamin D supplementation in pregnancy. *Cochrane Database of Systematic Reviews* 2000;(1).

83. Southwick FS, Purich DL. Intracellular pathogenesis of listeriosis. *New England Journal of Medicine* 1996;334:770–6.

84. Public Health Laboratory Service Press Release. Disease Facts: Salmonella. 2001.

85. British Nutrition Foundation. BNF Information. Diet through Life: Pregnancy. 2003. [www.nutrition.org.uk/] Accessed 20 August 2003.

86. Ledward RS. Drugs in pregnancy. In: Studd J, editor *Progress in Obstetrics and Gynaecology.* Edinburgh: Churchill Livingstone; 1998. p. 19–46.

87. Fugh-Berman A, Kronenberg F. Complementary and alternative medicine (CAM) in reproductive-age women: a review of randomized controlled trials. *Reproductive Toxicology* 2003;17:137–52.

88. Moore ML. Complementary and alternative therapies. *Journal of Perinatal Education* 2002;11:39–42.

89. Pinn G, Pallett L. Herbal medicine in pregnancy. *Complementary Therapies in Nursing and Midwifery* 2002;8:77–80.

90. Leung K-Y, Lee Y-P, Chan H-Y, Lee C-P, Tang MHY. Are herbal medicinal products less teratogenic than Western pharmaceutical products? *Acta Pharmacologica Sinica* 2002;23:1169–72.

91. Hepner DL, Harnett M, Segal S, Camann W, Bader AM, Tsen LC. Herbal medicine use in parturients. *Anesthesia and Analgesia* 2002;94:690–3.

92. Maats FH, Crowther CA. Patterns of vitamin, mineral and herbal supplement use prior to and during pregnancy. *Australian and New Zealand Journal of Obstetrics and Gynaecology* 2002;42:494–6.

93. Tsui B, Dennehy CE, Tsourounis C. A survey of dietary supplement use during pregnancy at an academic medical center. *American Journal of Obstetrics and Gynecology* 2001;185:433–7.

94. Medicines Control Agency. *Safety of Herbal Medicinal Products.* London; 2002. p. 22–23.

95. Ernst E. Herbal medicinal products during pregnancy: are they safe? *BJOG* 2002;109:227–35.

96. Dove D, Johnson P. Oral evening primrose oil: Its effect on length of pregnancy and selected intrapartum outcomes in low-risk nulliparous women. *Journal of Nurse-Midwifery* 1999;44:320–4.

97. Simpson M. Raspberry leaf in pregnancy; its safety and efficacy in labor. *Journal of Midwifery and Women's Health* 2001;46(2):51–9.

98. Gallo M, Sarkar M, Au W, Pietrzak K, Comas B, Smith M, *et al.* Pregnancy outcome following gestational exposure to Echinacea: a prospective controlled study. *Archives of Internal Medicine* 2000;160:3141–3.

99. Goldman RD, Koren G, Motherisk Team. Taking St John's wort during pregnancy. *Canadian Family Physician* 2003;49:29–30.

100. Clapp JF III, Simonian S, Lopez B, Appleby-Wineberg S, Harcar-Sevcik R. The one-year morphometric and neurodevelopmental outcome of the offspring of women who continued to exercise regularly throughout pregnancy. *American Journal of Obstetrics and Gynecology* 1998;178:594–9.

101. Kramer MS. Aerobic exercise for women during pregnancy. *Cochrane Database of Systematic Reviews* 2002;(4).

102. Camporesi EM. Diving and pregnancy. *Seminars in Perinatology* 1996;20:292–302.

103. Read JS, Klebanoff MA. Sexual intercourse during pregnancy and preterm delivery: effects of vaginal microorganisms. *American Journal of Obstetrics and Gynecology* 1993;168:514–19.

104. Klebanoff MA, Nugent RP, Rhoads GG. Coitus during pregnancy: is it safe? *Lancet* 1984;2:914–7.

105. Berghella V, Klebanhoff M, McPherson C. Sexual intercourse association with asymptomatic bacterial vaginosis and *Trichomonas vaginalis* treatment in relationship to preterm birth. *American Journal of Obstetrics and Gynecology* 2002;187:1277–82.

106. Walpole I, Zubrick S, Pontre J. Is there a fetal effect with low to moderate alcohol use before or during pregnancy? *Journal of Epidemiology and Community Health* 1990;44:297–301.

107. Borges G, Lopez-Cervantes M, Medina-Mora ME, Tapia-Conyer R, Garrido F. Alcohol consumption, low birth weight, and preterm delivery in the national addiction survey (Mexico). *International Journal of the Addictions* 1993;28(4):355–68.

108. Holzman C, Paneth N, Little R, Pinto-Martin J. Perinatal brain injury in premature infants born to mothers using alcohol in pregnancy. *Pediatrics* 1995;95:66–73.

109. Aronson M, Hagberg B, Gillberg C. Attention deficits and autistic spectrum problems in children exposed to alcohol during gestation: A follow-up study. *Developmental Medicine and Child Neurology* 1997;39:583–7.

110. Abel EL. Fetal alcohol syndrome: the 'American Paradox'. *Alcohol and Alcoholism* 1998;33:195–201.

111. Royal College of Obstetricians and Gynaecologists. *Alcohol consumption in pregnancy*. Guideline No. 9. London: RCOG; 1999.

112. Lumley J, Oliver S, Waters E. Interventions for promoting smoking cessation during pregnancy. *Cochrane Database of Systematic Reviews* 2001;(2). 2001.

113. Owen L, McNeill A, Callum C. Trends in smoking during pregnancy in England, 1992–7: quota sampling surveys. *British Medical Journal* 1998;317:728.

114. DiFranza JR, Lew, RA. Effect of maternal cigarette smoking on pregnancy complications and sudden infant death syndrome. *Journal of Family Practice* 1995;40(4):385–394.

115. Ananth CV, Smulian JC, Vintzileos AM. Incidence of placental abruption in relation to cigarette smoking and hypertensive disorders during pregnancy: A meta-analysis of observational studies. *Obstetrics and Gynecology* 1999;93:622–8.

116. Castles A, Adams EK, Melvin CL, Kelsch C, Boulton ML. Effects of smoking during pregnancy: Five meta-analyses. *American Journal of Preventive Medicine* 1999;16:208–15.

117. Shah NR, Bracken MB. A systematic review and meta-analysis of prospective studies on the association between maternal cigarette smoking and preterm delivery. *American Journal of Obstetrics and Gynecology* 2000;182:465–72.

118. Wyszynski DF, Duffy DL, Beaty TH. Maternal cigarette smoking and oral clefts: a meta – analysis. *Cleft Palate-Craniofacial Journal* 1997;34:206–10.

119. Conde-Agudelo A, Althabe F, Belizan JM, Kafury-Goeta AC. Cigarette smoking during pregnancy and risk of preeclampsia: a systematic review. *American Journal of Obstetrics and Gynecology* 1999;181:1026–35.

120. Clausson B, Cnattingius S, Axelsson O. Preterm and term births of small for gestational age infants: A population-based study of risk factors among nulliparous women. *British Journal of Obstetrics and Gynaecology* 1998;105:1011–7.

121. Raymond EG, Cnattingius S, Kiely JL. Effects of maternal age, parity and smoking on the risk of stillbirth. *British Journal of Obstetrics and Gynaecology* 1994;101:301–6.

122. Kleinman JC, Pierre MB Jr, Madans JH, Land GH, Schramm WF. The effects of maternal smoking on fetal and infant mortality. *American Journal of Epidemiology* 1988;127:274–82.

123. Lumley J. Stopping smoking. *British Journal of Obstetrics and Gynaecology* 1987;94:289–92.

124. MacArthur C, Knox EG, Lancashire RJ. Effects at age nine of maternal smoking in pregnancy: experimental and observational findings. *BJOG* 2001;108:67–73.

125. von Kries R, Toschke AM, Koletzko B, Slikker W Jr. Maternal smoking during pregnancy and childhood obesity. *American Journal of Epidemiology* 2002;156:954–61.

126. Faden VB, Graubard BI. Maternal substance use during pregnancy and developmental outcome at age three. *Journal of Substance Abuse* 2000;12:329–40.

127. Thorogood M, Hillsdon M, Summerbell C. Changing behaviour: cardiovascular disorders. *Clinical Evidence* 2002;8:37–59.

128. Law M, Tang JL. An analysis of the effectiveness of interventions intended to help people stop smoking. *Archives of Internal Medicine* 1995;155:1933–41.

129. Wisborg K, Henriksen TB, Jespersen LB, Secher NJ. Nicotine patches for pregnant smokers. *Obstetrics and Gynecology* 2000;96:967–71.

130. Hajek P, West R, Lee A, Foulds J, Owen L, Eiser JR, *et al.* Randomized controlled trial of a midwife-delivered brief smoking cessation intervention in pregnancy. *Addiction* 2001;96:485–94.

131. Stotts A, DiClemente CC, Dolan-Mullen P. One-to-one. A motivational intervention for resistant pregnant smokers. *Addictive Behaviors* 2002;27:275–92.

132. Moore L, Campbell R, Whelan A, Mills N, Lupton P, Misselbrook E, *et al.* Self help smoking cessation in pregnancy: cluster randomised controlled trial. *British Medical Journal* 2002;325:1383–6.

133. Li C, Windsor R, Perkins L, Lowe J, Goldenberg R. The impact on birthweight and gestational age of cotinine validated smoking reduction during pregnancy. *JAMA* 1993;269:1519–24.

134. Windsor R, Li C, Boyd N, Hartmann K. The use of significant reduction rates to evaluate health education methods for pregnant smokers: a new harm reduction – behavioral indicator. *Health Education and Behavior* 1999;26:648–62.

135. Fergusson DM, Horwood LJ, Northstone K, ALSPAC Study Team, Avon Longitudinal Study of Pregnancy and Childhood. Maternal use of cannabis and pregnancy outcome. *BJOG* 2002;109:21–7.

136. English DR, Hulse GK, Milne E, Holman CD, Bower CI. Maternal cannabis use and birth weight: a meta-analysis. *Addiction* 1997;92:1553–60.

137. Royal College of Obstetricians and Gynaecologists. Advice on preventing deep vein thrombosis for pregnant women travelling by air. Scientific Advisory Committee Opinion paper No. 1. London: RCOG; 2001.

138. James KV, Lohr JM, Deshmukh RM, Cranley JJ. Venous thrombotic complications of pregnancy. *Cardiovascular Surgery* 1996;4:777–82.

139. McColl MD, Ramsay JE, Tait RC, Walker ID, McCall F, Conkie JA, et al. Risk factors for pregnancy associated venous thromboembolism. *Thrombosis and Haemostasis* 1997;78:1183–8.

140. Kierkegaard A. Incidence and diagnosis of deep vein thrombosis associated with pregnancy. *Acta Obstetricia et Gynecologica Scandinavica* 1983;62:239–43.

141. Scurr JH, Machin SJ, Bailey-King S, Mackie IJ, McDonald S, Coleridge Smith PD. Frequency and prevention of symptomless deep-vein thrombosis in long-haul flights: a randomised trial. *Lancet* 2001;357:1485–9.

142. World Health Organization. Travellers with special needs. In: Martinez L, editor. *International Travel and Health*. Geneva: World Health Organization; 2002.

143. Lewis G, Drife J, editors. *Why mothers die 1997–1999: The fifth report of the Confidential Enquiries into Maternal Deaths in the United Kingdom*. London: RCOG Press; 2001.

144. Johnson HC, Pring DW. Car seatbelts in pregnancy: the practice and knowledge of pregnant women remain causes for concern. *BJOG* 2000;107:644–7.

145. Chang A, Magwene K, Frand E. Increased safety belt use following education in childbirth classes. *Birth* 1987;14:148–52.

146. Klinich KD, Schneider LW, Moore JL, Pearlman MD. Investigations of crashes involving pregnant occupants. *Annual Proceedings, Association for the Advancement of Automotive Medicine* 2000;44:37–55.

147. Crosby WM, Costiloe JP. Safety of lap-belt restraint for pregnant victims of automobile collisions. *New England Journal of Medicine* 1971;284:632–6.

148. Crosby WM, King AI, Stout LC. Fetal survival following impact: improvement with shoulder harness restraint. *American Journal of Obstetrics and Gynecology* 1972;112:1101–6.

149. Wolf ME, Alexander BH, Rivara FP, Hickok DE, Maier RV, Starzyk PM. A retrospective cohort study of seatbelt use and pregnancy outcome after a motor vehicle crash. *Journal of Trauma-Injury Infection and Critical Care* 1993;34:116–19.

150. World Health Organization. Special groups. In: Martinez L, editor. *International Travel and Health*. Geneva: World Health Organization; 2002.

151. Hurley PA. International travel and the pregnant women. In: Studd J, editor. *Progress in Obstetrics and Gynaecology*. Edinburgh: Churchill Livingstone; 2003. p. 45–55.

152. Hurley P. Vaccination in pregnancy. *Current Obstetrics and Gynaecology* 1998;8:169–75.

153. Jothivijayarani A. Travel considerations during pregnancy. *Primary Care Update for Ob/Gyns* 2002;9:36–40.

154. World Health Organization. Treatment of P. vivax, P. ovale and P. malariae infections. In: Martinez L, editor. *International Travel and Health*. Geneva: World Health Organization; 2002. [www.who.int/ith/chapter07_04.html] Accessed 4 September 2003.

155. Luxemburger C, McGready R, Kham A, Morison L, Cho T, Chongsuphajaisiddhi T, et al. Effects of malaria during pregnancy on infant mortality in an area of low malaria transition. *American Journal of Epidemiology* 2001;154:459–65.

156. World Health Organization. World malaria situation in 1993, Part 1. *Weekly Epidemiological Record* 1996;71:17–24.

157. Linday S, Ansell J, Selman C, Cox V, Hamilton K, Walraven G. Effect of pregnancy on exposure to malaria mosquitoes. *Lancet* 2000;355:1972.

158. Schaefer C, Peters PW. Intrauterine diethyltoluamide exposure and fetal outcome. *Reproductive Toxicology* 1992;6:175–6.

159. Dolan G, ter Kuile FO, Jacoutot V. Bed nets for the prevention of malaria and anaemia in pregnancy. *Transactions of the Royal Society of Tropical Medicine and Hygiene* 1993;87:620–6.

160. Pearce G. Travel insurance and the pregnant woman. *MIDIRS Midwifery Digest* 1997;7:164.

161. Brown H, Campbell H. Special considerations for pregnant travellers. *Modern Medicine of Australia* 1999;42:17–20.

162. Tucker R. Ensure pregnant travellers know the risks. *Practice Nurse* 1999;18:458–66.

163. Rose SR. Pregnancy and travel. *Emergency Medicine Clinics of North America* 1997;15:93–111.

164. Baron TH, Ramirez B, Richter JE. Gastrointestinal motility disorders during pregnancy. *Annals of Internal Medicine* 1993;118:366–75.

165. Weigel RM, Weigel MM. Nausea and vomiting of early pregnancy and pregnancy outcome. A meta-analytical review. *British Journal of Obstetrics and Gynaecology* 1989;96:1312–8.

166. Whitehead SA, Andrews PL, Chamberlain GV. Characterisation of nausea and vomiting in early pregnancy: a survey of 1000 women. *Journal of Obstetrics and Gynaecology* 1992;12:364–9.

167. Gadsby R, Barnie-Adshead AM, Jagger C. A prospective study of nausea and vomiting during pregnancy. *British Journal of General Practice* 1993;43:245–8.

168. Feldman M. Nausea and vomiting. In: Sleisenger MH, Fordtran JS, editors. *Gastrointestinal disease*. Philadelphia: WB Saunders; 1989. p. 229–31.

169. Klebanoff MA, Mills JL. Is vomiting during pregnancy teratogenic? *British Medical Journal* 1986;292:724–6.

170. Smith C, Crowther C, Beilby J, Dandeaux J. The impact of nausea and vomiting on women: a burden of early pregnancy. *Australian and New Zealand Journal of Obstetrics and Gynaecology* 2000;40:397–401.

171. Attard CL, Kohli MA, Coleman S, Bradley C, Hux M, Atanackovic G, et al. The burden of illness of severe nausea and vomiting of pregnancy in the United States. *American Journal of Obstetrics and Gynecology* 2002;186:S220–7.

172. Vutyavanich T, Kraisarin T, Ruangsri R. Ginger for nausea and vomiting in pregnancy: randomized, double-masked, placebo-controlled trial. *Obstetrics and Gynecology* 2001;97:577–82.

173. Jewell D, Young G. Interventions for nausea and vomiting in early pregnancy. *Cochrane Database of Systematic Reviews* 2001;(2).

174. Murphy PA. Alternative therapies for nausea and vomiting of pregnancy. *Obstetrics and Gynecology* 1998;91:149–55.

175. Keating A, Chez RA. Ginger syrup as an antiemetic in early pregnancy. *Alternative Therapies in Health and Medicine* 2002;8:89–91.

176. Vickers AJ. Can acupuncture have specific effects on health? A systematic review of acupuncture antiemesis trials. *Journal of the Royal Society of Medicine* 1996;89:303–11.

177. Norheim AJ, Pedersen EJ, Fonnebo V, Berge L. Acupressure treatment of morning sickness in pregnancy. A randomised, double-blind, placebo-controlled study. *Scandinavian Journal of Primary Health Care* 2001;19:43–7.

178. Knight B, Mudge C, Openshaw S, White A, Hart A. Effect of acupuncture on nausea of pregnancy: a randomized, controlled trial. *Obstetrics and Gynecology* 2001;97:184–8.

179. Werntoft E, Dykes AK. Effect of acupressure on nausea and vomiting during pregnancy: a randomized, placebo-controlled, pilot study. *Journal of Reproductive Medicine* 2001;46:835–9.

180. Smith C, Crowther C, Beilby J. Acupuncture to treat nausea and vomiting in early pregnancy: a randomized controlled trial. *Birth* 2002;29:1–9.

181. Smith C, Crowther C, Beilby J. Pregnancy outcome following womens' participation in a randomised controlled trial of acupuncture to treat nausea and vomiting in early pregnancy. *Complementary Therapies in Medicine* 2002;10:78–83.

182. Mazzotta P, Magee LA. A risk – benefit assessment of pharmacological and nonpharmacological treatments for nausea and vomiting of pregnancy. *Drugs* 2000;59:781–800.

183. Magee LA, Mazzotta P, Koren G. Evidence-based view of safety and effectiveness of pharmacologic therapy for nausea and vomiting of pregnancy (NVP). *American Journal of Obstetrics and Gynecology* 2002;186:S256–61.

184. Marrero JM, Goggin PM, Caestecker JS. Determinants of pregnancy heartburn. *British Journal of Obstetrics and Gynaecology* 1992;99:731–4.

185. Knudsen A, Lebech M, Hansen M. Upper gastrointestinal symptoms in the third trimester of the normal pregnancy. *European Journal of Obstetrics Gynecology and Reproductive Biology* 1995;60(1):29–33.

186. Bainbridge ET, Temple JG, Nicholas SP, Newton JR, Boriah V. Symptomatic gastro-esophageal reflux in pregnancy. A comparative study of white Europeans and Asians in Birmingham. *British Journal of Clinical Practice* 1983;37:53–7.

187. Shaw RW. Randomized controlled trial of Syn-Ergel and an active placebo in the treatment of heartburn of pregnancy. *Journal of International Medical Research* 1978;6:147–51.

188. Lang GD, Dougall A. Comparative study of Algicon suspension and magnesium trisilicate mixture in the treatment of reflux dyspepsia of pregnancy. *British Journal of Clinical Practice* 1989;66:48–51.

189. Association of the British Pharmaceutical Industry. *ABPI Compendium of Data Sheets and Summaries of Product Characteristics. Medicines Compendium.* London: Datapharm Communications; 2001.

190. Atlay RD, Parkinson DJ, Entwistle GD, Weekes AR. Treating heartburn in pregnancy: comparison of acid and alkali mixtures. *British Medical Journal* 1978;2:919–20.

191. Rayburn W, Liles E, Christensen H, Robinson M. Antacids vs. antacids plus non-prescription ranitidine for heartburn during pregnancy. *International Journal of Gynaecology and Obstetrics* 1999;66:35–7.

192. Larson JD, Patatanian E, Miner PB Jr, Rayburn WF, Robinson MG. Double-blind, placebo-controlled study of ranitidine for gastroesophageal reflux symptoms during pregnancy. *Obstetrics and Gynecology* 1997;90:83–7.

193. Magee LA, Inocencion G, Kamboj L, Rosetti F, Koren G. Safety of first trimester exposure to histamine H2 blockers. A prospective cohort study. *Digestive Diseases and Sciences* 1996;41:1145–9.

194. Nikfar S, Abdollahi M, Moretti ME, Magee LA, Koren G. Use of proton pump inhibitors during pregnancy and rates of major malformations: a meta-analysis. *Digestive Diseases and Sciences* 2002;47:1526–9.

195. Meyer LC, Peacock JL, Bland JM, Anderson HR. Symptoms and health problems in pregnancy: their association with social factors, smoking, alcohol, caffeine and attitude to pregnancy. *Paediatric and Perinatal Epidemiology* 1994;8:145–55.

196. Jewell DJ, Young G. Interventions for treating constipation in pregnancy. *Cochrane Database of Systematic Reviews* 2003;(1).

197. Abramowitz L, Sobhani I, Benifla JL, Vuagnat A, Darai E, Mignon M, *et al.* Anal fissure and thrombosed external hemorrhoids before and after delivery. *Diseases of the Colon and Rectum* 2002;45:650–5.

198. Wijayanegara H, Mose JC, Achmad L, Sobarna R, Permadi W. A clinical trial of hydroxyethylrutosides in the treatment of haemorrhoids of pregnancy. *Journal of International Medical Research* 1992;20:54–60.

199. Buckshee K, Takkar D, Aggarwal N. Micronized flavonoid therapy in internal hemorrhoids of pregnancy. *International Journal of Gynecology and Obstetrics* 1997;57:145–51.

200. Saleeby RG Jr, Rosen L, Stasik JJ, Riether RD, Sheets J, Khubchandani IT. Hemorrhoidectomy during pregnancy: risk or relief? *Diseases of the Colon and Rectum* 1991;3445:260–1.

201. Thaler E, Huch R, Huch A, Zimmermann R. Compression stockings prophylaxis of emergent varicose veins in pregnancy: A prospective randomised controlled study. *Swiss Medical Weekly* 2001;131:659–62.

202. Gulmezoglu, AM. Interventions for trichomoniasis in pregnancy. *Cochrane Database of Systematic Reviews* 2002;(3). CD000220.

203. French JI, McGregor JA, Draper D, Parker R, McFee J. Gestational bleeding, bacterial vaginosis, and common reproductive tract infections: risk for preterm birth and benefit of treatment. *Obstetrics and Gynecology* 1999;93:715–24.

204. Young GL, Jewell MD. Topical treatment for vaginal candidiasis in pregnancy. *Cochrane Database of Systematic Reviews* 2001;(2).

205. Greenwood CJ, Stainton MC. Back pain/discomfort in pregnancy: invisible and forgotten. *Journal of Perinatal Education* 2001;10:1–12.

206. Kristiansson P, Svardsudd K, von Schoultz B. Back pain during pregnancy: A prospective study. *Spine* 1996;21:702–9.

207. Ostgaard HC, Andersson GBJ, Karlsson K. Prevalence of back pain in pregnancy. *Spine* 1991;16:549–52.

208. Fast A, Shapiro D, Ducommun EJ, Friedman LW, Bouklas T, Floman Y. Low-back pain in pregnancy. *Spine* 1987;12:368–71.

209. Stapleton DB, MacLennan AH, Kristiansson P. The prevalence of recalled low back pain during and after pregnancy: A South Australian population survey. *Australian and New Zealand Journal of Obstetrics and Gynaecology* 2002;42:482–5.

210. Mantle MJ, Greenwood RM, Currey HL. Backache in pregnancy. *Rheumatology and Rehabilitation* 1977;16:95–101.

211. Young G, Jewell, D. Interventions for preventing and treating pelvic and back pain in pregnancy. *Cochrane Database of Systematic Reviews* 2003;(1).

212. Field T, Hernandez-Reif M, Hart S, Theakston H, Schanberg S, Kuhn C. Pregnant women benefit from massage therapy. *Journal of Psychosomatic Obstetrics and Gynecology* 1999;20:31–8.

213. Ostgaard HC, Zetherstrom G, Roos-Hansson E, Svanberg B. Reduction of back and posterior pelvic pain in pregnancy. *Spine* 1994;19:894–900.

214. Noren L, Ostgaard S, Nielsen TF, Ostgaard HC. Reduction of sick leave for lumbar back and posterior pelvic pain in pregnancy. *Spine* 1997;22:2157–60.

215. Tesio L, Raschi A, Meroni M. Autotraction treatment for low-back pain in pregnancy: A pilot study. *Clinical Rehabilitation* 1994;8:314–19.

216. Guadagnino MR III. Spinal manipulative therapy for 12 pregnant patients suffering from low back pain. *Chiropractic Technique* 1999;11:108–11.

217. McIntyre IN, Broadhurst NA. Effective treatment of low back pain in pregnancy. *Australian Family Physician* 1996;25:S65–7.

218. Requejo SM, Barnes R, Kulig K, Landel R, Gonzalez S. The use of a modified classification system in the treatment of low back pain during pregnancy: A case report. *Journal of Orthopaedic and Sports Physical Therapy* 2002;32:318–26.

219. Owens K, Pearson A, Mason G. Symphysis pubis dysfunction: a cause of significant obstetric morbidity. *European Journal of Obstetrics Gynecology and Reproductive Biology* 2002;105:143–6.

220. Fry D, Hay-Smith J, Hough J, McIntosh J, Polden M, Shepherd J, *et al.* National clinic guideline for the care of women with symphysis pubis dysfunction. *Midwives* 1997;110:172–3.

221. Gould JS, Wissinger HA. Carpal tunnel syndrome in pregnancy. *Southern Medical Journal* 1978;71:144–5,154.

222. Voitk AJ, Mueller JC, Farlinger DE, Johnston RU. Carpal tunnel syndrome in pregnancy. *Canadian Medical Association Journal* 1983;128:277–81.

223. Padua L, Aprile I, Caliandro P, Carboni T, Meloni A, Massi S, *et al.* Symptoms and neurophysiological picture of carpal tunnel syndrome in pregnancy. *Clinical Neurophysiology* 2001;112:1946–51.

224. Courts RB. Splinting for symptoms of carpal tunnel syndrome during pregnancy. *Journal of Hand Therapy* 1995;8:31–4.

225. Ekman-Ordeberg G, Salgeback S, Ordeberg G. Carpal tunnel syndrome in pregnancy. A prospective study. *Acta Obstetricia et Gynecologica Scandinavica* 1987;66:233–5.

226. Stahl S, Blumenfeld Z, Yarnitsky D. Carpal tunnel syndrome in pregnancy: Indications for early surgery. *Journal of the Neurological Sciences* 1996;136:182–4.

227. Dawes MG, Grudzinskas JG. Repeated measurement of maternal weight during pregnancy. Is this a useful practice? *British Journal of Obstetrics and Gynaecology* 1991;98:189–94.

228. National Academy of Sciences, Institute of Medicine, Food and Nutrition Board, Committee on Nutritional Status During Pregnancy and Lactation, Subcommittee on Dietary Intake and Nutrient Supplements During Pregnancy, Subcommittee on Nutritional Status and Weight Gain During Pregnancy. *Nutrition during pregnancy*. Washington DC: National Academy Press; 1990.

229. Siega-Riz AM, Adair LS, Hobel CJ. Maternal underweight status and inadequate rate of weight gain during the third trimester of pregnancy increases the risk of preterm delivery. *Journal of Nutrition* 1996;126:146–53.

230. Bergmann MM, Flagg EW, Miracle-McMahill HL, Boeing H. Energy intake and net weight gain in pregnant women according to body mass index (BMI) status. *International Journal of Obesity and Related Metabolic Disorders* 1997;21:1010–7.

231. Alexander JM, Grant AM, Campbell MJ. Randomised controlled trial of breast shells and Hoffman's exercises for inverted and non-protractile nipples. *British Medical Journal* 1992;304:1030–2.

232. Pattinson RE. Pelvimetry for fetal cephalic presentations at term. *Cochrane Database of Systematic Reviews* 2001;(3). 2001.

233. Lenihan JP Jr. Relationship of antepartum pelvic examinations to premature rupture of the membranes. *Obstetrics and Gynecology* 1984;83:33–7.

234. Goffinet F. [Ovarian cyst and pregnancy]. [French]. *Journal de Gynecologie, Obstetrique et Biologie de la Reproduction* 2001;30:4S100–8.

235. O'Donovan P, Gupta JK, Savage J, Thornton JG, Lilford RJ. Is routine antenatal booking vaginal examination necessary for reasons other than cervical cytology if ultrasound examination is planned? *British Journal of Obstetrics and Gynaecology* 1988;95:556–9.

236. World Health Organization. *Female genital mutilation.* WHO Information Fact Sheet No. 241. Geneva: World Health Organization; 2000.

237. British Medical Association. *Female genital mutilation: caring for patients and child protection.* London: BMA; 2001.

238. Momoh C, Ladhani S, Lochrie DP, Rymer J. Female genital mutilation: Analysis of the first twelve months of a southeast London specialist clinic. *BJOG* 2001;108:186–91.

239. World Health Organization. *A systematic review of the health complications of female genital mutilation including sequelae in childbirth.* Geneva: WHO; 2000.

240. McCaffrey M, Jankowska A, Gordon H. Management of female genital mutilation: The Northwick Park Hospital experience. *British Journal of Obstetrics and Gynaecology* 1995;102:787–90.

241. Jordan JA. Female genital mutilation (female circumcision). *British Journal of Obstetrics and Gynaecology* 1994;101:94–5.

242. British Medical Association. *Domestic violence: a health care issue?* London: BMA; 1998.

243. Tjaden P, Thoennes N. *Full report of the prevalence, incidence, and consequences of violence against women. Findings from the National Violence Against Women Survey. NCJ 183781, 1–61*. Washington DC: US Department of Justice, National Institute of Justice; 2000.

244. Canadian Centre for Justice Statistics. *Family violence in Canada: A statistical profile 2002*. 85-224-XIE. Ottawa: Statistics Canada; 2002. [www.statcan.ca/english/IPS/Data/85-224-XIE.htm] Accessed 20 August 2003.

245. Jones AS, Carlson Gielen A, Campbell JC. Annual and lifetimes prevalence of partner abuse in a sample of female HMO enrollees. *Women's Health Issues* 1999;9:295–305.

246. Ballard TJ, Saltzman LE, Gazmararian JA, Spitz AM, Lazorick S, Marks JS. Violence during pregnancy: measurement issues. *American Journal of Public Health* 1998;88:274–6.

247. Royal College of Obstetricians and Gynaecologists. *Violence against women*. London: RCOG Press; 1997.

248. Johnson JK, Haider F, Ellis K, Hay DM, Lindow SW. The prevalence of domestic violence in pregnant women. *BJOG* 2003;110:272–5.

249. Newberger EH, Barkan SE, Lieberman ES, McCormick MC, Yllo K, Gary LT, *et al*. Abuse of pregnant women and adverse birth outcome: current knowledge and implications for practice. *Journal of the American Medical Association* 1992;267:2370–2.

250. Murphy CC, Schei B, Myhr TL, Du MJ. Abuse: a risk factor for low birth weight? A systematic review and meta-analysis. [see comments]. *Canadian Medical Association Journal* 2001;164:1567–72.

251. Cokkinides VE, Coker AL, Sanderson M, Addy C, Bethea L. Physical violence during pregnancy: maternal complications and birth outcomes. *Obstetrics and Gynecology* 1999;93:661–6.

252. Janssen PA, Holt VL, Sugg NK, Emanuel I, Critchlow CM, Henderson AD. Intimate partner violence and adverse pregnancy outcomes: A population-based study. *American Journal of Obstetrics and Gynecology* 2003;188:1341–7.

253. Royal College of Midwives. *Domestic abuse in pregnancy*. London: RCM; 1999.

254. Royal College of Psychiatrists. *Domestic violence*. CR102. London: RCPsych; 2002.

255. Wathen CN, MacMillan HL. Interventions for violence against women. Scientific review. *JAMA* 2003;289:589–600.

256. Ramsay J, Richardson J, Carter YH, Davidson LL, Feder G. Should health professionals screen women for domestic violence? Systematic review. *British Medical Journal* 2002;325:314–18.

257. Cann K, Withnell S, Shakespeare J, Doll H, Thomas J. Domestic violence: a comparative survey of levels of detection, knowledge, and attitudes in healthcare workers. *Public Health* 2001;115:89–95.

258. Department of Health. *Domestic violence: A resource manual for health care professionals*. London: Department of Health; 2000.

259. Wilson LM, Reid AJ, Midmer DK, Biringer A, Carroll JC, Stewart DE. Antenatal psychosocial risk factors associated with adverse postpartum family outcomes. *Canadian Medical Association Journal* 1996;154:785–99.

260. Perkin MR, Bland JM. The effect of anxiety and depression during pregnancy on obstetric complications. *British Journal of Obstetrics and Gynaecology* 1993;100:629–34.

261. Dayan J, Creveuil C, Herlicoviez M. Role of anxiety and depression in the onset of spontaneous preterm labor. *American Journal of Epidemiology* 2002;155:293–301.

262. Lundy BL, Jones NA, Field T. Prenatal depression effects on neonates. *Infant Behavior and Development* 1999;22:119–29.

263. Murray D, Cox JL. Screening for depression during pregnancy with the Edinburgh Depression Scale (EPDS). *Journal of Reproductive and Infant Psychology* 1990;8:99–107.

264. Bolton HL, Hughes PM, Turton P. Incidence and demographic correlates of depressive symptoms during pregnancy in an inner London population. *Journal of Psychosomatic Obstetrics and Gynecology* 1998;19:202–9.

265. Evans J, Heron J, Francomb H, Oke S, Golding J. Cohort study of depressed mood during pregnancy and after childbirth. *British Medical Journal* 2001;323:257–60.

266. Austin M-P, Lumley J. Antenatal screening for postnatal depression: a systematic review. *Acta Psychiatrica Scandinavica* 2003;107:10–17.

267. Hayes BA, Muller R, Bradley BS. Perinatal depression: a randomized controlled trial of an antenatal education intervention for primiparas. *Birth* 2001;28:28–35.

268. Brugha TS, Wheatly S, Taub NA, Culverwell A, Friedman T, Kirwan P. Pragmatic randomized trial of an antenatal intervention to prevent post-natal depression by reducing psychosocial risk factors. *Psychological Medicine* 2000;30:1273–81.

269. Hytten F. Blood volume changes in normal pregnancy. *Clinical Haematology* 1985;14:601–12.

270. Ramsey M, James D, Steer P, Weiner C, Gornik B. *Normal values in pregnancy*. 2nd ed. London: WB Saunders; 2000.

271. Steer P, Alam MA, Wadsworth J, Welch A. Relation between maternal haemoglobin concentration and birth weight in different ethnic groups. *British Medical Journal* 1995;310:489–91.

272. Zhou LM, Yang WW, Hua JZ, Deng CQ, Tao X, Stoltzfus RJ. Relation of hemoglobin measured at different times in pregnancy to preterm birth and low birth weight in Shanghai, China. *American Journal of Epidemiology* 1998;148:998–1006.

273. Breymann C. Iron supplementation during pregnancy. *Fetal and Maternal Medicine Review* 2002;13:1–29.

274. Cuervo LG, Mahomed K. Treatments for iron deficiency anaemia during pregnancy. *Cochrane Database of Systematic Reviews* 2001;(2).

275. Davies SC, Cronin E, Gill M, Greengross P, Hickman M, Normand C. Screening for sickle cell disease and thalassaemia: a systematic review with supplementary research. *Health Technology Assessment* 2000;4:1–119.

276. Modell B, Harris R, Lane B, Khan M, Darlison M, Petrou M, *et al*. Informed choice in genetic screening for thalassaemia during pregnancy: audit from a national confidential inquiry. *British Medical Journal* 2000;320:337–41.

277. Modell B, Petrou M, Layton M, Varnavides L, Slater C, Ward RH, *et al*. Audit of prenatal diagnosis for haemoglobin disorders in the United Kingdom: the first 20 years. [see comments]. *British Medical Journal* 1997;315:779–84.

278. Department of Health. *Sickle cell, thalassaemia and other haemoglobinopathies. Report of a Working Party of the Standing Medical Advisory Committee*. London: DoH; 1999.

279. Zeuner D, Ades AE, Karnon J, Brown JE, Dezateux C, Anionwu EN. Antenatal and neonatal haemoglobinopathy screening in the UK: review and economic analysis. *Health Technology Assessment* 1999;3(11):1–186.

280. Streetly A. A national screening policy for sickle cell disease and thalassaemia major for the United Kingdom. Questions are left after two evidence based reports. *British Medical Journal* 2000;320:1353–4.

281. Aspinall PJ, Dyson SM, Anionwu EN. The feasibility of using ethnicity as a primary tool for antenatal selective screening for sickle cell disorders: pointers from the research evidence. *Social Science and Medicine* 2003;56:285–97.

282. Petrou M, Brugiatelli M, Ward RHT, Modell B. Factors affecting the uptake of prenatal diagnosis for sickle cell disease. *Journal of Medical Genetics* 1992;29:820–3.

283. Modell B, Ward RH, Fairweather DV. Effect of introducing antenatal diagnosis on reproductive behaviour of families at risk for thalassaemia major. *British Medical Journal* 1980;280:1347–50.

284. Ahmed S, Saleem M, Sultana N, Raashid Y, Waqar A, Anwar M, *et al.* Prenatal diagnosis of beta-thalassaemia in Pakistan: experience in a Muslim country. *Prenatal Diagnosis* 2000;20:378–83.

285. UK Blood Transfusion Services. Guidelines for the Blood Transfusion Service. 6th ed. London; TSO; 2002. [www.transfusionguidelines.org.uk/uk_guidelines/ukbts6_$01.html] Accessed 20 August 2003.

286. Whittle MJ. Antenatal serology testing in pregnancy. *British Journal of Obstetrics and Gynaecology* 1996;103:195–6.

287. Brouwers HA, Overbeeke MA, van E, I, Schaasberg W, Alsbach GP, van der HC, *et al.* What is the best predictor of the severity of ABO-haemolytic disease of the newborn? *Lancet* 1988;2:641–4.

288. Mollison PL, Engelfriet CP, Contreras M. *Haemolytic disease of the fetus and newborn. Blood transfusion in clinical medicine.* Oxford: Blackwell Science. 1997. p. 390–424.

289. Shanwell A, Sallander S, Bremme K, Westgren M. Clinical evaluation of a solid-phase test for red cell antibody screening of pregnant women. *Transfusion* 1999;39:26–31.

290. Filbey D, Hanson U, Wesstrom G. The prevalence of red cell antibodies in pregnancy correlated to the outcome of the newborn: a 12 year study in central Sweden. *Acta Obstetrica et Gynecologica Scandinavica* 1995;74:687–92.

291. British Committee for Standards in Haematology, Blood Transfusion Task Force. Guidelines for blood grouping and red cell antibody testing during pregnancy. *Transfusion Medicine* 1996;6:71–4.

292. National Institute for Clinical Excellence. *Guidance on the use of routine antenatal anti-D prophylaxis for RhD-negative women.* Technology Appraisal Guidance, No. 41. London: National Institute for Clinical Excellence; 2002. [www.nice.org.uk/pdf/prophylaxisFinalguidance.pdf] Accessed 20 August 2003.

293. Royal College of Obstetricians and Gynaecologists. *Ultrasound screening for fetal abnormalities: report of the RCOG working party.* London: RCOG Press; 1997.

294. Jepsen RG, Forbes CA, Sowden AJ, Lewis RA. Increasing informed uptake and non-uptake of screening: evidence from a systematic review. *Health Expectations* 2001;4:116–26.

295. Department of Health, social Services and Public Safety, Northern Ireland, National Assembly for Wales, Scottish Executive, Department of Health. *Second report of the UK National Screening Committee.* London: DoH; 2000. [www.nsc.nhs.uk/pdfs/secondreport.pdf] Accessed 21 August 2003.

296. Royal College of Obstetricians and Gynaecologists. *Report of the RCOG working party on biochemical markers and the detection of Down's syndrome.* London: Royal College of Obstetricians and Gynaecologists; 1993.

297. Bricker L, Garcia J, Henderson J, Mugford M, Neilson J, Roberts T, *et al.* Ultrasound screening in pregnancy: a systematic review of the clinical effectiveness, cost-effectiveness and women's views. *Health Technology Assessment* 2000;4:1–193.

298. Williamson P, Alberman E, Rodeck C, Fiddler M, Church S, Harris R. Antecedent circumstances surrounding neural tube defect births in 1990–1991. *British Journal of Obstetrics and Gynaecology* 1997;104:51–6.

299. Saari-Kemppainen A, Karjalainen O, Ylostalo P, Heinonen OP. Fetal anomalies in a controlled one-stage ultrasound screening trial. A report from the Helsinki Ultrasound Trial. *Journal of Perinatal Medicine* 1994;22(4):279–289.

300. Whitlow BJ, Chatzipapas IK, Lazanakis ML, Kadir RA, Economides DL. The value of sonography in early pregnancy for the detection of fetal abnormalities in an unselected population. *British Journal of Obstetrics and Gynaecology* 1999;106:929–36.

301. National Assembly for Wales/Velindre NHS Trust Antenatal Project Team Steering Board. *Choices: Recommendations for the provision and management of antenatal screening in Wales.* Cardiff: Velindre NHS Trust; March 2002. [www.velindre-tr.wales.nhs.uk/antenatal/consult_doc/choices.pdf] Accessed 21 August 2003.

302. Royal College of Obstetricians and Gynaecologists. *Routine ultrasound screening in pregnancy, protocols, standards and training. Supplement to ultrasound screening for fetal abnormalities. Report of the RCOG Working Party.* London: RCOG Press; 2000.

303. Office for National Statistics. *Child health statistics.* London: National Statistics; 2000. p. 1–26.

304. Noble J. Natural history of Down's syndrome: a brief review for those involved in antenatal screening. *Journal of Medical Screening* 1998;5:172–7.

305. Marteau TM, Dormandy E. Facilitating informed choice in prenatal testing: how well are we doing? *American Journal of Medical Genetics* 2001;106:185–90.

306. Smith DK, Shaw RW, Marteau TM. Informed consent to undergo serum screening for Down's syndrome: the gap between policy and practice. *British Medical Journal* 1994;309:776.

307. Royal College of Obstetricians and Gynaecologists. *Amniocentesis.* Guideline No. 8. London: Royal College of Obstetricians and Gynaecologists; 2000.

308. Deeks JJ. Systematic reviews of evaluations of diagnostic and screening tests. *British Medical Journal* 2001;323:157–62.

309. Lijmer JG, Mol BW, Heisterkamp S, Bonsel GJ, Prins MH, van der Meulen JH, *et al.* Empirical evidence of design-related bias in studies of diagnostic tests. *JAMA* 1999;282:1061–6.

310. Hook EB. Spontaneous deaths of fetuses with chromosomal abnormalities diagnosed prenatally. *New England Journal of Medicine* 1978;299:1036–8.

311. Morris JK, Mutton DE, Alberman E. Revised estimates of the maternal age specific live birth prevalence of Down's syndrome. *Journal of Medical Screening* 2002;9:2–6.

312. Paranjothy S, Thomas J. National Sentinel Caesarean Section Audit. *MIDIRS Midwifery Digest* 2001;11:S13–15.

313. Wald NJ, Huttly WJ, Hennessy CF. Down's syndrome screening in the UK in 1998. *Lancet* 1999;354:1264.

314. Youings S, Gregson N, Jacobs P. The efficacy of maternal age screening for Down's syndrome in Wessex. *Prenatal Diagnosis* 1991;11:419–25.

315. Smith-Bindman R, Hosmer W, Feldstein VA, Deeks JJ, Goldberg JD. Second-trimester ultrasound to detect fetuses with Down's syndrome. *JAMA* 2001;285:1044–55.

316. Wald NJ, Rodeck C, Hackshaw AK, Walters J, Chitty L, Mackinson AM. First and second trimester antenatal screening for Down's syndrome: the results of the serum, urine and ultrasound screening study (SURUSS). *Health Technology Assessment* 2003;7:1–88.

317. Bindra R, Heath V, Nicolaides KH. Screening for chromosomal defects by fetal nuchal translucency at 11 to 14 weeks. *Clinical Obstetrics and Gynecology* 2002;45:661–70.

318. Niemimaa M, Suonpaa M, Perheentupa A, Seppala M, Heinonen S, Laitinen P, *et al.* Evaluation of first trimester maternal serum and ultrasound screening for Down's syndrome in Eastern and Northern Finland. *European Journal of Human Genetics* 2001;9:404–8.

319. Wald NJ, Kennard A, Hackshaw A, McGuire A. Antenatal screening for Down's syndrome. *Health Technology Assessment* 1998;2:1–112.

320. Conde-Agudelo A, Kafury-Goeta AC. Triple-marker test as screening for Down syndrome: a meta-analysis. *Obstetrical and Gynecological Survey* 1998;53:369–76.

321. Wald NJ, Huttly WJ, Hackshaw AK. Antenatal screening for Down's syndrome with the quadruple test. *Lancet* 2003;361:835–6.

322. Spencer K, Spencer CE, Power M, Dawson C, Nicolaides KH. Screening for chromosomal abnormalities in the first trimester using ultrasound and maternal serum biochemistry in a one-stop clinic: a review of three years prospective experience. *BJOG* 2003;110:281–6.

323. Alfirevic Z, Gosden C, Neilson, JP. Chorion villus sampling versus amniocentesis for prenatal diagnosis. *Cochrane Database of Systematic Reviews* 1998;(4):1–8.

324. Alfirevic, Z. Early amniocentesis versus transabdominal chorion villus sampling. *Cochrane Database of Systematic Reviews* 2000;(1), 1.

325. Tercyak KP, Johnson SB, Roberts SF, Cruz AC. Psychological response to prenatal genetic counseling and amniocentesis. *Patient Education and Counseling* 2001;43:73–84.

326. Green JM. Women's experiences of prenatal screening and diagnosis. In: Abramsky L, Chapple J, editors. Prenatal diagnosis: the human side. London: Chapman and Hall; 1994. p. 37–53.

327. Liu S, Joseph KS, Kramer MS, Allen AC, Sauve R, Rusen ID, *et al.* Relationship of prenatal diagnosis and pregnancy termination to overall infant mortality in Canada. *JAMA* 2002;287:1561–7.

328. Whalley P. Bacteriuria of pregnancy. *American Journal of Obstetrics and Gynecology* 1967;97:723–38.

329. Little PJ. The incidence of urinary infection in 5000 pregnant women. *Lancet* 1966;2:925–8.

330. Campbell-Brown M, McFadyen IR, Seal DV, Stephenson ML. Is screening for bacteriuria in pregnancy worth while? *British Medical Journal* 1987;294:1579–82.

331. Foley ME, Farquharson R, Stronge JM. Is screening for bacteriuria in pregnancy worthwhile? *British Medical Journal* 1987;295:270.

332. LeBlanc AL, McGanity WJ. The impact of bacteriuria in pregnancy: a survey of 1300 pregnant patients. *Biologie Medicale* 1964;22:336–47.

333. Kincaid-Smith P, Bullen M. Bacteriuria in pregnancy. *Lancet* 1965;395–9.

334. Thomsen AC, Morup L, Hansen KB. Antibiotic elimination of group-B streptococci in urine in prevention of preterm labour. *Lancet* 1987;591–3.

335. Elder HA, Santamarina BAG, Smith S, Kass EH. The natural history of asymptomatic bacteriuria during pregnancy: the effect of tetracycline on the clinical course and the outcome of pregnancy. *American Journal of Obstetrics and Gynecology* 1971;111:441–62.

336. Gold EM, Traub FB, Daichman I, Terris M. Asymptomatic bacteriuria during pregnancy. *Obstetrics and Gynecology* 1966;27:206–9.

337. Mulla N. Bacteriuria in Pregnancy. *Obstetrics and Gynecology* 1960;16:89–92.

338. Savage WE, Hajj SN, Kass EH. Demographic and prognostic characteristics of bacteriuria in pregnancy. *Medicine* 1967;46:385–407.

339. Mittendorf R, Williams MA, Kass EH. Prevention of preterm delivery and low birth weight associated with asymptomatic bacteriuria. *Clinical Infectious Diseases* 1992;14:927–32.

340. Patterson TF, Andriole VT. Bacteriuria in pregnancy. *Infectious Disease Clinics of North America* 1987;1:807–22.

341. Screening for asymptomatic bacteriuria, hematuria and proteinuria. The US Preventive Services Task Force. *American Family Physician* 1990;42:389–95.

342. Etherington IJ, James DK. Reagent strip testing of antenatal urine specimens for infection. *British Journal of Obstetrics and Gynaecology* 1993;100:806–8.

343. Shelton SD, Boggess KA, Kirvan K, Sedor F, Herbert WN. Urinary interleukin-8 with asymptomatic bacteriuria in pregnancy. *Obstetrics and Gynecology* 2001;97:583–6.

344. Millar L, Debuque L, Leialoha C, Grandinetti A, Killeen J. Rapid enzymatic urine screening test to detect bacteriuria in pregnancy. *Obstetrics and Gynecology* 2000;95:601–4.

345. McNair RD, MacDonald SR, Dooley SL, Peterson LR. Evaluation of the centrifuged and Gram-stained smear, urinalysis, and

reagent strip testing to detect asymptomatic bacteriuria in obstetric patients. *American Journal of Obstetrics and Gynecology* 2000;182:1076–9.

346. Robertson AW, Duff P. The nitrite and leukocyte esterase tests for the evaluation of asymptomatic bacteriuria in obstetric patients. *Obstetrics and Gynecology* 1988;71:878–81.

347. Bachman JW, Heise RH, Naessens JM, Timmerman MG. A study of various tests to detect asymptomatic urinary tract infections in an obstetric population. *JAMA* 1993;270:1971–4.

348. Tincello DG, Richmond DH. Evaluation of reagent strips in detecting asymptomatic bacteriuria in early pregnancy: prospective case series. *British Medical Journal* 1998;316:435–7.

349. Abyad A. Screening for asymptomatic bacteriuria in pregnancy: urinalysis vs. urine culture. *Journal of Family Practice* 1991;33:471–4.

350. Graninger W, Fleischmann D, Schneeweiss B, Aram L, Stockenhuber F. Rapid screening for bacteriuria in pregnancy. *Infection* 1992;20:9–11.

351. Smaill, F. Antibiotic treatment for symptomatic bacteriuria: antibiotic vs. no treatment for asymptomatic bacteriuria in pregnancy. *Cochrane Database of Systematic Reviews* 2002;(3):1–5.

352. Villar J, Lydon-Rochelle MT, Gulmezoglu AM. Duration of treatment for asymptomatic bacteriuria during pregnancy. *Cochrane Database of Systematic Reviews* 2001;(2).

353. Centers for Disease Control and Prevention. Sexually transmitted diseases treatment guidelines 2002. *Morbidity and Mortality Weekly Report* 2002;51:1–80.

354. Joesoef M, Schmid G. Bacterial vaginosis. *Clinical Evidence* 2002;7:1400–8.

355. Goldenberg RL, Klebanoff MA, Nugent R, Krohn MA, Hilliers S, Andrews WW. Bacterial colonization of the vagina during pregnancy in four ethnic groups. Vaginal Infections and Prematurity Study Group. *American Journal of Obstetrics and Gynecology* 1996;174:1618–21.

356. Hay PE, Morgan DJ, Ison CA, Bhide SA, Romney M, McKenzie P, *et al.* A longitudinal study of bacterial vaginosis during pregnancy. *British Journal of Obstetrics and Gynaecology* 1994;101:1048–53.

357. Flynn CA, Helwig AL, Meurer LN. Bacterial vaginosis in pregnancy and the risk of prematurity: a meta-analysis. *Journal of Family Practice* 1999;48:885–92.

358. Gratacos E, Figueras F, Barranco M, Vila J, Cararach V, Alonso PL, *et al.* Spontaneous recovery of bacterial vaginosis during pregnancy is not associated with an improved perinatal outcome. *Acta Obstetricia et Gynecologica Scandinavica* 1998;77:37–40.

359. Amsel R, Totten PA, Spiegel CA. Nonspecific vaginitis: diagnostic criteria and microbial and epidemiological associations. *American Journal of Medicine* 1983;74:14–22.

360. Nugent RP, Krohn MA, Hillier SL. Reliability of diagnosing bacterial vaginosis is improved by a standardised methods of Gram stain interpretation. *Journal of Clinical Microbiology* 1991;29:297–301.

361. Thiagarajan M. Evaluation of the use of yogurt in treating bacterial vaginosis in pregnancy. *Journal of Clinical Epidemiology* 1998;51:22S.

362. McDonald H, Brocklehurst P, Parsons J, Vigneswaran R. Interventions for treating bacterial vaginosis in pregnancy. *Cochrane Database of Systematic Reviews* 2003;(2):1–30.

363. Ugwumadu A, Manyonda I, Reid F, Hay P. Effect of early oral clindamycin on late miscarriage and preterm delivery in asymptomatic women with abnormal vaginal flora and bacterial vaginosis: a randomised controlled trial. *Lancet* 2003;361:983–8.

364. Stary A. European guideline for the management of chlamydial infection. *International Journal of STD and AIDS* 2001;12:30–3.

365. Preece PM, Ades A, Thompson RG, Brooks JH. Chlamydia trachomatis infection in late pregnancy: A prospective study. *Paediatric and Perinatal Epidemiology* 1989;3:268–77.

366. Goh BT, Morgan-Capner P, Lim KS. Chlamydial screening of pregnant women in a sexually transmitted diseases clinic. *British Journal of Venereal Diseases* 1982;58:327–9.

367. Association of chlamydia trachomatis and mycoplasma hominis with intrauterine growth restriction and preterm delivery. The John Hopkins Study of Cervicitis and Adverse Pregnancy Outcome. *American Journal of Epidemiology* 1989;129:1247–51.

368. Ryan GM, Jr, Abdella TN, McNeeley SG, Baselski VS, Drummond DE. Chlamydia trachomatis infection in pregnancy and effect of treatment on outcome. [see comments.]. *American Journal of Obstetrics and Gynecology* 1990;162:34–9.

369. Brocklehurst P, Rooney G. Interventions for treating genital chlamydia trachomatis infection in pregnancy. *Cochrane Database of Systematic Reviews* 2002;(3).

370. Preece PM, Anderson JM, Thompson RG. Chlamydia trachomatis infection in infants: A prospective study. *Archives of Disease in Childhood* 1989;64:525–9.

371. Schachter J, Grossman M, Sweet RL, Holt J, Jordan C, Bishop E. Prospective study of perinatal transmission of Chlamydia trachomatis. *JAMA* 1986;255:3374–7.

372. FitzGerald MR, Welch J, Robinson AJ, Ahmed-Jushuf IH. Clinical guidelines and standards for the management of uncomplicated genital chlamydial infection. *International Journal of STD and AIDS* 1998;9:253–62.

373. Scottish Intercollegiate Guidelines Network. *Management of genital Chlamydia trachomatis Infection.* SIGN Publication No. 42. Edinburgh: Scottish Intercollegiate Guideline Network; 2000.

374. Ryan M, Miller E, Waight P. Cytomegalovirus infection in England and Wales: 1992 and 1993. *Communicable Diseases Report* 1995;5:R74–6.

375. Preece PM, Tookey P, Ades A, Peckham CS. Congenital cytomegalovirus infection: predisposing maternal factors. *Journal of Epidemiology and Community Health* 1986;40:205–9.

376. Peckham CS, Coleman JC, Hurley R, Chin KS, Henderson K, Preece PM. Cytomegalovirus infection in pregnancy: preliminary findings from a prospective study. *Lancet* 1983;1352–5.

377. Bolyard EA, Tablan OC, Williams WW, Pearson ML, Shapiro CN, Deitchmann SD. Guideline for infection control in health care personnel. Centers for Disease Control and Prevention. *Infection Control and Hospital Epidemiology* 1998;19:407–63. Erratum 1998;19:493

378. Stagno S, Whitley RJ. Herpesvirus infections of pregnancy. Part 1: Cytomegalovirus and Epstein-Barr virus infections. *New England Journal of Medicine* 1985;313:1270–4.

379. Boxall E, Skidmore S, Evans C, Nightingale S. The prevalence of hepatitis B and C in an antenatal population of various ethnic origins. *Epidemiology and Infection* 1994;113:523–8.

380. Brook MG, Lever AM, Kelly D, Rutter D, Trompeter RS, Griffiths P, *et al.* Antenatal screening for hepatitis B is medically and economically effective in the prevention of vertical transmission: three years experience in a London hospital. *Quarterly Journal of Medicine* 1989;71:313–7.

381. Chrystie I, Sumner D, Palmer S, Kenney A, Banatvala J. Screening of pregnant women for evidence of current hepatitis B infection: selective or universal? *Health Trends* 1992;24:13–5.

382. Derso A, Boxall EH, Tarlow MJ, Flewett TH. Transmission of HBsAg from mother to infant in four ethnic groups. *British Medical Journal* 1978;15(6118):949–952.

383. Beasley RP, Trepo C, Stevens CE, Szmuness W. The e antigen and vertical transmission of hepatitis B surface antigen. *American Journal of Epidemiology* 1977;105:94–8.

384. Beasley RP, Hwang L-Y. Epidemiology of hepatocellular carcinoma. In: Vyas GN, Dienstag JL, Hoofnagle JH, editors. *Viral hepatitis and liver disease.* Orlando, FL: Grune and Stratton; 1984. p. 209–24.

385. Ramsay M, Gay N, Balogun K, Collins M. Control of hepatitis B in the United Kingdom. *Vaccine* 1998;16 Suppl:S52–5.

386. Sehgal A, Sehgal R, Gupta I, Bhakoo ON, Ganguly NK. Use of hepatitis B vaccine alone or in combination with hepatitis B immunoglobulin for immunoprophylaxis of perinatal hepatitis B infection. *Journal of Tropical Pediatrics* 1992;38:247–51.

387. Wong VC, Ip HM, Reesink HW, Lelie PN, Reerink-Brongers EE, Yeung CY, *et al.* Prevention of the HBsAg carrier state in newborn infants of mothers who are chronic carriers of HBsAg and HBeAg by administration of hepatitis-B vaccine and hepatitis-B immunoglobulin. Double-blind randomised placebo – controlled study. *Lancet* 1984;1:921–6.

388. Zhu Q. A preliminary study on interruption of HBV transmission in uterus. *Chinese Medical Journal* 1997;110:145–7.

389. Lo K, Tsai Y, Lee S, Yeh C, Wang J, Chiang BN, *et al.* Combined passive and active immunization for interruption of perinatal transmission of hepatitis B virus in Taiwan. *Hepato-gastroenterology* 1985;32:65–8.

390. Beasley RP, Hwang LY, Lee GC, Lan CC, Roan CH, Huang FY, *et al.* Prevention of perinatally transmitted hepatitis B virus infections with hepatitis B virus infections with hepatitis B immune globulin and hepatitis B vaccine. *Lancet* 1983;2:1099–102.

391. Nair PV, Weissman JY, Tong MJ, Thursby MW, Paul RH, Henneman CE. Efficacy of hepatitis B immune globulin in prevention of perinatal transmission of the hepatitis B virus. *Gastroenterology* 1984;87:293–8.

392. Xu Z-Y, Liu C-B, Francis DP. Prevention of perinatal acquisition of hepatitis B virus carriage using vaccine: preliminary report of a randomized, double-blind placebo-controlled and comparative trial. *Pediatrics* 1985;76:713–18.

393. Balmer S, Bowens A, Bruce E, Farrar H, Jenkins C, Williams R. *Quality management for screening: report to the National Screening Committee.* Leeds: Nuffield Institute for Health; 2000.

394. Summers PR, Biswas MK, Pastorek JG, Pernoll ML, Smith LG, Bean BE. The pregnant hepatitis B carrier: evidence favoring comprehensive antepartum screening. *Obstetrics and Gynecology* 1987;69:701–4.

395. Chaita TM, Graham SM, Maxwell SM, Sirivasin W, Sabchareon A, Beeching NJ. Salivary sampling for hepatitis B surface antigen carriage: a sensitive technique suitable for epidemiological studies. *Annals of Tropical Paediatrics* 1995;15:135–9.

396. Pembrey L, Newell ML, Tovo PA. Hepatitis C virus infection in pregnant women and their children. *Italian Journal of Gynaecology and Obstetrics* 2000;12:21–8.

397. Whittle M, Peckham C, Anionwu E, *et al.* Antenatal screening for hepatitis C. Working party report on screening for hepatitis C in the UK. January 2002. [www.nelh.nhs.uk/screening/antenatal_pps/Hep_C_NSC.pdf] Accessed 4 September 2003.

398. Ades AE, Parker S, Walker J, Cubitt WD, Jones R. HCV prevalence in pregnant women in the UK. *Epidemiology and Infection* 2000;125:399–405.

399. Okamoto M, Nagata I, Murakami J, Kaji S, Iitsuka T, Hoshika T, *et al.* Prospective reevaluation of risk factors in mother-to-child transmission of hepatitis C virus: high virus load, vaginal delivery, and negative anti-NS4 antibody. *Journal of Infectious Diseases* 2000;182:1511–4.

400. Tajiri H, Miyoshi Y, Funada S, Etani Y, Abe J, Onodera T, *et al.* Prospective study of mother-to-infant transmission of hepatitis C virus. *Pediatric Infectious Disease Journal* 2001;20:10–4.

401. Paccagnini S, Principi N, Massironi E, Tanzi E, Romano L, Muggiasca ML, *et al.* Perinatal transmission and manifestation of hepatitis C virus infection in a high risk population. *Pediatric Infectious Disease Journal* 1995;14:195–9.

402. Tovo PA, Pembrey L, Newell M-L. Persistence rate and progression of vertically acquired hepatitis C infection. *Journal of Infectious Diseases* 2001;181:419–24.

403. Ketzinel-Gilad M, Colodner SL, Hadary R, Granot E, Shouval D, Galun E. Transient transmission of hepatitis C virus from mothers to newborns. *European Journal of Clinical Microbiology and Infectious Diseases* 2000;19:267–74.

404. Lin HH, Kao J-H. Effectiveness of second- and third-generation immunoassays for the detection of hepatitis C virus infection in pregnant women. *Journal of Obstetrics and Gynaecology Research* 2000;26:265–70.

405. Vrielink H, Reesink HW, van den Burg PJ. Performance of three generations of anti-hepatitis C virus enzyme-linked immunosorbent assays in donors and patients. *Vox Sanguinis* 1997;72:67–70.

406. Zaaijer HL, Vrielink H, Van Exel-Oehlers PJ, Cuypers HT, Lelie PN. Confirmation of hepatitis C infection: a comparison of five immunoblot assays. *Transfusion* 1993;33:634–8.

407. Unlinked Anonymous Surveys Steering Group. *Prevalence of HIV and hepatitis infections in the United Kingdom 2001. Annual report of the Unlinked Anonymous Prevalence Monitoring Programme.* London: Department of Health; 2002. [www.doh.gov.uk/hivhepatitis/hivhepatitis2001.pdf] Accessed 21 August 2003.

408. Unlinked Anonymous Surveys Steering Group. *Prevalence of HIV and hepatitis infections in the United Kingdom 2000. Annual report of the Unlinked Anonymous Prevalence Monitoring Programme.* London: Department of Health; 2001. p. 5, 7, 24–30.

409. Connor EM, Sperling RS, Gelber R, Kiselev P, Scott G, O'Sullivan MJ, et al. Reduction of maternal – infant transmission of human immunodeficiency virus type 1 with zidovudine treatment. Pediatric AIDS Clinical Trials Group Protocol 076 Study Group. *New England Journal of Medicine* 1994;331:1173–80.

410. Mandelbrot L, Le Chenadec J, Berrebi A, Bongain A, Benifla J-L, Delfraissy JF, et al. Perinatal HIV-1 transmission. Interaction between zidovudine prophylaxis and mode of delivery in the French perinatal cohort. *JAMA* 1998;280:55–60.

411. Duong T, Ades AE, Gibb DM, Tookey PA, Masters J. Vertical transmission rates for HIV in the British Isles: estimates based on surveillance data. *British Medical Journal* 1999;319:1227–9.

412. AIDS and HIV infection in the United Kingdom: monthly report. *CDR Weekly* 2001;11(17):10–15. [www.phls.org.uk/publications/cdr/PDFfiles/2001/cdr1701.pdf] Accessed 4 September 2003.

413. Samson L, King S. Evidence-based guidelines for universal counselling and offering of HIV testing in pregnancy in Canada. *Canadian Medical Association Journal* 1998;158:1449–57 [erratum appears in *CMAJ* 1999;159(1):22.

414. Van Doornum GJJ, Buimer M, Gobbers E, Bindels PJ, Coutinho RA. Evaluation of an expanded two-ELISA approach for confirmation of reactive serum samples in an HIV-screening programme for pregnant women. *Journal of Medical Virology* 1998;54:285–90.

415. Public Health Laboratory Service AIDS Diagnosis Working Group. Towards error free HIV diagnosis: notes on laboratory practice. *PHLS Microbiology Digest* 1992;9:61–4.

416. Brocklehurst P, Volmink J. Antiretrovirals for reducing the risk of mother-to-child transmission of HIV infection. *Cochrane Database of Systematic Reviews* 2002;(3).

417. European Mode of Delivery Collaboration. Elective caesarean-section versus vaginal delivery in prevention of vertical HIV-1 transmission: a randomised clinical trial. The European Mode of Delivery Collaboration. *Lancet* 1999;353:1035–9. [published erratum appears in *Lancet* 1999;353:1714].

418. Ricci E, Parazzini F. Caesarean section and antiretroviral treatment. *Lancet* 2000;355:496.

419. Cunningham CK, Chaix ML, Rekacewicz C, Britto P, Rouzioux C, Gelber RD, et al. Development of resistance mutations in women receiving standard antiretroviral therapy who received intrapartum nevirapine to prevent perinatal human immunodeficiency virus type 1 transmission: a substudy of pediatric AIDS clinical trials group protocol 316. *Journal of Infectious Diseases* 2002;186:181–8.

420. Palumbo P, Holland B, Dobbs T, Pau CP, Luo CC, Abrams EJ, et al. Antiretroviral resistance mutations among pregnant human immunodeficiency virus type 1-infected women and their newborns in the United States: vertical transmission and clades. *Journal of Infectious Diseases* 2001;184:1120–6.

421. Control and prevention of rubella: evaluation and management of suspected outbreaks, rubella in pregnant women, and surveillance for congenital rubella syndrome. *Morbidity and Mortality Weekly Report* 2001; 50:1–23.

422. Tookey P. Antenatal screening for rubella. Personal communication; 2002.

423. Miller E, Waight P, Gay N, Ramsay M, Vurdien J, Morgan-Capner P, et al. The epidemiology of rubella in England and Wales before and after the 1994 measles and rubella vaccination campaign: fourth joint report from the PHLS and the National Congenital Rubella Surveillance Programme. *Communicable Diseases Report* 1997;7:R26–32.

424. Tookey PA, Corina-Borja M, Peckham CS. Rubella susceptibility among pregnant women in North London, 1996–1999. *Journal of Public Health Medicine* 2002;24:211–6.

425. Miller E, Cradock-Watson JE, Pollock TM. Consequences of confirmed maternal rubella at successive stages of pregnancy. *Lancet* 1982;2:781–4.

426. Grangeot-Keros L, Enders G. Evaluation of a new enzyme immunoassay based on recombinant Rubella virus-like particles for detection of immunoglobulin M antibodies to Rubella virus. *Journal of Clinical Microbiology* 1997;35:398–401.

427. Morgan-Capner P, Crowcroft NS. Guidelines on the management of, and exposure to, rash illness in pregnancy (including consideration of relevant antibody screening programmes in pregnancy). On behalf of the PHLS joint working party of the advisory committees of virology and vaccines and immunisation. *Communicable Disease and Public Health/PHLS* 2002;5(1):59–71.

428. Grillner L, Forsgren M, Barr B. Outcome of rubella during pregnancy with special reference to the 17th–24th weeks of gestation. Scandinavian Journal of Infectious Diseases 1983;Vol 15:321–5.

429. Morgan-Capner P, Hodgson J, Hambling MH. Detection of rubella-specific IgM in subclinical rubella reinfection in pregnancy. *Lancet* 1985;1:244–6.

430. Revised ACIP recommendation for avoiding pregnancy after receiving a rubella-containing vaccine. *MMWR–Morbidity and Mortality Weekly Report* 2001;50:1117.

431. Health Protection Agency. Incidence of Group B streptococcal disease in infants aged less than 90 days old. *CDR Weekly* 2002;12(16):3. [http://193.129.245.226/publications/cdr/archive02/News/news1602.html gpB] Accessed 21 August 2003.

432. Merenstein GB, Todd WA, Brown G. Group B beta-hemolytic streptococcus: Randomized controlled treatment study at term. *Obstetrics and Gynecology* 1980;55:315–8.

433. Regan JA, Klebanoff MA, Nugent RP. The epidemiology of Group B streptococcal colonization in pregnancy. *Obstetrics and Gynecology* 1991;77:604–10.

434. Hastings MJ, Easmon CS, Neill J, Bloxham B, Rivers RP. Group B streptococcal colonisation and the outcome of pregnancy. *Journal of Infection* 1986;12:23–9.

435. Oddie S, Embleton ND. Risk factors for early onset neonatal group B streptococcal sepsis: case–control study. *British Medical Journal* 2002;325:308.

436. Centers for Disease Control and Prevention. Prevention of perinatal group B streptococcal disease. Revised Guidelines from CDC. *Morbidity and Mortality Weekly Report* 2002;51(RR11):1–25. [www.cdc.gov/mmwr/preview/mmwrhtml/rr5111a1.htm] Accessed 21 August 2003.

437. Fey R, Stuart J, George R. Neonatal group B streptococcal disease in England and Wales 1981–1997. *Archives of Disease in Childhood* 1999;80:A70.

438. Bignardi GE. Surveillance of neonatal group B streptococcal infection in Sunderland. *Communicable Disease and Public Health/PHLS* 1999;2(1):64–5.

439. Yancey MK, Schuchat A, Brown LK, Ventura VL, Markenson GR. The accuracy of late antenatal screening cultures in predicting genital group B streptococcal colonization at delivery. *Obstetrics and Gynecology* 1996;88:811–5.

440. Boyer KM, Gadzala CA, Kelly PD, Burd LI, Gotoff SP. Selective intrapartum chemoprophylaxis of neonatal group B streptococcal early-onset disease. II. Predictive value of prenatal cultures. *Journal of Infectious Diseases* 1983;148:802–9.

441. Molnar P, Biringer A, McGeer A, McIsaac W. Can pregnant women obtain their own specimens for group B streptococcus? A comparison of maternal versus physician screening. The Mount Sinai GBS Screening Group. *Family Practice* 1997;14:403–6.

442. Spieker MR, White DG, Quist BK. Self-collection of group B Streptococcus cultures in pregnant women. *Military Medicine* 1999;164:471–4.

443. Schrag SJ, Zell ER, Lynfield R, Roome A, Arnold KE, Craig AS, et al. A population-based comparison of strategies to prevent early-onset group B streptococcal disease in neonates. *New England Journal of Medicine* 2002;347:233–9.

444. Smaill, F. Intrapartum antibiotics for group B streptococcal colonisation. *Cochrane Database of Systematic Reviews* 1999;(3):1–5.

445. Benitz WE, Gould JB, Druzin ML. Antimicrobial prevention of early-onset group B streptococcal sepsis: estimates of risk reduction based on a critical literature review. *Pediatrics* 1999;103:e78.

446. Gibbs RS, McNabb F. Randomized clinical trial of intrapartum clindamycin cream for reduction of group B streptococcal maternal and neonatal colonization. *Infectious Disease in Obstetrics and Gynecology* 1996;41:25–7.

447. Schrag SJ, Zywicki S, Farley MM, Reingold AL. Group B streptococcal disease in the era of intrapartum antibiotic prophylaxis. *New England Journal of Medicine* 2000;342:15–20.

448. Jeffery HE, Moses LM. Eight-year outcome of universal screening and intrapartum antibiotics for maternal group B streptococcal carriers. *Pediatrics* 1998;101:E2.

449. Egglestone SI, Turner AJL. Serological diagnosis of syphilis. *Communicable Disease and Public Health/PHLS* 2000;3:158–62.

450. Doherty L, Fenton KA, Jones J, Paine TC, Higgins SP, Williams D, et al. Syphilis: old problem, new strategy. *British Medical Journal* 2002;325:153–6.

451. Division of STD/HIV Prevention. *Sexually Transmitted Disease Surveillance 1993.* Atlanta, GA: Centers for Disease Control and Prevention;1994.

452. Flowers J, Camilleri-Ferrante. *Antenatal screening for syphilis in East Anglia: a cost-benefit analysis.* Cambridge: Institute of Public Health; 1996.

453. STD Section, HIV and STD Division, PHLS Communicable Disease Surveillance Centre, with the PHLS Syphilis Working Group. *Report to the National Screening Committee. Antenatal Syphilis Screening in the UK: A Systematic Review and National Options Appraisal with Recommendations.* London: PHLS; 1998.

454. Public Health Laboratory Service, DHSS & PS, Scottish ISD D 5 Collaborative Group. *Sexually transmitted infections in the UK: new episodes seen at Genitourinary Medicine Clinics, 1995–2000.* London: PHLS; 2001.

455. Ingraham NR Jr. The value of penicillin alone in the prevention and treatment of congenital syphilis. *Acta Dermato-Venereologica* 1951;31:60–88.

456. Association of Genitourinary Medicine and the Medical Society for the Study of Venereal Diseases, Clinical Effectiveness Group. *UK national guidelines on the management of early syphilis.* London: Medical Society for the Study of Venereal Diseases; 2002. p. 1–18.

457. Goh BT, van Voorst Vader PC. European guideline for the management of syphilis. *International Journal of STD and AIDS* 2001;12:14–26.

458. Fiumara NJ, Fleming WL, Downing JG, Good FL. The incidence of prenatal syphilis at the Boston City Hospital. *New England Journal of Medicine* 1952;247:48–52.

459. Rotchford K, Lombard C, Zuma K, Wilkinson D. Impact on perinatal mortality of missed opportunities to treat maternal syphilis in rural South Africa: baseline results from a clinic randomized controlled trial. *Tropical Medicine and International Health* 2000;5:800–4.

460. Young H, Moyes A, McMillan A, Patterson J. Enzyme immunoassay for anti-treponemal IgG: Screening of confirmatory test? *Journal of Clinical Pathology* 1992;45:37–41.

461. Young H, Moyes A, McMillan A, Robertson DHH. Screening for treponemal infection by a new enzyme immunoassay. *Genitourinary Medicine* 1989;65:72–8.

462. Walker, GJA. Antibiotics for syphilis diagnosed during pregnancy [protocol]. *Cochrane Database of Systematic Reviews* 2001;(2).

463. Alexander JM, Sheffield JS, Sanchez PJ, Mayfield J, Wendel GD Jr. Efficacy of treatment for syphilis in pregnancy. *Obstetrics and Gynecology* 1999;93:5–8.

464. Watson-Jones D, Gumodoka B, Weiss H, Changalucha J, Todd J, Mugeye K, et al. Syphilis in pregnancy in Tanzania. II. The effectiveness of antenatal syphilis screening and single-dose benzathine penicillin treatment for the prevention of adverse pregnancy outcomes. *Journal of Infectious Diseases* 2002;186:948–57.

465. Hashisaki P, Wertzberger GG, Conrad GL, Nicholes CR. Erythromycin failure in the treatment of syphilis in a pregnant woman. *Sexually Transmitted Diseases* 1983;10:36–8.

466. Eskild A, Oxman A, Magnus P, Bjorndal A, Bakketeig LS. Screening for toxoplasmosis in pregnancy: what is the evidence of reducing a health problem? *Journal of Medical Screening* 1996;3:188–94.

467. Ades AE, Parker S, Gilbert R, Tookey PA, Berry T, Hjelm M, et al. Maternal prevalence of toxoplasma antibody based on anonymous neonatal serosurvey: a geographical analysis. *Epidemiology and Infection* 1993;110:127–33.

468. Allain JP, Palmer CR, Pearson G. Epidemiological study of latent and recent infection by toxoplasma gondii in pregnant women from a regional population in the UK. *Journal of Infection* 1998;36:189–96.

469. Lebech M, Andersen O, Christensen NC, Hertel J, Nielsen HE, Peitersen B, *et al.* Feasibility of neonatal screening for toxoplasma infection in the absence of prenatal treatment. *Lancet* 1999;353:1834–7.

470. Cook AJ, Gilbert RE, Buffolano W, Zufferey J, Petersen E, Jenum PA, *et al.* Sources of toxoplasma infection in pregnant women: European multicentre case–control study. European Research Network on Congenital Toxoplasmosis. *British Medical Journal* 2000;321:142–7.

471. Pratlong F, Boulot P, Villena I, Issert E, Tamby I, Cazenave J *et al.* Antenatal diagnosis of congenital toxoplasmosis: evaluation of the biological parameters in a cohort of 286 patients. *British Journal of Obstetrics and Gynaecology* 1996;103:552–7.

472. Dunn D, Wallon M, Peyron F, Petersen E, Peckham C, Gilbert R. Mother-to-child transmission of toxoplasmosis: risk estimates for clinical counselling. *Lancet* 1999;353:1829–33.

473. Foulon W, Villena I, Stray-Pedersen B, Decoster A, Lappalainen M, Pinon JM, *et al.* Treatment of toxoplasmosis during pregnancy: a multicenter study of impact on fetal transmission and children's sequelae at age 1 year. *American Journal of Obstetrics and Gynecology* 1999;180:410–5.

474. Cubitt WD, Ades AE, Peckham CS. Evaluation of five commercial assays for screening antenatal sera for antibodies to Toxoplasma gondii. *Journal of Clinical Pathology* 1992;45:435–8.

475. Gilbert RE, Peckham CS. Congenital toxoplasmosis in the United Kingdom: to screen or not to screen? *Journal of Medical Screening* 2002;9:135–41.

476. Peyron, F, Wallon, M, Liou, C, and Garner, P. Treatments for toxoplasmosis in pregnancy. *Cochrane Database of Systematic Reviews* 2002;(3).

477. Wallon M, Liou C, Garner P, Peyron F. Congenital toxoplasmosis: systematic review of evidence of efficacy of treatment in pregnancy. *British Medical Journal* 1999;318:1511–14.

478. Garland SM, O'Reilly MA. The risks and benefits of antimicrobial therapy in pregnancy. *Drug Safety* 1995;13:188–205.

479. Bader TJ, Macones GA, Asch DA. Prenatal screening for toxoplasmosis. *Obstetrics and Gynecology* 1997;90:457–64.

480. Scottish Intercollegiate Guidelines Network. Management of diabetes: a national clinical guideline. SIGN Publication No. 55Edinburgh: SIGN; 2001. [www.sign.ac.uk/guidelines/fulltext/55/index.html] Accessed 21 August 2003.

481. World Health Organization, Department of Noncommunicable Disease Surveillance. *Definition, diagnosis and classification of diabetes mellitus and its complications. Report of a WHO consultation. Part 1: diagnosis and classification of diabetes mellitus.* Geneva: World Health Organization; 1999.

482. Alberti KGMM, Zimmet PZ. Definition, diagnosis and classification of diabetes mellitus and its complications. Part 1: Diagnosis and classification of diabetes mellitus. Provisional report of a WHO consultation. *Diabetic Medicine* 1998;15:539–53.

483. Scott DA, Loveman E, McIntyre L, Waugh N. Screening for gestational diabetes: a systematic review and economic evaluation. *Health Technology Assessment* 2002;6:1–172.

484. World Health Organization. *Prevention of diabetes mellitus: report of a WHO study group.* WHO Technical Report Series No. 844. Geneva: WHO; 1994.

485. Mestman JH, Anderson GV, Guadalupe V. Follow-up study of 360 subjects with abnormal carbohydrate metabolism during pregnancy. *Obstetrics and Gynecology* 1972;39:421–5.

486. Jensen DM, Sorensen B, Feilberg-Jorgensen N, Westergaard JG, Beck-Neilsen H. Maternal and perinatal outcomes in 143 Danish women with gestational diabetes mellitus and 143 controls with a similar risk profile. *Diabetic Medicine* 2000;17:281–6.

487. O'Sullivan JB, Charles D, Mahan CM, Dandrow RV. Gestational diabetes and perinatal mortality rate. *American Journal of Obstetrics and Gynecology* 1973;116:901–4.

488. Essel JK, Opai-Tetteh ET. Macrosomia: maternal and fetal risk factors. *South African Medical Journal* 1995;85(1):43–6.

489. Vogel N, Burnand B, Vial Y, Ruiz J, Paccaud F, Hohlfeld P. Screening for gestational diabetes: variation in guidelines. *European Journal Obstetrics, Gynecology and Reproductive Biology* 2000;91:29–36.

490. Marquette GP, Klein VR, Niebyl JR. Efficacy of screening for gestational diabetes. *American Journal of Perinatology* 1985;2:7–9.

491. O'Sullivan JB, Mahan CM, Charles D, Dandrow RV. Screening criteria for high-risk gestational diabetic patients. *American Journal of Obstetrics and Gynecology* 1973;116:895–900.

492. Wen SW, Liu S, Kramer MS, Joseph KS, Levitt C, Marcoux S, *et al.* Impact of prenatal glucose screening on the diagnosis of gestational diabetes and on pregnancy outcomes. *American Journal of Epidemiology* 2000;152:1009–14.

493. Watson WJ. Screening for glycosuria during pregnancy. *Southern Medical Journal* 1990;83:156–8.

494. Gribble RK, Meier PR, Berg RL. The value of urine screening for glucose at each prenatal visit. *Obstetrics and Gynecology* 1995;86:405–10.

495. Hooper DE. Detecting GD and preeclampsia. Effectiveness of routine urine screening for glucose and protein. *Journal of Reproductive Medicine* 1996;41:885–8.

496. McElduff A, Goldring J, Gordon P, Wyndham L. A direct comparison of the measurement of a random plasma glucose and a post-50 g glucose load glucose, in the detection of gestational diabetes. *Australian and New Zealand Journal of Obstetrics and Gynaecology* 1994;34:28–30.

497. Jowett NI, Samanta AK, Burden AC. Screening for diabetes in pregnancy: is a random blood glucose enough? *Diabetic Medicine* 1987;4:160–3.

498. Reichelt AJ, Spichler ER, Branchtein L, Nucci LB, Franco LJ, Schmidt MI. Fasting plasma glucose is a useful test for the detection of gestational diabetes. Brazilian Study of Gestational Diabetes (EBDG) Working Group. *Diabetes Care* 1998;21:1246–9.

499. Perucchini D, Fischer U, Spinas GA, Huch R, Huch A, Lehmann R. Using fasting plasma glucose concentrations to screen for gestational diabetes mellitus: prospective population based study. *British Medical Journal* 1999;319:812–5.

500. Lewis GF, McNally C, Blackman JD, Polonsky KS, Barron WM. Prior feeding alters the response to the 50-g glucose challenge test in pregnancy. The Staub-Traugott Effect revisited. *Diabetes Care* 1993;16:1551–6.

501. Watson WJ. Serial changes in the 50-g oral glucose test in pregnancy: implications for screening. *Obstetrics and Gynecology* 1989;74:40–3.

502. Jovanovic L, Peterson CM. Screening for gestational diabetes. Optimum timing and criteria for retesting. *Diabetes* 1985;34:21–3.

503. Expert Committee on the Diagnosis and Classification of Diabetes Mellitus Report of the expert committee on the diagnosis and classification of diabetes mellitus. *Diabetes Care 2000*;26 Supplement 1:S5–S20.

504. Walkinshaw SA. Dietary regulation for 'gestational diabetes'. *Cochrane Database of Systematic Reviews* 2000;(2).

505. Persson B, Stangenberg M, Hansson U, Nordlander E. Gestational diabetes mellitus (GDM). Comparative evaluation of two treatment regimens, diet versus insulin and diet. *Diabetes* 1985;34:101–4.

506. Naylor CD, Sermer M, Chen E, Sykora K. Cesarean delivery in relation to birth weight and gestational glucose tolerance. Pathophysiology or practice style? *JAMA* 1996;275:1165–70.

507. Avery MD, Leon AS, Kopher RA. Effects of a partially home-based exercise program for women with gestational diabetes. *Obstetrics and Gynecology* 1997;89:10–5.

508. Goldberg JD, Franklin B, Lasser D, Jornsay DL, Hausknecht RU, Ginsberg-Fellner F, *et al.* Gestational diabetes: impact of home glucose monitoring on neonatal birth weight. *American Journal of Obstetrics and Gynecology* 1986;154:546–50.

509. Roberts JM, Redman CW. Pre-eclampsia: more than pregnancy-induced hypertension. *Lancet* 1993;341:1447–51.

510. Douglas KA, Redman CW. Eclampsia in the United Kingdom. *British Medical Journal* 1994;309:1395–400.

511a. National High Blood Pressure Education Programme. *Working Group Report on high blood pressure in pregnancy.* NIH Publication 00-3029. Bethesda, MD: National Institutes of Health, National Heart, Lung and Blood Institute; 2000.

511b. National High Blood Pressure Education Program Working Group. Report on high blood pressure in pregnancy. *American Journal of Obstetrics and Gynecology* 1990;163:1691–712.

512. Duckitt, K. Risk factors for pre-eclampsia that can be assessed at the antenatal booking visit: a systematic review. Presented at the International Society for the Study of Hypertension in Pregnancy Conference, 24–25 July 2003, Glasgow. 2003.

513. Friedman EA. *Blood pressure, edema and proteinuria in pregnancy.* Oxford: Elsevier Scientific; 1976.

514. Redman CW. Hypertension in pregnancy. pp 182–225. 1995.

515. Barton JR, O'Brien JM, Bergauer NK, Jacques DL, Sibai BM. Mild gestational hypertension remote from term: progression and outcome. American Journal of *Obstetrics and Gynaecology* 2001;184:979–83.

516a. Page EW, Christianson R. The impact of mean arterial pressure in the middle trimester upon the outcome of pregnancy. *American Journal of Obstetrics and Gynecology* 1976;125:740–6.

516b. Page EW, Christianson R. Influence of blood pressure changes with and without proteinuria upon outcome of pregnancy. *American Journal of Obstetrics and Gynecology* 1976;126:821–33.

517. Greer IA. Hypertension. In Dunlop W, Calder AA, editors. *High risk pregnancy.* Oxford: Butterworth Heinemann; 1992. p. 30–93.

518. Redman CW, Jefferies M. Revised definition of pre-eclampsia. *Lancet* 1988;1:809–12.

519. North RA, Taylor RS, Schellenberg JC. Evaluation of a definition of pre-eclampsia. *British Journal of Obstetrics and Gynaecology* 1999;106:767–73.

520. Levine RJ. Should the definition of preeclampsia include a rise in diastolic blood pressure > 15 mmHg to a level < 90 mmHg in association with proteinuria? *American Journal of Obstetrics and Gynecology* 2000;183:787–92.

521. Perry IJ, Wilkinson LS, Shinton RA, Beevers DG. Conflicting views on the measurement of blood pressure in pregnancy. *British Journal of Obstetrics and Gynaecology* 1991;98:241–3.

522. Frohlich ED, Grim C, Labarthe DR, Maxwell MH, Perloff D, Weidman WH. Recommendations for human blood pressure determination by sphygmomanometers: Report of a special task force appointed by the Steering Committee, American Heart Association. *Hypertension* 1988;11:210A–22A.

523. Petrie JC, O'Brien ET, Littler WA, de Swiet M. Recommendations on blood pressure measurement. *British Medical Journal* 1986;293:611–5.

524. Shennan AH, Halligan AWF. Measuring blood pressure in normal and hypertensive pregnancy. *Baillieres Clinical Obstetrics and Gynaecology* 1999;13(1):1–26.

525. Cuckson AC, Golara M, Reinders A, Shennan AH. Accuracy of automated devices in pregnancy and pre-eclampsia: a meta-analysis. *Journal of Obstetrics and Gynaecology* 2002;22:S43.

526. Mattoo TK. Arm cuff in the measurement of blood pressure. *American Journal of Hypertension* 2002;15:675–85.

527. Brown MA, Buddle ML, Farrell T, Davis G, Jones M. Randomised trial of management of hypertensive pregnancies by Korotkoff phase IV or phase V. *Lancet* 1998;352:777–81.

528. Shennan A, Gupta M, Halligan A, Taylor DJ, de Swiet M. Lack of reproducibility in pregnancy of Korotkoff phase IV as measured by mercury sphygmomanometry. *Lancet* 1996;347:139–42.

529. MacGillivray I. *Pre-eclampsia. The hypertensive disease of pregnancy.* London: WB Saunders; 1983.

530. Stamilio DM, Sehdev HM, Morgan MA, Propert K, Macones GA. Can antenatal clinical and biochemical markers predict the development of severe preeclampsia? *American Journal of Obstetrics and Gynecology* 2000;182:589–94.

531. Skjaerven R, Wilcox AJ, Lie RT. The interval between pregnancies and the risk of preeclampsia. *New England Journal of Medicine* 2002;346:33–8.

532. Taylor DJ. The epidemiology of hypertension during pregnancy. In: Rubin PC, editor. *Hypertension in pregnancy.* Amsterdam: Elsevier Science; 1988. p. 223–40.

533. Salonen-Ros H, Lichtenstein P, Lipworth W. Genetic effects on the liability of developing pre-eclampsia and gestational hypertension. *American Journal of Medical Genetics* 2000;91:256–60.

534. Sibai BM, Caritis S, Hauth J. Risks of preeclampsia and adverse neonatal outcomes among women with progestational diabetes mellitus. *American Journal of Obstetrics and Gynecology* 2000;182:364–9.

535. Davey DA, MacGillivray I. The classification and definition of the hypertensive disorders of pregnancy. *American Journal of Obstetrics and Gynecology* 1988;158(4):892–898.

536. Murray N, Homer LS, Davis GK, Curtis J, Manzos G, Brown MA. The clinical utility of routine urinalysis in pregnancy: a prospective study. *Medical Journal of Australia* 2002;177:477–80.

537. Shennan AH, Waugh JJS. The measurement of blood pressure and proteinuria. In: Critchley H, MacLean AB, Poston L, Walker JJ, editors. *Pre-eclampsia*. London: RCOG Press; 2003. p. 305–24.

538. Rodriguez-Thompson D, Lieberman ES. Use of a random urinary protein-to-creatinine ratio for the diagnosis of significant proteinuria during pregnancy. *American Journal of Obstetrics and Gynecology* 2001;185:808–11.

539. Ferrazzani S, Caruso A, De Carolis S, Martino IV, Mancuso S. Proteinuria and outcome of 444 pregnancies complicated by hypertension. *American Journal of Obstetrics and Gynecology* 1990;162:366–71.

540. Waugh JJS, Clark TJ, Divakaran TG, Khan KS, Kilby MD. A systematic review and meta-analysis comparing protein/creatinine ratio measurements and dipstick urinalysis in predicting significant proteinuria in pregnancy. Presented at the British Maternal and Fetal Medicine Society, University of York, 20–21 March 2003.

541. Chamberlain G, Morgan M. *ABC of Antenatal Care*. London: BMJ Publishing; 2002.

542. Buekens P, Alexander S, Boutsen M, Blondel B, Kaminski M, Reid M. Randomised controlled trial of routine cervical examinations in pregnancy. European Community Collaborative Study Group on Prenatal Screening. *Lancet* 1994;344:841–4.

543. Iams JD, Goldenberg RL, Meis PJ. The length of the cervix and the risk of spontaneous premature delivery. *New England Journal of Medicine* 1996;334:567–72.

544. Goldenberg RL, Klebanoff M, Carey JC. Vaginal fetal fibronectin measurements from 8 to 22 weeks' gestation and subsequent spontaneous preterm birth. *American Journal of Obstetrics and Gynecology* 2000;183:469–75.

545. Goldenberg RL, Mercer BM, Meis PJ, Copper RL, Das A, McNellis D. The preterm prediction study: fetal fibronectin testing predicts early spontaneous birth. *Obstetrics and Gynecology* 1996;87:643–8.

546. Mercer BM, Goldenberg RL, Das A. The preterm prediction study: a clinical risk assessment system. *American Journal of Obstetrics and Gynecology* 1996;174:1885–95.

547. Newton ER, Barss V, Cetrulo CL. The epidemiology and clinical history of asymptomatic midtrimester placenta previa. *American Journal of Obstetrics and Gynecology* 1984;148:743–8.

548. Lauria MR, Smith RS, Treadwell MC, Comstock CH, Kirk JS, Lee W, *et al.* The use of second-trimester transvaginal sonography to predict placenta previa. *Ultrasound in Obstetrics and Gynecology* 1996;8:337–40.

549. Leerentveld RA, Gilberts EC, Arnold MJ, Wladimiroff JW. Accuracy and safety of transvaginal sonographic placental localization. *Obstetrics and Gynecology* 1990;76:759–62.

550. Oppenheimer L, Holmes P, Simpson N, Dabrowski A. Diagnosis of low-lying placenta: can migration in the third trimester predict outcome? *Ultrasound in Obstetrics and Gynecology* 2001;18:100–2.

551. Sherman SJ, Carlson DE, Platt LD, Medearis AL. Transvaginal ultrasound: does it help in the diagnosis of placenta previa? *American Journal of Obstetrics and Gynecology* 1991;164:344.

552. Farine D, Peisner DB, Timor-Tritsch IE. Placenta previa: is the traditional diagnostic approach satisfactory? *Journal of Clinical Ultrasound* 1990;18:328–30.

553. Taipale P, Hiilesmaa V, Ylostalo P. Diagnosis of placenta previa by transvaginal sonographic screening at 12–16 weeks in a nonselected population. *Obstetrics and Gynecology* 1997;89:364–7.

554. Taipale P, Hiilesmaa V, Ylostalo P. Transvaginal ultrasonography at 18–23 weeks in predicting placenta previa at delivery. *Ultrasound in Obstetrics and Gynecology* 1998;12:422–5.

555. Hill LM, DiNofrio DM, Chenevey P. Transvaginal sonographic evaluation of first-trimester placenta previa. *Ultrasound in Obstetrics and Gynecology* 1995;5:301–3.

556. Dashe JS, McIntire DD, Ramus RM. Persistence of placenta previa according to gestational age at ultrasound detection. *Obstetrics and Gynecology* 2002;99:692–7.

557. Groo KM, Paterson-Brown S. Placenta praevia and placenta praevia accreta: A review of aetiology, diagnosis and management. *Fetal and Maternal Medicine Review* 2001;12:41–66.

558. Ananth CV, Smulian JC, Vintzileos AM. The association of placenta previa with history of cesarean delivery and abortion: a metaanalysis. *American Journal of Obstetrics and Gynecology* 1997;177:1071–8.

559. Ananth CV, Demissie K, Smulian JC. Placenta previa in singleton and twin births in the United States, 1989 through 1998: a comparison of risk factor profiles and associated conditions. *American Journal of Obstetrics and Gynecology* 2003;188:275–81.

560. Royal College of Obstetricians and Gynaecologists. *Placenta praevia: diagnosis and management*. Guideline No. 27. London: RCOG; 2001.

561. Neilson JP. Interventions for suspected placenta praevia. *Cochrane Database of Systematic Reviews* 2003;(1):1–19.

562. McFarlin BL, Engstrom JL, Sampson MB, Cattledge F. Concurrent validity of Leopold's maneuvers in determining fetal presentation and position. *Journal of Nurse-Midwifery* 1985;30:280–4.

563. Vause S, Hornbuckle J, Thornton JG. Palpation or ultrasound for detecting breech babies? *British Journal of Midwifery* 1997;5:318–9.

564. Thorp JM Jr, Jenkins T, Watson W. Utility of Leopold maneuvers in screening for malpresentation. *Obstetrics and Gynecology* 1991;78:394–6.

565. Olsen K. Midwife to midwife. 'Now just pop up here, dear...' revisiting the art of antenatal abdominal palpation. *Practising Midwife* 1999;2:13–5.

566. Neilson JP. Symphysis-fundal height measurement in pregnancy. *Cochrane Database of Systematic Reviews* 2001;(2).

567. Gardosi J, Francis A. Controlled trial of fundal height measurement plotted on customised antenatal growth charts. *British Journal of Obstetrics and Gynaecology* 1999;106:309–317.

568. Macones GA, Depp R. Fetal monitoring. In: Wildschut HIJ, Weiner CP, Peters TJ, editors. *When to screen in obstetrics and gynaecology*. London: WB Saunders; 1996. p. 202–18.

569. Grant A, Elbourne D, Valentin L, Alexander S. Routine formal fetal movement counting and risk of antepartum late death in normally formed singletons. *Lancet* 1989;ii:345–9.

570. Divanovic E, Buchmann EJ. Routine heart and lung auscultation in prenatal care. *International Journal of Gynecology and Obstetrics* 1999;64:247–51.

571. Sharif K, Whittle M. Routine antenatal fetal heart rate auscultation: is it necessary? *Journal of Obstetrics and Gynaecology* 1993;13:111–3.

572. Garcia J, Corry M, MacDonald D, Elbourne D, Grant A. Mothers' views of continuous electronic fetal heart monitoring and intermittent auscultation in a randomized controlled trial. *Birth* 1985;12:79–86.

573. Pattison N, McCowan L. Cardiotocography for antepartum fetal assessment. *Cochrane Database of Systematic Reviews* 2001;(2).

574. Bricker L, Neilson JP. Routine ultrasound in late pregnancy (> 24 weeks gestation). *Cochrane Database of Systematic Reviews* 2001;(2).

575. Bricker L, Neilson JP. Routine Doppler ultrasound in pregnancy. *Cochrane Database of Systematic Reviews* 2001;(2).

576. Chien PF, Arnott N, Gordon A, Owen P, Khan KS. How useful is uterine artery Doppler flow velocimetry in the prediction of pre-eclampsia, intrauterine growth retardation and perinatal death? An overview. *BJOG* 2000;107:196–208.

577. Hilder L, Costeloe K, Thilaganathan B. Prolonged pregnancy: evaluating gestation-specific risks of fetal and infant mortality. *British Journal of Obstetrics and Gynaecology* 1998;105:169–73.

578. Crowley, P. Interventions for preventing or improving the outcome of delivery at or beyond term. *Cochrane Database of Systematic Reviews* 2003;(1).

579. Boulvain M, Fraser WD, Marcoux S, Fontaine JY, Bazin S, Pinault JJ, Blouin D. Does sweeping of the membranes reduce the need for formal induction of labour? A randomised controlled trial. *British Journal of Obstetrics and Gynaecology* 1998;105:34–40.

580. Melzack R. The short-form McGill pain questionnaire. *Pain* 1987;30:191–7.

581. Royal College of Obstetricians and Gynaecologists, Clinical Effectiveness Support Unit. *National Sentinel Caesarean Section Audit Report*. London: RCOG Press; 2001.

582. Nelson KB, Ellenberg JH. Antecedents of cerebral palsy. Multivariate analysis of risk. *New England Journal of Medicine* 1986;315:81–6.

583. Kitchen WH, Yu VY, Orgill AA, Ford G, Rickards A, Astbury J, et al. Infants born before 29 weeks gestation: survival and morbidity at 2 years of age. *British Journal of Obstetrics and Gynaecology* 1982;89:887–91.

584. Lau TK, Lo KW, Rogers M. Pregnancy outcome after successful external cephalic version for breech presentation at term. *American Journal of Obstetrics and Gynecology* 1997;176:218–23.

585. Brocks V, Philipsen T, Secher NJ. A randomized trial of external cephalic version with tocolysis in late pregnancy. *British Journal of Obstetrics and Gynaecology* 1984;91:653–6.

586. Van Veelan AJ, Van Cappellen AW, Flu PK, Straub MJPF, Wallenburg HC. Effect of external cephalic version in late pregnancy on presentation at delivery: a randomized controlled trial. *British Journal of Obstetrics and Gynaecology* 1989;96:916–21.

587. Dugoff L, Stamm CA, Jones OW, Mohling SI, Hawkins JL. The effect of spinal anesthesia on the success rate of external cephalic version: a randomized trial. *Obstetrics and Gynecology* 1999;93:345–9.

588. Van Dorsten JP, Schifrin BS, Wallace RL. Randomized control trial of external cephalic version with tocolysis in late pregnancy. *American Journal of Obstetrics and Gynecology* 1981;141:417–24.

589. Hofmeyer GJ. External cephalic version for breech presentation before term. *Cochrane Database of Systematic Reviews* 2001;(2).

590. Hofmeyer GJ. External cephalic version facilitation for breech presentation at term. *Cochrane Database of Systematic Reviews* 2001;(2).

591. Mahomed K, Seeras R, Coulson R. External cephalic version at term. A randomized controlled trial using tocolysis. *British Journal of Obstetrics and Gynaecology* 1991;98:8–13.

592. Hofmeyr GJ. Effect of external cephalic version in late pregnancy on breech presentation and caesarean section rate: a controlled trial. *British Journal of Obstetrics and Gynaecology* 1983;90:392–9.

593. Mushambi M. External cephalic version: new interest and old concerns. *International Journal of Obstetric Anesthesia* 2001;10:263–6.

594. Hofmeyr GJ. Interventions to help external cephalic version for breech presentation at term. *Cochrane Database of Systematic Reviews* 2002;(4).

595. van Loon AJ, Mantingh A, Serlier EK, Kroon G, Mooyaart EL, Huisjes HJ. Randomised controlled trial of magnetic-resonance pelvimetry in breech presentation at term. *Lancet* 1997;350:1799–804.

596. Walkinshaw SA. Pelvimetry and breech at term. *Lancet* 2002;350:1791–2.

597. Hofmeyr GJ, Kulier, R. Cephalic version by postural management for breech presentation. *Cochrane Database of Systematic Reviews* 2003;(1).

598. Cardini F, Weixin H. Moxibustion for correction of breech presentation: a randomized controlled trial. *JAMA* 1998;280:1580–4.

599. Li Q. Clinical observation on correcting malposition of fetus by electro-acupuncture. *Journal of Traditional Chinese Medicine* 1996;16:260–2.

600. Rouse DJ, Andrews WW, Goldenberg RL, Owen J. Screening and treatment of asymptomatic bacteriuria of pregnancy to prevent pyelonephritis: a cost-effectiveness and cost-benefit analysis. *Obstetrics and Gynecology* 1995;86:119–23.

601. Petrou S, Sach T, Davidson L. The long-term costs of preterm birth and low birth weight: results of a systematic review. *Child: Care, Health and Development* 2001;27:97–115.

602. Connor N, Roberts J, Nicoll A. Strategic options for antenatal screening for syphilis in the United Kingdom: a cost effectiveness analysis. *Journal of Medical Screening* 2000;7:7–13.

603. Read JS, Klebanoff MA. Sexual intercourse during pregnancy and preterm delivery: effects of vaginal microorganisms. *American Journal of Obstetrics and Gynecology* 1993;168:514–19.

604. Raymond EG, Cnattingius S, Kiely JL. Effects of maternal age, parity, and smoking on the risk of stillbirth. *British Journal of Obstetrics and Gynaecology* 1994;101:301–6.

605. Ho KY, Kang JY, Viegas OA. Symptomatic gastro-oesophageal reflux in pregnancy: a prospective study among Singaporean women. *Journal of Gastroenterology and Hepatology* 1998;13:1020–6.

606. Kovacs GT, Campbell J, Francis D, Hill D, Adena A. Is Mucaine an appropriate medication for the relief of heartburn during pregnancy? *Asia-Oceania Journal of Obstetrics and Gynaecology* 1990;16:357–62.

607. Briggs DW, Hart DM. Heartburn of pregnancy. A continuation study. *British Journal of Clinical Practice* 1972;26:167–9.

608. Dick PT, with the Canadian Task Force on the Periodic Health Examination. Prenatal screening and diagnosis of Down Syndrome. 84–98. 1994. [www.ctfphc.org/Full_Text/Ch08full.htm] Accessed 4 September 2003.

609. Bindra R, Heath V, Liao A, Spencer K, Nicolaides KH. One-stop clinic for assessment of risk for trisomy 21 at 11–14 weeks: a prospective study of 15030 pregnancies. *Ultrasound in Obstetrics and Gynecology* 2002;20:219–25.

610. Mastrobattista JM, Bishop KD, Newton ER. Wet smear compared with gram stain diagnosis of bacterial vaginosis in asymptomatic pregnant women. *Obstetrics and Gynecology* 2000;96:504–6.

611. Krohn MA, Hillier SL, Eschenbach DA. Comparison of methods of diagnosing bacterial vaginosis among pregnant women. *Journal of Clinical Microbiology* 1990;27:1266–71.

612. Royal College of Obstetricians and Gynaecologists. *Induction of labour.* Evidence-based Clinical Guideline No. 9. London: RCOG Press; 2001.

613. Department of Health. Unlinked Anonymous Prevalence Monitoring Programme in the United Kingdom. *Summary Report from the Unlinked Anonymous Surveys Steering Group. Data to the end of 1998.* London: DoH; 1999.

614. Balano K, Beckerman K, Ng V. Rapid HIV screening during labor. *JAMA* 1998;280:1664.

615. Postma MJ, Beck EJ, Mandalia S, Sherr L, Walters MDS, Houweling H, *et al.* Universal HIV screening of pregnant women in England: cost effectiveness analysis. *British Medical Journal* 1999;318:1656–60.

616. Shey Wiysonge CU, Brocklehurst P, Sterne JAC. Vaginal disinfection during labor for reducing the risk of mother-to-child transmission of HIV infection. *Cochrane Database of Systematic Reviews* 2002;(3).

617. Kind C, Rudin C, Siegrist C, Wyler C, Biedermann K, Lauper U, *et al.* Prevention of vertical HIV transmission: additive protective effect of elective cesarean section and zidovudine prophylaxis. *AIDS* 1998;12:205–10.

618. Shey Wiysonge CU, Brocklehurst P, Sterne, JAC. Vitamin A supplementation for reducing the risk of mother-to-child transmission of HIV infection. *Cochrane Database of Systematic Reviews* 2002;(3).

619. Stray-Pedersen B. Economic evaluation of different vaccination programmes to prevent congenital rubella. *NIPH Annals* 1982;5:69–83.

620. Hurtig AK, Nicoll A, Carne C, Lissauer T, Connor N, Webster JP, *et al.* Syphilis in pregnant women and their children in the United Kingdom: results from national clinician reporting surveys 1994–97. *British Medical Journal* 1998;317:1617–19.

621. Ryan M, Hall SM, Barrett NJ, Balfour AH, Holliman RE, Joynson DH. Toxoplasmosis in England and Wales 1981 to 1992. *CDR Review* 1995;5:R13–21.

622. Lappalainen M, Koskiniemi M, Hiilesmaa V, Ammala P, Teramo K, Koskela P, *et al.* Outcome of children after maternal primary Toxoplasma infection during pregnancy with emphasis on avidity of specific IgG. *Pediatric Infectious Disease Journal* 1995;14:354–61.

623. Danielian PJ, Wang J, Hall MH. Long-term outcome by method of delivery of fetuses in breech presentation at term: population based follow up. *British Medical Journal* 1996;312:1451–3.

624. Krebs L, Topp M, Langhoff-Roos, J. The relation of breech presentation at term to cerebral palsy. *British Journal of Obstetrics and Gynaecology* 1999;106:943–7.

625. Milsom I, Ladfors L, Thiringer K, Niklasson A, Odeback A, Thornberg E. Influence of maternal, obstetric and fetal risk factors on the prevalence of birth asphyxia at term in a Swedish urban population. *Acta Obstetricia et Gynecologica Scandinavica* 2002;81:907–17.

626. van Loon AJ, Mantingh A, Thijn CJP, Mooyaart EL. Pelvimetry by magnetic resonance imaging in breech presentation. *American Journal of Obstetrics and Gynecology* 1990;163:1256–60.

627. Hofmeyr GJ, Hannah ME. Planned caesarean section for term breech delivery. *Cochrane Database of Systematic Reviews* 2000;(2).

628. Hannah ME, Hannah WJ, Hewson SA, Hodnett ED, Saigal S, Willan AR. Planned caesarean section versus planned vaginal birth for breech presentation at term: a randomised multicentre trial. *Lancet* 2000;356:1375–83.

629. Gimovsky ML, Wallace RL, Schifrin BS, Paul RH. Randomized management of the nonfrank breech presentation at term: a preliminary report. *American Journal of Obstetrics and Gynecology* 1983;146:34–40.

630. Collea JV, Chein C, Quilligan EJ. The randomized management of term frank breech presentation: a study of 208 cases. *American Journal of Obstetrics and Gynecology* 1980;137:235–44.

631. Royal College of Obstetricians and Gynaecologists. *The Management of Breech Presentation.* Guideline No. 20. London: RCOG; April 2001. [www.rcog.org.uk/guidelines.asp?PageID=106&GuidelineID=19] Accessed 8 September 2003.

Index

abdominal palpation 18, 105
ABO typing 70
acoustic stimulation, in breech presentation 111
acupressure 44
    P6 54, 55
acupuncture 44
    for backache 59
    in breech presentation 112
African women, genital mutilation 63
AIDS 86
    see also HIV infection
air travel 49, 119
    future research 19, 49
    recommendation 13, 49
alcohol consumption 13, 46, 118
alginate preparations 56
algorithms, routine antenatal care 22–3, 126
alphafetoprotein (AFP) 76
alternative (complementary) therapies 13, 44–5, 119
amniocentesis 76–7
amoxicillin 82
Amsel's criteria, bacterial vaginosis 82
Anacal cream 57
anaemia 67–8, 120
    evidence tables 171–3
    recommendation 15, 68
    see also iron supplements
anencephaly 40, 41, 72
angury cut 63
antacids 14, 56
antenatal appointments 9–12
    first 10, 35
    16 weeks 10, 36
    18–20 weeks 10, 36
    25 weeks 10, 36
    28 weeks 11, 36
    31 weeks 11, 36
    34 weeks 11, 36
    36 weeks 11, 37
    38 weeks 11, 37
    40 weeks 11, 37
    41 weeks 12, 37
    algorithms 22–3, 126
    economic aspects 33
    frequency of *see* frequency of antenatal
      appointments
    information for women 117–18, 126
    place of 8–9, 30
    schedule and components 10–12, 35–7
antenatal care, information for women 116–17
Antenatal care: routine antenatal care for healthy
  pregnant women (NICE guideline) 115–26
    recommendations 116–24
    sources of further information 124–5
    summary of routine appointments 126

    versions 116
antenatal diagnosis *see* prenatal diagnosis
antenatal education/classes 8, 26
antenatal haemorrhage 2, 104
antibiotic treatment
    in asymptomatic bacteriuria 80, 192
    in bacterial vaginosis 82–3, 195
    in group B streptococcus infection 89
    in syphilis 91–2
anti-D prophylaxis 15, 16, 70–1, 120
antihistamines 54, 55
antimalarial drugs 52
antiphospholipid syndrome 2
antiretroviral therapy 86, 87
Anusol-HC cream 57
appointments, antenatal *see* antenatal appointments
aromatherapy 45
asthma, severe 2
asymptomatic bacteriuria (ASB) 79–81, 121
    economic analyses 80–1, 127–8
    evidence tables 184–92
    future research 20, 81
    methods of testing 79–80
    recommendation 16, 81
    treatment 80
atovaquone 52
auditable standards 113
auscultation, fetal heart 18, 107
autoimmune disorders 2
autotraction 60

backache 59–60, 123
    evidence tables 167–70
    future research 19–20, 60
    recommendations 14, 60
back-care classes 59, 60
bacterial vaginosis (BV) 58
    asymptomatic 16, 82–3, 123
    evidence tables 193–5
    sexual intercourse and 46
bacteriuria, asymptomatic *see* asymptomatic bacteriuria
BCG vaccine 51
bed nets, permethrin-impregnated 51
bed rest, for varicose veins 58
benzathine penicillin 91–2
bias xi
binge drinking 46
bioluminescence test, urine 80
biparietal diameter 34, 35
blinding xi
blood grouping 15–16, 70–1, 120
blood pressure
    automated devices for monitoring 101
    frequency of monitoring 101
    measurement 18, 20, 100–1, 122